GENERAL AND ORAL PATHOLOGY
FOR THE DENTAL HYGIENIST

GENERAL AND ORAL PATHOLOGY
FOR THE DENTAL HYGIENIST

Richard L. Miller, D.D.S., Ph.D.
Professor
Department of Pathology/Oral Pathology

Alan R. Gould, D.D.S., M.S.
Professor
Department of Pathology/Oral Pathology

Mark L. Bernstein, D.D.S.
Professor
Department of Pathology/Oral Pathology

Carol J. Read, R.D.H., B.S., M.Ed.
Associate Professor
Oral Health

all of
School of Dentistry
University of Louisville
Louisville, Kentucky

with 275 illustrations

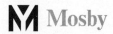 Mosby

St. Louis Baltimore Boston Carlsbad Chicago Naples New York Philadelphia Portland
London Madrid Mexico City Singapore Sydney Tokyo Toronto Wiesbaden

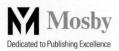

Dedicated to Publishing Excellence

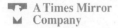

A Times Mirror
Company

Acquisitions Editor: Linda Duncan
Developmental Editor: Jo Salway
Project Manager: Mark Spann
Production and Editing: Carlisle Publishers Services
Designer: David Zielinski
Manufacturing Supervisor: Karen Lewis

Printed in the United States of America
Composition by Carlisle Communications Ltd.
Printing/binding by R.R. Donnelley & Sons Co.

Mosby–Year Book, Inc.
11830 Westline Industrial Drive
St. Louis, Missouri 63146

Library of Congress Cataloging-in-Publication Data

General and oral pathology for the dental hygienist / Richard L.
   Miller ... [et al.].
      p. cm.
    Includes bibliographical references.
    ISBN 0-8016-7024-1
    1. Mouth—Diseases. 2. Teeth—Diseases. 3. Dental hygienists.
 I. Miller, Richard L., D.D.S.
    [DNLM: 1. Mouth Diseases. 2. Tooth Diseases. 3. Dental
 Hygienists.   WU 140 1995]
 RK307.G46   1995
 617.5'22—dc20
 DNLM/DLC   94-48855

95 96 97 98 99 / 9 8 7 6 5 4 3 2 1

To our families, who have constantly encouraged us,
our teachers, who have guided us,
and our students, who have challenged us.

R.L.M.

A.R.G.

M.L.B.

C.J.R.

Preface

The primary objective of this book is to help prepare the reader for the role of a quality practitioner and as an important member of the dental team. This role includes the acquisition of skills in recognizing, diagnosing, treating, and preventing oral diseases and those manifestations and complications associated with systemic diseases. This book is intended as a text for the dental hygiene student and as an update and review source for the practicing dental hygienist. On occasion, it should also provide a reference for the practicing dentist, dental student, and other members of the dental team.

The book deals with major aspects of pathology as they impact on patient care. Several chapters acquaint the dental hygienist with the basic principles of pathology. Special care should be taken to understand these fundamental concepts and their application to the oral treatment plan. The reader is also encouraged to learn and recognize the significance of common systemic diseases and to apply this knowledge to patient care. In addition, numerous specific oral diseases and conditions that are common, quite morbid, contagious, or illustrative of basic disease concepts are presented. The signs, symptoms, demographic and epidemiologic data, and sequelae of these oral and systemic conditions are described. An attempt is made to provide clinical relevance to all basic principles and diseases discussed. Once readers have acquired the skills of understanding these basic and specific principles, they can better comprehend future changes in the treatment of diseases, including new preventive techniques, therapies, and even future alterations in the basic theory of cause and development of disease. Clinical knowledge of and research in disease development of almost every condition have evolved considerably in the past decade in such areas, for example, as autoimmunity, the significance of oncogenes in cancer, the role of the immune system in infection and transplantation, and genetic predisposition to diseases. Using these concepts as a base, the graduate hygienist is encouraged to pursue life-long continuing education for review of the disease process and to remain current.

It is hoped that the reader will further be motivated to better detect disease and recognize the impact of diseases and abnormal conditions on patient health. The hygienist is encouraged to aid the dentist by all possible and legal means to produce a proper result. This aid includes pertinent data collection and interpretation of relevant information. The graduate hygienist is thereby encouraged to function as an informed, safe, and effective member of the dental team.

It is also important for the hygienist to learn nomenclature and terminology in order to better communicate with members of the team and other health care workers. Familiarization with the basic concepts and the terminology of disease further aids comprehension of the medical and dental literature and successful completion of national and regional licensure boards. A chapter on forensic dentistry is included to familiarize you with this important component of dentistry and pathology, to inform you of legal ramifications associated with dental diagnosis and treatment, and to encourage you to properly chart and record the oral conditions you detect.

The nature of pathology is often complex, and the development of disease is often complicated. We have attempted to simplify the etiology and pathogenesis of disease in a manner that will more clearly delineate the process. We have chosen to use analogies and examples to help clarify some of the more difficult concepts, while trying not to understate the significance of these disease processes. Illustrations are further used to clarify and simplify the text material. Instructors are encouraged to use similar techniques in student instruction and evaluation.

We consider the case reports and corresponding questions as one of the most important assets of the text. The case reports are, in most instances, representative of actual situations. The data in these case reports are significant and represent clinical situations that the graduate can be expected to face. You are encouraged to analyze each case report, cross-reference the information with the text material, and answer each question to the best of your ability. In some instances, there is no single "correct" answer. Alternative approaches or choices exist. Group discussion of the case reports and questions is encouraged.

The reader will notice that important terminology is italicized in the text for emphasis and reference. In addition, summaries at the end of the chapter are intended to serve as points of emphasis. It is suggested that students concentrate on the objectives and summary material.

Finally, an instructor's manual is intended to accompany this text. This manual includes sample evaluation material and comments on the questions from the case reports. Instructors are encouraged to write new and different case reports and questions while using the included material as a guideline.

We wish to express our appreciation to Ms. Maurine S. Fisher and Ms. Sherry L. Roark for their assistance and patience in preparation of the written and illustrative portions of this manuscript. Without their support we could not have accomplished this project.

Richard L. Miller
Alan R. Gould
Mark L. Bernstein
Carol J. Read

Contents

GENERAL AND ORAL PATHOLOGY

FOR THE DENTAL HYGIENIST

1

Introduction to Disease

IN THIS CHAPTER

1. Health and disease
2. Functions of the oral cavity
3. The oral cavity and systemic disease
4. The role of the dental auxiliary in oral health
5. The diagnostic process
6. Disease management
7. Case studies

After studying this chapter, you should be able to meet the following objectives and define the key terms:

- Compare the state of disease to the state of health.
- Define *lesion* in terms of morphologic and functional change.
- Recognize that the pathogenesis of a disease is dependent on etiologic factors and inherent susceptibility of the patient.
- Discuss the relationship between oral health and systemic diseases.
- Recognize that oral diseases often have a pathogenesis similar to that of systemic diseases.
- List the functions of the oral cavity and the importance of the loss of these functions.
- Define the role of the auxiliary in evaluation and treatment of oral diseases.
- List the procedures necessary for the correct diagnosis, treatment, and prevention of disease.
- Recognize the need to protect patients and staff from iatrogenic disease.

- Develop and complete the diagnostic process.
- Help develop and understand treatment plans that include sound principles of disease management.

HEALTH AND DISEASE

Disease can be defined as a malady, disorder, or deviation from normal health. Normal health, in turn, is a state of well-being, soundness, and vigor with freedom from disease. Both conditions are subjective. Health usually is characterized in terms of baseline cellular or tissue function. An individual who cannot run a mile in 4 minutes certainly is not diseased; however, an individual who is unable to walk a continuous mile probably has some disease. Disease, then, might best be described as a functional deviation from the normal where an individual cannot achieve minimal baseline function of an organ or a tissue. However, some states of disease are associated with excessive function of organs or tissues— which in turn leads to dysfunction of the organ *systems*. For example, if the salivary glands fail to function, the individual may not be able to swallow. If the salivary gland over-functions, the individual may choke or drool—events that indicate disease.

Virchow (1821-1902) was one of the first to realize that most diseases occur because of deviation from normal at a cellular basis. The functional and/or morphologic focus of change within cells and tissues is frequently termed a *lesion*. The lesion is usually morphologic and can be detected by looking at the tissues grossly, microscopically, or ultrastructurally. Virchow is considered the father of pathology because he realized that these changes allowed one the opportunity to diagnose and study the disease process. (Pathology is defined as the study of the essential nature of diseases and especially of the structural and functional changes produced by them.) Since that time, we have come to the realization that the lesion caused by disease is biochemical and functional as well as morphologic. In fact, some lesions are predominately biochemical and/or functional (phenylketonuria, schizophrenia) and are not manifested as morphologic lesions. As health care practitioners, we must be aware that disease is represented by biochemical, functional, and anatomic disorders that frequently involve the oral tissues.

The degree of malady or disorder caused by a disease is dependent on the cause (*etiology*) of the disease, the series of events (*pathogenesis*) responsible for the malfunction, the *course* of the deviation from normal, and the effects (*sequelae*) of the disease on other organs and the patient as a whole. The etiology, pathogenesis, course, and sequelae are in turn affected by the host's total health and

resistance to disease and by the injurious agent's strength, concentration, and ability to injure cells (Fig. 1-1). For example, although a concentration of infectious organisms may not be able to cause disease in a healthy individual, the same concentration might cause fatal disease in an unhealthy individual. Likewise, a small concentration of radiation may not cause any tissue damage, whereas double the concentration might cause a significant lesion. Finally, a certain injurious agent may cause disease in one healthy individual, whereas the same concentration of agent at a similar site may not injure another healthy individual.

The etiology of disease may be and frequently is of outside origin (exogenous). Microbial organisms, physical damage, radiation, chemical injury, nutritional deficiency and nutritional excess, and thermal injury are all common causes of disease. Bugs, bangs, bullets, and burns account for numerous deaths and diseases. Other diseases are caused by internal (endogenous) etiologic events. Genetic disease can be fatal or lead to a dysfunctional course. Aging itself seems at least partially endogenous and can lead to dysfunction. A genetic disorder such as Tay-Sachs disease causes a metabolic defect that ultimately in-

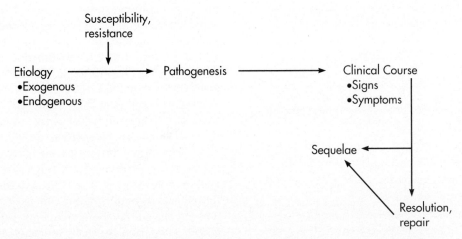

Fig. 1-1   The normal progression of disease.

jures the cells and causes direct cellular death; other genetic diseases, such as cystic fibrosis, may lead to other sequelae that cause death. There is even a rare genetic disease (progeria) that is characterized by premature aging and early patient death.

In many instances, exogenous and endogenous factors both play a role in the etiology and pathogenesis of disease. Some genetic populations of individuals seem immune to certain microbial diseases (dental caries), whereas other genetic populations are especially susceptible. Nevertheless, neither population will develop caries if the etiologic agent (bacterium) is not present. Identical-twin studies and environmentally separated–twin studies have shown that many diseases—including many bacterial infections, diabetes, hardening of the arteries, some cancers, and even some viral infections—are dependent on the interplay and interrelationship of exogenous and endogenous factors (Fig. 1-2).

The knowledge of basic disease processes is an essential part of the practice of dentistry and affects almost every facet of the dental care given. The mouth is functionally and psychologically a most important organ system. Disorders of the mouth can have a profound impact on the patient's overall health, appearance, and self-respect. As health care providers, we must have knowledge of all common disease processes and the ability to accurately recognize systemic and oral disease. Oral diseases are frequently a manifestation of systemic problems. In addition, systemic conditions and diseases may have a major impact on oral treatment. Fortunately, disease confined to the oral cavity almost always follow the "rules" of basic disease processes; therefore, understanding of the major disease processes (infection, neoplasia, hemostasis) has a direct relationship to the understanding of oral conditions. For example, if we generally understand how cancers form and behave, we will know much about oral cancer. If we understand the mechanisms of infections, we can better diagnose, treat, and prevent oral infections. Some conditions of the oral cavity, however, are quite specific, and knowledge of these conditions is essential to a quality dental health care practice. Either way, it is necessary for the dental health care provider to have a basic knowledge of systemic and oral disease and a specific knowledge of oral conditions that have an impact upon the treatment plans and care of our patients.

FUNCTIONS OF THE ORAL CAVITY

The oral cavity is the opening or portal to both the digestive and respiratory tracts; therefore, oral diseases can result in disorders of these systems (see the box on page 5). The maintenance of healthy oral tissues contributes to the optimal function of these systems, whereas the neglect or disorder of oral tissues can lead to patient *morbidity* (sickness) or *mortality* (death). For example, individuals who suffer from obstruction of the mouth or oropharynx will soon asphyxiate if the tract is not reopened or an alternate tract is not established (tracheostomy). Patients with persistent oral obstruction (growths, swellings) may become dehydrated or demonstrate starvation due to the obstruction. Patients with missing, broken, or infected teeth may suffer indigestion or poor nutrition because of failure to chew foods; patients with very dry mouths may be unable to chew food, enjoy food, or swallow food and therefore must suffer the consequences.

The oral cavity provides a first line of protection from exogenous elements that may cause disease. Oral mucous membranes are impervious to most infectious organisms. Saliva is antimicrobial, dilutes toxins, and transports noxious agents either to the outside or to the site of neutralizing stomach acids. Both the sense of taste and the sense of oral touch have protective functions. For example, many poisons are bitter and are expectorated by reflex

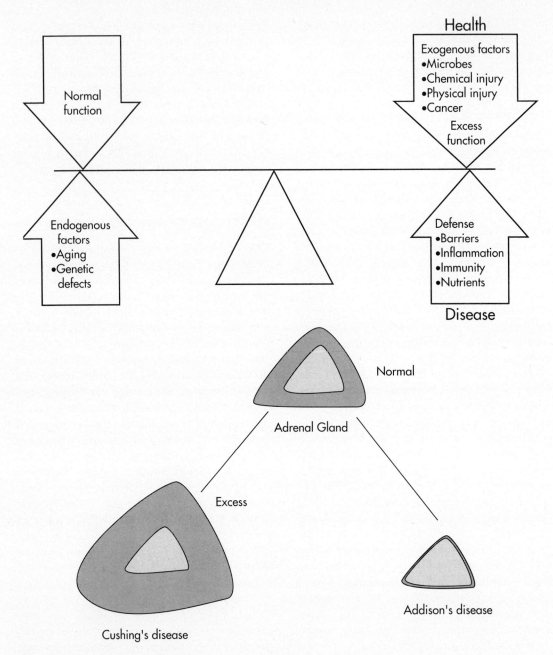

Fig. 1-2 Exogenous and endogenous factors contribute to disease. Normal function and defensive mechanisms contribute to health. Disease may result from reduced function or excessive function of tissue.

Functions of the oral cavity

Digestion

Mastication of solids for digestion

Beginning of digestion by salivary enzymes

Respiration

Passage of air and exchange of gases

Moistening and warming of air

Protection

Taste rejection of toxins

Tactile rejection of solids

Antimicrobial activity

Diluting and buffering activity

Transportation of injurious agents

Speech

Composition

Inflection

Esthetics

Physical appearance of lips and teeth

Odor

Gratification

Taste

Erogenous gratification

Habitual gratification (smoking)

---

when encountered. Similarly, hard foreign bodies (fish bone) are immediately rejected—almost by tactile reflex. Patients who exhibit oral numbness (anesthesia) can easily aspirate material into the lungs and respiratory tract, with resultant morbidity or mortality.

The oral cavity is regarded as being psychologically important, esthetic, and even erogenous by many people. Straight white teeth, pleasant breath, well-formed and well-colored lips, pleasant smiles, and healthy oral soft tissues are gratification areas long recognized by the salesmen and advertisers of the world as areas of extreme concern. More money is spent on oral esthetic agents such as mouthwash, lipstick, esthetic toothpaste, esthetic dentistry, and breath freshener than is spent on all other forms of dentistry. Patients with stained, missing, or malaligned teeth, un-

sightly lips, obvious periodontal gum disease, or halitosis frequently become socially introverted or even reclusive. You are sure to encounter the dental emergency where a patient needs a fractured tooth repaired "so I can go to the party" or a denture repaired "before the business meeting." Concerts, weddings, and even funerals have been postponed so that someone's oral esthetic problems might be corrected.

The oral cavity serves as a zone of self-gratification. The erogenous qualities are well documented, and kissing remains a very popular activity. Would you kiss someone with a cold sore of the lip or a brown unsightly tongue? Taste represents another form of sensation and gratification. Billions of dollars a year are spent on chocolates, wines, and other specialized foods and desserts to provide this gratification. Disappearance of taste associated with diseases or aging can have an impact upon an individual's habits, desires, and even personality.

Finally, the oral tissues are essential for verbal communication between individuals. Both the composition and the inflection of speech are dependent on the synthesis of words by the interaction of teeth, palate, tongue, and lips. Defects or disease of any of these structures can result in miscommunications, misunderstanding, and the perception of individuals as being socially inadequate. Speech disorders resulting from ankyloglossia (tongue-tie), clefting (lip or palate), and edentulism are not uncommon and are usually correctable.

THE ORAL CAVITY AND SYSTEMIC DISEASE

Because of the relationship of oral health and disease to the health of the individual, the oral cavity may serve as an indicator (barometer) of a person's systemic health. Many common and potentially morbid systemic conditions—such as diabetes, acquired immunodeficiency syndrome (AIDS), leukemia, nutritional deficiencies, and other diseases—may show early associated oral effects. The oral manifestations of systemic conditions can be useful in both the diagnosis and monitoring of a patient's systemic condition. On the other hand, many patients will have either diagnosed or undiagnosed systemic conditions, without oral manifestations, that might have a profound impact on oral therapy. For example, invasive periodontal treatment of a patient with a systemic bleeding problem (drug induced), a healing problem (vascular disease), or immune suppression (AIDS) will probably result in severe morbidity from hemorrhage, infection, or both. We certainly must be aware of these conditions in the course of treatment planning. The dental care team must therefore work closely with and communicate with the rest of the patient's health care providers to ensure optimal patient care and health.

THE ROLE OF THE DENTAL AUXILIARY IN ORAL HEALTH

The dental hygienist plays a most important role in evaluation and treatment. Within the confines of the regulatory statutes, auxiliaries may perform oral examinations; assist in history taking and evaluation; perform certain diagnostic tests, such as radiography; assist the practitioner in examination, evaluation, and therapy; and in some instances, perform irreversible procedures on oral tissues. Each and every one of these procedures necessitates a basic understanding of systemic and oral disease. The term *auxiliary* is defined as "someone who affords aid" to the dental practitioner. When the hygienist notes changes indicative of disease, it is important for the hygienist to alert the practitioner to these changes. It is appropriate for the hygienist to present an opinion concerning the observation and to suggest intervention or prevention. Final decision making is usually reserved for the practitioner, and optimal patient care is rendered when the decision is based on practitioner judgment with aid from the auxiliary.

As stated previously, disease is frequently demonstrable orally. The dental hygienist frequently has the responsibility of first-line disease detection. In a sound dental practice, a thorough systematic oral examination is mandatory on a regular basis. Often it is the auxiliary who is initially responsible for this procedure. Patients are frequently unaware of early—and therefore less morbid—signs of disease. That means that the examiner must become a detective searching for signs or changes indicative of disease. As we will see in later chapters, some of the most serious diseases tend to occur in areas of the mouth that are the least accessible. Unless we compress the tongue to examine the oropharynx, take radiographs to examine the dental hard tissues and bones, probe the periodontal crevices, palpate the salivary tissues and nodes, and measure the blood pressure, we will surely fail to detect significant disease. Dental practitioners who have never "seen" oral cancer, hypertension, salivary tumors, or incipient periodontal problems probably have failed to look for them.

Once changes have been detected by thorough systematic examination, it is most important that abnormal changes be recognized. This recognition is based on knowledge of normal morphology, function, and biochemistry. If a red pathologic area of the lateral surface of the tongue is detected but is considered normal and is therefore neglected, then the disease process may continue and intervention will not occur. Likewise, if a "normal" yellow glandular area of the buccal mucosa is detected and assumed incorrectly to be diseased, excessive and unnecessary intervention with associated discomfort, expense, and worry may result. The auxiliary must therefore learn to recognize a range of normal characteristics and follow up where characteristics are detected that fall outside of this range.

A correct diagnosis is most important for a successful outcome. You should be familiar with the different possibilities when addressing a detected disorder. Once the differential diagnosis is developed, additional tests, measures, and information can be assembled and a correct diagnosis can be established. Failure to correctly diagnose a lesion will almost invariably result in incorrect intervention, even if the lesion was properly detected. In most instances, diagnosis is not the responsibility of a dental hygienist. However, as a health care provider, member of the dental team, and one who gives aid, you should be concerned with the correct diagnosis. The treatment plan, mode of therapy, and patient education program will depend on the diagnosis.

Needless to say, success in patient care is highly dependent on the prescription and provision of the correct treatment for the diagnosed condition. The treatment is often provided by the dental hygienist, even though the prescription or treatment plan originates with the dentist. For example, it would be ludicrous to treat dental decay (caries) with antibiotics, even after superior detection and diagnosis. Therefore, we must have knowledge of the best therapies and apply this knowledge to our clinical situations. When we detect disease, we must predict the outcome (make a prognosis) of the disorder and thus inform the patient. In many cases, therapy is partially dictated by prognosis. If patient A has a 99% chance of suffering no significant effects from his or her disease, we should so inform the patient and treat conservatively. On the other hand, if patient B has only a 50% chance of surviving the disease, our treatment plan should be influenced by this prognosis, and therapy will most likely be quite aggressive—even destructive to surrounding tissue if necessary.

Additional reasons for understanding the principles of and relationships between basic pathology and oral disease may be less apparent. As health care providers, we are pledged to try our best not to create diseases. *Iatrogenic* (practitioner-induced) diseases are not uncommon. Burns, caustic necrosis, physical trauma, medication reactions, infections, and many other forms of injury can result from dental

treatment. We must detect, diagnose, and understand diseases in order to avoid creating them. Failure to detect an allergy to a dental medication might result in a morbid or even mortal result. Failure to realize the potential of a dental instrument to puncture or sever tissue at a particular site might well create traumatic disease as a consequence of dental treatment. Failure to practice adequate infection control or to appreciate the impact of iatrogenic infections might result in patient infection.

We must also detect, recognize, and understand disease in order to protect ourselves. Infectious organisms can be transferred from patient to practitioner. Such transfer can usually be prevented using barriers, sterilants, vaccines, or other protective measures. In some instances, upon detecting highly contagious diseases, we may wish to defer elective therapy or increase our barriers to infection. Sometimes the materials of dentistry can cause practitioner disease. We must therefore understand these substances and their potential for injury, and protect ourselves from them. If your neighbor's dog bites, you would want to know this before you opened the gate. Likewise, if your patient has tuberculosis, you need to have knowledge of this before you open the oral gate to infection.

Many patients will have a disease when they have a dental appointment. This disease may or may not be diagnosed. We must detect and diagnose such disease so that we avoid complicating the patient's condition. We surely want to know if a patient has a bleeding problem before we perform invasive scaling procedures. We certainly want to know if a patient has a heart murmur before we probe the periodontal sulcus or pocket. We need to know if a patient is hypertensive before we submit him or her to a highly stressful procedure. Again, the need to "do no harm" should prevail.

If we understand the etiology and pathogenesis of a disease, we may better understand how to prevent that disease from occurring in our patients. A patient may be susceptible to a gingival infection that is related to a nutritional defect. By correctly detecting, diagnosing, and understanding the mechanism of this disorder, we might be able to prevent the condition from occurring or escalating. If we understand the association of plaque with dental caries, then we can help patients to avoid plaque formation or accumulation and to prevent the decay. In many practices, prevention is a primary responsibility of the hygienist and an area in which you can have an enormous impact on the patient's health.

Finally, knowledge of disease contributes to observations, data collection, and conclusions that can be useful in future detection, diagnosis, treatment, or prevention. This research should occur constantly in every health care setting. Why do our female patients have better plaque scores after home care instruction than our male patients? Why do all members of this family have white patches on the tongue? Why do cigarette smokers never complain of mouth sores? Why do people who eat onions have worn teeth? All these types of observations may lead to conclusions or at least to related intelligent questions. If the last 10 patients you treated with a certain technique responded poorly, you need to research and evaluate that technique and its (your) effectiveness.

THE DIAGNOSTIC PROCESS

A correct clinical diagnosis leads to proper care and prevention. The more information we can accumulate about a patient's condition, the more successful the diagnosis and outcome. How is data collection accomplished? The dental team must obtain from all patients a comprehensive, thorough, and up-to-date health history. The patient should provide a health history and the dental practitioner or auxiliary should review and discuss it with the patient. Patients do not always understand historical questions and their significance; therefore, such a review is mandatory. The health history should include a drug and medication history, documentation of current and recent disease, an update of previous

diseases, and information concerning certain conditions (murmur, hepatitis, immune deficiency) that are of special interest to the dental team. The health history should be referred to and updated at each visit. "Has your health or medication changed since our last appointment?" This takes minimal time and effort and can usually be done while the patient is waiting to be treated.

When a condition or disorder is detected, the patient should be questioned for additional information. Clinical *symptoms* are changes noticeable to the patient that can be used as determinants of a disease. Symptoms noted may include pain, swelling, texture changes, color change, loss or increase in function, and other characteristics apparent to the patient. Clinical *signs* are changes detected by the practitioner and may include all of the above changes and the results of clinical tests (radiopacity, nonvital tooth, percussion sensitivity). Most diseases present a specific combination of signs and symptoms related to the organ or tissue involved with the disease and the causative injurious agent. A patient who has red, swollen, pus-filled periodontal structures probably has a bacterial infection (cause) of the periodontal ligament (tissue), based on the clinical signs and symptoms. A pale patient who appears with a bald red tongue and has a health history of long-term weakness and malaise (tiredness) should be suspect for anemia, based on signs and symptoms.

Once we accumulate the data concerning our patients, we must sort and synthesize this data in order to arrive at a clinical diagnosis. In many instances, we must consider a number of diseases that can present similar combinations of signs and symptoms. A nonpainful, rough, slightly raised white patch on the lateral surface of the tongue may represent numerous diseases—some of which are of little consequence, and others of which can be fatal. When confronted with this situation, the dental practitioner must develop a list (differential diagnosis) of all the possible lesions. This list is usually prioritized from most likely to least likely, based on the data available. The differential diagnosis can then be further constricted by performing appropriate tests that will give evidence for or against those conditions listed. If we think the pus-coated periodontitis is caused by a specific organism of genus *Actinomyces,* then the disease actinomycosis should be included in our differential diagnosis. If, however, all tests (culture, biopsy, cytologic test) are negative for the organism, then we should remove the disease from the differential diagnostic list. The tests performed must be appropriate for the diseases listed in our differential diagnosis. There is no reason to perform a cancer test if all the diseases in our differential diagnosis are infectious. There is no sense in performing a bacterial culture if all the diseases listed are viral. Therefore, high levels of skill are necessary in compiling a differential diagnosis and in narrowing it to a final diagnosis. The entire process is similar to the technique used by a detective at the site of the crime. An examination of the crime site (lesion) reveals physical evidence such as weapon, location, and evidence of struggle. Interrogation follows—of those in proximity to the crime and of the victim—revealing what people saw, heard, and know about the crime (history, signs, and symptoms of the disease). A list of suspects (the differential diagnosis) is assembled. Further tests exclude (because of alibi or lack of proximity) or include (because of motive or smoking gun) suspects until finally an arrest (final diagnosis) is made based on all the data.

DISEASE MANAGEMENT

In most cases, disease can be managed by treatment and elimination of the cause or by interference with, and inhibition of the pathogenic mechanisms. Treatment may involve surgical elimination of diseased tissues, medical destruction of the injurious agent, support of defensive mechanisms, or other physical or chemical interference with the etiologic factors. Frequently, further investigation of the

pathogenic mechanism and fortification and support of the injured tissues are necessary. For example, a patient with severe periodontal disease with resultant bone destruction may need surgical treatment, antibiotics, and hygienic treatment to eliminate the cause of the disease, as well as splinting of teeth and nutritional supplementation to promote healing. In addition, bone-growth stimulants might be used to reverse the pathogenesis of the disease. Once a disease has reached the stage of treatment, psychologic and preventive measures should accompany and facilitate treatment. Patients should be educated regarding the cause of the disease and informed of the pathogenesis and sequelae. A prognosis (prediction of the outcome of the disease) based on the diagnosis and course of treatment is necessary—as discussed previously. This communication must be understandable to your patient. If your patient understands the cause and course of the disease, he or she will usually better accept both the treatment and the preventive measures that are needed.

Case Studies

Case 1
P. B. is a 53-year-old woman who was referred to her physician for a slow-growing ulcer of the skin of her right cheek. The physician, using appropriate tests, determined that the lesion was a mild skin cancer (basal cell carcinoma) and prescribed a chemical salve known to cure the condition. The patient was not informed of the diagnosis, prognosis, or rationale of therapy, but simply told to apply salve 4 times a day. The patient substituted Vaseline for the chemical salve to save money. Three years later the patient went to her dentist for routine dental care with an ulcer of the cheek 5 times larger than the original ulcer. There was some destruction of the eye socket. She was referred to a dermatologist who performed surgical cancer therapy. P. B. was then educated on the cause of her condition (sunlight) and now uses sun shields and avoidance techniques to prevent further cancer from developing.

Case 2
J. B. is a 46-year-old man who was being treated for kidney failure secondary to a developmental defect (polycystic disease). He was receiving dialysis 3 times a week and had an intravenous line in his arm used for dialysis and irrigated with heparin—an anticoagulant adjunct to dialysis. When J. B. went to the dentist for scaling and cleaning of his teeth, the health interview revealed the preceding as new information. After physician consultation, the dental procedure was deferred and subsequently performed in a hospital dental setting.

Case 1

1. Should the dental team be concerned about detecting a lesion on the patient's face?
2. Why did the patient not follow her physician's instructions?
3. What might be the significance of sun-avoidance techniques in the pathogenesis of skin cancer (basal cell carcinoma)?
4. What do you think is the cause of the skin cancer?

Case 2

1. What might have happened if the health history had not been updated?
2. Why was a physician consultation necessary? Why not just defer treatment?
3. Is it necessary to perform dental hygiene procedures in a hospital setting?
4. Do you think this patient might have any other problems that would impact dental treatment?

SUMMARY

- Disease indicates a departure in tissue morphology and function from normally expected values.
- By understanding the etiology, pathogenesis, and course of disease, one can best anticipate treatment and prevention.
- Dentistry must be concerned with basic diseases that can impact on dental care or be manifest in the oral cavity.
- The oral cavity is multifunctional; therefore, oral diseases may affect patients' function, anatomy, and even perception of social adequacy.
- Dental auxiliaries have the responsibility to assist in diagnosis, treatment, and prevention of diseases that may affect the dental treatment plan.
- The diagnostic process involves adequate data collection and evaluation of evidence to arrive at a clinical diagnosis. The differential diagnosis can be restricted further by using specific tests and questioning to rule in or rule out possible causes of disease.
- Disease management includes elimination of the cause, interference with pathogenic mechanisms, and support of defense mechanisms and healing mechanisms.
- Dental auxiliaries should explain the etiology and pathogenesis of a disease to the patient so the patient will accept treatment and preventive procedures.

Suggested readings

1. Grisham JW and Nopanitaya W: Cellular basis of disease. In Kissane JM, editor: Anderson's pathology, St Louis, 1985, Mosby.
2. Kiple KF, editor: The Cambridge world history of human disease, New York, 1993, Cambridge University Press.
3. Sheldon H: Boyd's introduction to the study of disease, ed 11, Philadelphia, 1992, Lea & Febiger, chapters 1-3.

2

Developmental and Retrogressive Tissue Changes

After studying this chapter, you should be able to meet the following objectives and define the key terms:

- List types of developmental defects by degree of failure of development.
- Explain the interaction of genetic factors, acquired factors, time, and space in the formation of developmental defects.
- List the types of injury that lead to atrophy and give several common examples not listed in the chapter.
- Explain the morphologic and functional changes that reflect cell injury.
- Discuss the morphologic changes that reflect cell necrosis.
- Recognize that cell necrosis causes reactions that help control disease and initiate repair.
- Recognize that morphologic changes of cell necrosis reflect the cause of the tissue injury.

When a tissue has been injured by either exogenous or endogenous mechanisms, it re-

sponds to that injury. The cells and tissues injured will demonstrate functional, biochemical, and anatomic changes that may be detected by symptoms, signs, and laboratory observations. Such changes may be either developmental or acquired.

DEVELOPMENTAL DEFECTS

Developmental defects occur when there is interference with organ or tissue formation. Since most tissues develop during embryogenesis, these defects usually occur in the fetus and are frequently apparent at birth. However, since tissue development continues after birth (teeth, immune system, secondary sexual characteristics), some of these defects show up following birth. Birth defects are often termed *congenital* (con: with, genital: formation), whereas defects that occur in adult life are termed *tardive* (delayed). An organ or tissue may fail to develop or fully mature for numerous reasons. Exogenous agents such as viruses, drugs, or trauma can damage developing tissues and arrest maturation. When organs and tissues develop, there is a complicated interaction between cells or between adjacent tissues. This interaction occurs over both space and time. To make an analogy, if a class of dental auxiliary students embarks on a community fluoride program, they might agree to meet with needy patients at a specific place at a certain time. Each student would be assigned a task (application, rinsing, instruction, disposal), and the coordinated project should result in a positive outcome. If, however, the project is uncoordinated and the fluoride arrives too late, or the patients visit the wrong clinic, or the instructional materials are not understandable (exogenous or endogenous agents), the project will either fail or not give an optimal result. Likewise, if developing tissues are insufficient, late in forming, or displaced during development, organ formation will be aborted or diminished. During palate formation, the palate can only fuse if the developing tongue drops out of the plane of formation. The tongue can drop only when the mandible becomes large enough to allow the tongue sufficient space to move. If the pregnant female takes certain drugs that inhibit mandibular growth in the fetus, the tongue will not drop and the palate will not close—hence, cleft palate will occur because of failure of the palatal shelves to fuse. This series of events must be coordinated. Therefore, later growth of the mandible will not correct the problem; the cleft will remain.

The failure of an organ or tissue to form is termed *agenesis* (a: without, genesis: formation). Agenesis may result from a genetic defect (as with hereditary missing maxillary lateral incisors) or from exogenous injury (as with failure of the palate to fuse when a pregnant woman takes certain medications). *Aplasia* (a: without, plasia: growth) can occur in similar circumstances and implies that only nonfunctional rudimentary tissue develops (a flipper rather than fingers on a hand). *Hypoplasia* (hypo: less than normal, plasia: growth) also may occur, due to similar exogenous or endogenous injury in a time-and-space relationship. Hypoplastic tissue will be small and will not attain a normal level of function (Fig. 2-1). During the 1960s the drug thalidomide was widely used in Europe as a sedative or tranquilizer. This drug was not approved by the Food and Drug Administration (FDA) for use in the United States; however, some pregnant American women traveled to Europe and received thalidomide treatments. Unfortunately, this drug caused developmental defects whereby the infants were born without arms and legs (agenesis), with rudimentary flippers (aplasia, phocomelia), or with very short appendages (hypoplasia). The incidence of phocomelia seemed to depend on thalidomide dosage levels, the time during pregnancy at which the drug was used, and patient susceptibility—some neonates were normal. Thousands of European births resulted in phocomelia.

ACQUIRED DEFECTS

Retrogressive defects are usually acquired. The term *atrophy* is used to designate acquired retrogressive loss of size of tissues or organs due to injury. Fully developed organs and tissues begin to shrink in size and decrease in function in response to exogenous injury or genetic and metabolic injury (Fig. 2-2). For example, mucosal atrophy—manifested as thin, red, nonkeratinized mucosa—can result from chronic vitamin or iron deficiencies. The number of cells within the mucosal epithelium decreases, and the amount of keratin is reduced. The patient complains of irritation caused by acid or spicy foods and burning caused by warm beverages. As another example, brown atrophy of the heart is a fairly frequent complication of aging. The heart (cardiac) muscle cells shrink due to endogenous aging changes and loss of circulation, resulting in accumulation of metabolic byproducts (brown pigments). The cardiac muscle decreases in both size and number of cells. This chronic atrophy results in a small and somewhat weakened heart. Atrophic changes such as these usually occur over a lengthy period of time (are chronic) and arise from very low grade injury.

CELL DEGENERATION AND NECROSIS

The term *degeneration* is used to designate a reversible acquired change of cells and tissues in response to injury. Degenerating tissues become biochemically and functionally diminished and often show morphologic alterations at the gross and/or microscopic levels. These

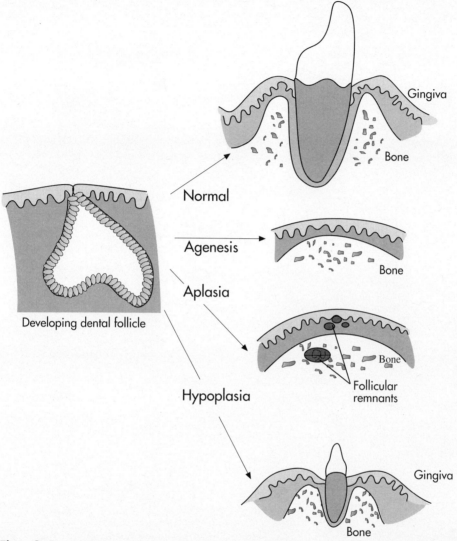

Fig. 2-1 Examples of agenesis, aplasia, and hypoplasia of a tooth. In agenesis there is a failure of tooth formination. In aplasia only remnants are formed. In hypoplasia a small tooth develops.

tissues are still alive but are injured. Marked degeneration of a tissue or organ can cause severe illness or even death. For example, ethyl alcohol is a hepatotoxin that causes degeneration of the liver cells. High-dosage alcoholism may result in liver degeneration to such a degree that an alcoholic patient will be jaundiced, hemorrhagic, or toxic as a result of decreased liver function—becoming a consid-

erable therapeutic risk. If the patient discontinues alcohol intake and associated injurious practices (malnutrition), the degenerated liver cells should recover their functions and the liver should revert to normal.

Necrosis denotes irreversible cell death. Injury occurs at such a magnitude that the cellular nuclear and cytoplasmic components are functionally and morphologically destroyed.

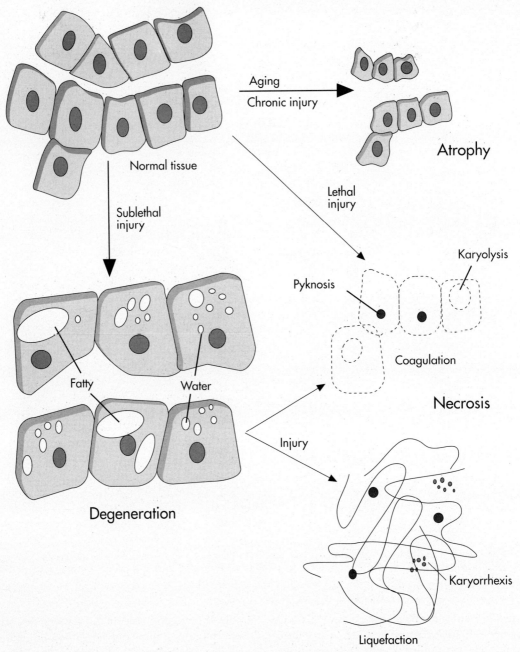

Fig. 2-2 Retrogressive changes caused by injury include atrophy from chronic injury or aging, degeneration from sublethal injury, and types of necrosis from lethal injury.

The injury may be of acute concentration (such as a burn) or long-term repetition (such as chronic lack of oxygen). Therefore, long-term degeneration often may precede necrosis. The necrotic cells show microscopic nuclear changes. The nuclei of the dead cells may shrink (pyknosis), dissolve (karyolysis), or disintegrate (karyorrhexis) (Fig. 2-2). The end result is nuclear death and cell death. Not only do necrotic cells cease to function; they also release intracellular products that may irritate, injure, or stimulate surviving tissues. Cell necrosis therefore usually initiates secondary reactions (inflammation, blood coagulation, healing) that help to limit injury and repair the damaged tissue.

When we as health care practitioners detect, evaluate, and diagnose injured tissues, we look for morphologic, functional, and biochemical changes (lesions) indicative of degeneration and necrosis. Some tissues react to an injurious agent in a specific way, and certain injurious agents tend to cause very specific types of injuries that are recognizable to the practitioner. When we become acquainted with these specific changes, we can recognize "fingerprints" in patterns of necrosis, degeneration, and subsequent inflammation that help us to diagnose the cause.

Cloudy swelling, hydropic degeneration, and fatty degeneration represent morphologic and biochemical alterations of cells that indicate injury and degeneration.

Cloudy Swelling and Hydropic Degeneration

Tissues that transport water frequently lose that function shortly after injury. The injured cells do not have the energy necessary to transport water to the outside of the cell, and therefore they begin to swell up. Microscopically, the cytoplasm appears watery, indistinct, and cloudy—hence the designation *cloudy swelling*. In mildly injured tissues that are highly active in water transport (kidney tubules) or in tissues that are severely injured,

large water droplets may accumulate within the cytoplasm—hence the designation *hydropic degeneration*. (See Fig. 2-3.) Remember, these are reversible processes and the nuclei of these cells are alive and intact. The tissues or organs will appear swollen, pale, or parboiled to the clinical eye, and biochemical dysfunction is expected.

Fatty Degeneration

Tissues that transport complex fats will frequently accumulate large amounts of lipid when injured. The metabolic mechanism that releases fats from such tissue operates at a reduced level, therefore, the injured cell does not have the energy to move lipid complexes out of the cell. Fatty acids, however, still may enter the cell, and fats therefore accumulate in the injured tissue. As a result, cells of certain tissues—such as liver cells, kidney cells, and cardiac muscle cells—may accumulate fat (*fatty degeneration*) when injured. This fat is detectable within the cells microscopically and biochemically (Fig. 2-3). The organ will swell, appear yellow, and feel greasy or fatty. The previous example of alcoholic liver generation frequently is manifest as fatty degeneration, with the hypofunctional liver 2 to 3 times its normal weight, markedly increased in size, and yellow in color. Again, it is stressed that these changes are reversible, that the cells are viable, and that removal of the stimulus should correct the problem.

Liquefactive Necrosis

Necrotic cells and tissues also assume a certain morphologic pattern that may be apparent grossly or microscopically. This appearance frequently gives an indication of the type of injurious agent responsible for the cell death and so serves as a clue for diagnosis. Frequently, tissues liquefy when they become necrotic (*liquefactive necrosis*). This is especially common in tissues that have a high water content (such as the brain) and in cell necrosis involving microorganisms which elaborate dissolving enzymes (infections). This liquefactive necrosis involves both nuclear and cytoplasmic components of cells; therefore, the tissue literally dissolves. Tissue architecture is lost and a defective tissue filled with fluid and debris remains. Grossly and microscopically, the tissue bears no resemblance to its living counterpart, with only putrified liquid material remaining. Karyolysis is usually the indicator of nuclear death

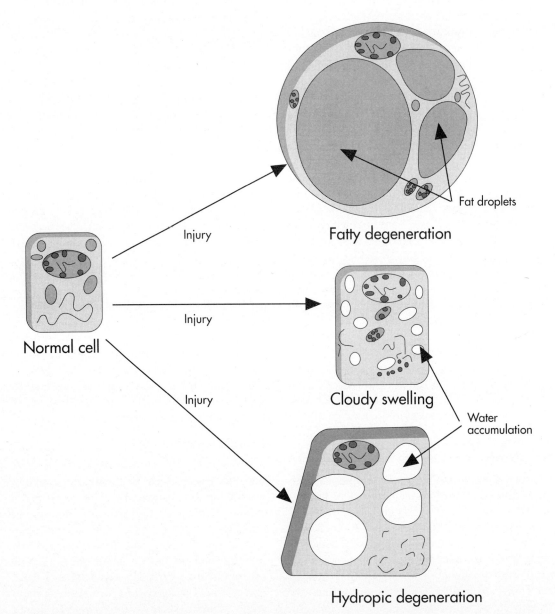

Fig. 2-3 Three types of morphologic changes that reflect cell necrosis. Notice that the nucleus remains vital.

ture of degenerating tissues (cloudy swelling, hydropic degeneration) and necrotic debris (liquefaction). The body will not tolerate necrotic tissues, and therefore, a reaction to remove this debris and repair the damage functionally and structurally is necessary. An efficient inflammatory process is triggered by the byproducts of liquefaction, coagulation, caseation, or gumma formation.

Case Studies

Case 1

A.K. is a 48-year-old woman who has been treated for chronic alcoholism 3 times in the past 5 years. She is divorced, has lost her job, and drinks 14 ounces of liquor a day. Although she appears emaciated, her liver has increased to 3 times its normal size. She recently was hospitalized for hemorrhage following dental extraction. Liver tests revealed remarkable fatty degeneration and decreased circulating clotting factors. Subsequent to arrest for writing bad checks, A.K. was incarcerated for 2 years. During that time, her liver shrank to a size slightly greater than normal and results of her liver enzyme and clotting tests returned to normal.

Case 2

D.J. was a 67-year-old diabetic male smoker who had a history of heart disease and high blood pressure. During dental examination, his blood pressure was 180/120 and he was advised to see his physician. Three weeks later he had a heart attack while playing golf. He died 4 days later. Autopsy revealed coagulation necrosis of most of the heart muscle of the anterior left ventricle and intraventricular septum. Blockage of the left circumflex coronary artery was complete.

Case 1

1. Explain the cause of the increased size of the patient's liver.
2. Name some important functions of the liver that might relate to dental treatment.

3. Why do you think she hemorrhaged after tooth extraction?
4. Why do you think her liver returned to normal while she was incarcerated, based on the information available?

Case 2

1. What might be the etiology of vascular heart disease?
2. Is the dental team responsible for monitoring blood pressure on routine patients?
3. Why did the dentist refer D.J. to a physician? Why refer at all? Why not just treat the high blood pressure?
4. What do you think is the pathogenesis of coagulation necrosis resulting from blockage of the supplying coronary vessel?

SUMMARY

- Injuries to tissues may be caused by developmental defects or outside agents, or by a combination of the two.
- Developmental defects can result from direct interference with tissue formation, from uncoordinated tissue interaction, or from failure of developing tissue to mature.
- Once tissues are fully developed, injurious circumstance can cause degeneration, necrosis or atrophy. Such injured tissues show functional and anatomic changes that reflect both the type of tissue injured and the cause of injury.
- Tissue death usually stimulates an inflammatory reaction in a living patient.

Suggested readings

1. Chandrasoma P and Taylor CR: Concise pathology, East Norwalk, Conn, 1991, Appleton & Lange, pp 1-2, 12-16.
2. Cotran RS, Kumar V, and Robbins SL: Robbins pathologic basis of disease, ed 4, Philadelphia, 1989, WB Saunders Co, pp 17-22.

3. Goldstein S: The biology of aging, N Engl J Med 285:1120, 1971.
4. Rubin E and Farber JL: Pathology, Philadelphia, 1988, JB Lippincott Co, chapter 1.
5. Trump BF, McDowell EM, and Arstila AU: Cellular reaction to injury. In Hill RB and LaVia MF, editors: Principles of pathology, ed 3, London, 1980, Oxford Press, pp 20-80.

3 Inflammation and Repair

IN THIS CHAPTER

1. Inflammation
   - The vascular response
   - The early cellular phase
   - The late cellular stage
2. Repair
   - Tissue regeneration
   - Connective tissue substitution—scarring
3. Complications of inflammation
4. Chronic inflammation
   - Nonspecific chronic inflammation
   - Granulomatous inflammation
5. Nomenclature of inflammation
6. Discussion
7. Case Studies

After studying this chapter, you should be able to meet the following objectives and define the key terms:

- Discuss the function of the inflammatory process.
- Relate the interactions of the inflammatory process to the hemostatic and immune reactions.
- List and discuss the roles of common inflammatory mediators.
- Discuss the origin of the common inflammatory mediators.
- Explain the function of the vascular response in initiating the inflammatory process.
- Draw a permeable vessel, showing the manner of margination and emigration.
- List the inflammatory phagocytes and discuss their functions.

- Define chemotaxis and list the common mediators.
- Distinguish lymphocytes by type and function.
- Identify the types of exudate in acute inflammation.
- Recognize the association between type of exudate and etiology of the inflammatory process.
- Explain how factors repress and stimulate cell growth and repair.
- Categorize tissues by their potential to repair.
- Distinguish regeneration from scarring by tissue affected and size of injury.
- Define granulation tissue and comment on the role of granulation tissue in repair.
- Categorize chronic inflammation by type and cause.
- Categorize inflammatory lesions by symptoms, exudation, duration, and morphology.
- List common complications that prolong inflammation and inhibit repair.
- Name common causes of granulomatous inflammation.

INFLAMMATION

The inflammatory process consists of a coordinated series of events that is designed to neutralize, destroy, isolate, and remove any injurious agent from tissue, clean out necrotic debris, and initiate tissue repair. Repair is necessary to restore the anatomic and functional integrity of injured tissue. The processes of inflammation and repair are intertwined and depend on each other. A delayed inflammatory process will almost assuredly delay or even prevent repair, leading to morbid consequences.

We have already seen that at least some of the injurious agents that cause tissue necrosis may directly attack tissues and continue to kill cells unless intervention occurs. Microbial organisms, injurious chemicals, cancerous cells, and even necrotic cellular products may have a continued injurious effect on surrounding tissues and must be isolated, neutralized, and destroyed. We have also noted that necrotic cells become coagulated, liquefied, or caseous, and that the resultant debris occupies space in the damaged tissue. This debris must be removed before new growth can proceed correctly. The inflammatory process is responsible for these functions.

The inflammatory reaction is a very efficient process. It is usually triggered by byproducts of necrosis. Occasionally the inflammatory process is activated by the injurious agents themselves (microbes). The entire process of inflammation and repair can be compared to that of war—that is, the injurious agent is the enemy that destroys native tissue. Offensive and defensive battles result in destruction of the enemy and the rebuilding of the war-torn tissues.

We will discuss uncomplicated inflammation for purposes of clarity. As we will see later, this process is frequently complicated by either external or internal factors. Uncomplicated inflammation can be conveniently divided into three chronologic stages: the vascular stage, the early cellular response, and the late cellular response. Each stage has a specific purpose in isolating, neutralizing, or destroying the injurious agent.

The Vascular Response

The vascular response is triggered by the injurious agent itself, or by necrotic products of cell death. When a tissue is injured the sensory nerve endings of that tissue will be stimulated and will send a reflex signal (axon reflex) to the arterioles of the local area, causing them to constrict. This constriction is necessary for hemorrhage control (hemostasis). In fact, hemostasis is interwoven with the inflammatory process in several other ways, as we will see later. Vasoconstriction of arterioles limits flow of blood to the area for seconds. The smooth muscle of the arterioles then fatigues and the exhausted arterioles dilate. This allows for increased blood flow into the capillaries of the area of damage. At the same time, biochemical byproducts of tissue necrosis are activated.

Mast cells reside near capillaries and venules in most tissues. When injured, mast cells release several vasoactive substances, including *histamine*. Histamine is a potent short-acting vasodilator that causes venules and capillaries to increase markedly in diameter. This allows still more blood to accumulate within the area of tissue injury. In addition, the kinin system in the blood is activated. Inactive kinin precursors, such as blood factor XII, circulate in normal blood. When injury to tissue occurs, that injury will most likely involve some vascular components. Blood factor XII is activated by such vessel injury (exposure to collagen). Activated factor XII initiates a series of intravascular events that ultimately results in *bradykinin* production in the area of necrosis. Bradykinin is a potent short-term vasodilator of capillaries and venules. Activated factor XII also helps initiate blood clot formation. Again, the inflammatory and hemostatic processes efficiently share pathways and precursors.

Other vasodilators are formed that are longer acting. These include products of arachidonic acid. Arachidonic acid is released from necrotic cellular membranes and is biochemically transformed within the necrotic area to form prostaglandins, leukotrienes, and thromboxanes. The prostaglandin PGE is a potent medium-action vasodilator. Thromboxane is responsible for platelet aggregation—another important component of hemostasis and clot formation. The formation of both thromboxane and PGE is inhibited by aspirin. Therefore, aspirin may have an antiinflammatory effect but also may promote bleeding in injured tissues.

The result of arteriole fatigue, histamine release, bradykinin and PGE formation, and other events of lesser consequence is remarkable vasodilation with congestion of blood in the injured area (hyperemia) (Fig. 3-1). The congested vessels allow increased blood fluids and cells to concentrate within the damaged area to help isolate, neutralize, and destroy the agent and to clean up the necrotic debris.

The dilated blood vessels soon become permeable, and fluids begin to leak out into the tissues. These fluids are termed *exudates,* since they leak from intact vessel pores. Vasodilation itself allows pores to form between the endothelial cells that line the vessels. Activated substances such as histamine, bradykinin, and leukotrienes (arachidonic acid products) increase vascular permeability. In addition, the *complement system* supports and

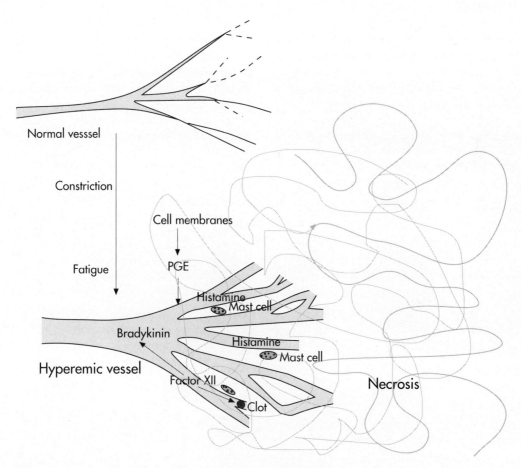

Fig. 3-1 A normal vessel is transformed into a dilated vessel in the region of necrosis. Vasodilation factors activated include histamine, bradykinin, and prostaglandins. Clotting begins by activation of factor XII in blood.

sustains vascular hyperemia and permeability. Inactive complement precursors circulate in the blood. A complement cascade can be activated by certain microbial toxins and polysaccharides (alternative pathway) or by antigen-antibody complexes (classical pathway). Activated complement is a potent permeability agent and will function in other roles as part of the inflammatory process. Notice that complement can be activated (fixed) directly by microbes and as a sequela of the immune response. We will discuss complement further in the context of the immune response.

The exudates resulting from the hyperemia and vascular permeability escape into the tissues, where they dilute toxins and help wash away or entrap offending injurious agents (Fig. 3-2). Certain white blood cells (PMNs, monocytes) are also necessary for the removal of particulate injurious agents and removal of the necrotic debris. Hyperemia aids the movement of these cells and concentrates them in the area of inflammation. Since exudation is occurring, the hyperemic blood is thick and moves slowly because of loss of fluids to the tissues.

The Early Cellular Phase

An efficient system exists to maximize the function of the white cells. This mechanism is called *chemotaxis*—which means, literally, chemical attraction. Chemotactic agents work like a fire siren that attracts volunteer firemen to extinguish a fire and clean the debris. Chemicals activated by necrotic cells or by the injurious agent are efficiently utilized and function to attract white cells to the area of chemical concentration—which is also the area of injury. The first cells chemotactically attracted to the area of inflammation are the *polymorphonuclear neutrophils* (PMNs). Cell membrane products, such as specific leukotrienes, and activated complement components are important and potent chemotactic agents for neutrophils. We have already seen

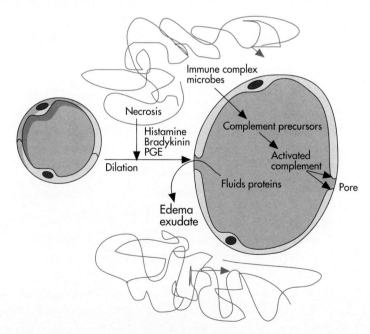

Fig. 3-2 Dilated vessels develop pores and begin to leak exudates into the surrounding injured tissues.

how these chemotactic agents are activated. Bacterial products also attract neutrophils chemotactically. Since complement is easily activated by bacteria, and bacterial products are also chemotactic for neutrophils, most bacterial infections result in marked aggregation of neutrophils. The neutrophils that are attracted to the area of inflammation must escape from the blood vessels. Several of the chemotactic agents percolate into the surrounding congested vessels and alter the endothelium in such a way that the neutrophils stick to the vessel wall—a circumstance that does not occur in vessels free of inflammation, where flow is rapid. The sticking phenomenon is termed *margination* or *pavementing*. The margination allows the neutrophils to locate pores and escape the vessel. Remember, the vascular pores have already formed and dilated secondary to activated permeability agents (kinin, PGE, complement). Neutro-

phils have the ability to physically change portions of their cytoplasm from a liquid (sol) to a more solid (gel) state. This change allows the cell to flow and then solidify in such a manner that they can penetrate the endothelial pores and move (*emigrate*) through tissues toward the greater concentration of chemotactic agents (Fig. 3-3). The volunteer firemen have responded to the siren and are ready to help isolate or neutralize the fire and clear the debris.

Once neutrophils encounter particulate matter—be it injurious agent or debris—the cells surround and engulf the particles. If the particles are very small, dissolved, or slippery, they must first be precipitated, agglutinated, or opsonized (made sticky) by antibodies (Ab's) and activated complement in order for the neutrophils to engulf the substance. Once again, the immune system may come into play and aid the inflammatory process. Immune

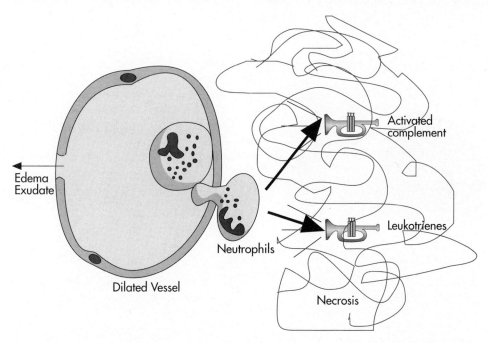

Fig. 3-3 Neutrophils marginate and are attracted to the area of necrosis and inflammation by activated complement and leukotrienes.

antibodies (if present) facilitate agglutination, precipitation, and opsonization of particles bearing antigen (Ag). The process of engulfing particles is termed phagocytosis (cell eating) and consumes much of the energy of the neutrophil (Fig. 3-4).

Once engulfed, the substance is digested within the neutrophil by several methods. Neutrophils contain numerous neutral staining lysosomes—from which they derive their name. The lysosomes are packets of enzymes that may digest lipids, proteins, and other organic substances. Shortly after phagocytosis, the lysosomes combine with the engulfed particles and digestion begins. This process is referred to as oxygen-independent digestion, since oxygen is not necessary for the reaction to occur. Neutrophilic cell membranes also contain enzymes that convert water and oxygen to *peroxide*. The peroxide combines with cellular chlorine ions to form *hypochlorite*. Hypochlorite and peroxide are highly antibacterial and are therefore responsible for destruction of engulfed bacteria. Because of their

antibacterial efficiency, hypochlorite granules are used to purify drinking water and swimming pools. Because oxygen is required, this process is designated the oxygen-dependent mechanism of digestion. Some microorganisms have evolved protective measures such as polysaccharide capsules to protect them from phagocytosis and oxygen-independent digestion. Other microbes produce enzymes that inhibit or break down peroxide and hypochlorite formation. These organisms must be isolated and destroyed by other methods, or they persist and thrive during inflammation.

Neutrophils are formed in the bone marrow and circulate in the blood in normal circumstances. Neutrophils do not contain mitochondria and therefore depend on anaerobic glycolysis for energy. Normally neutrophils survive for 2 to 7 days; however, the life span is shortened considerably when they function in the cellular phase of inflammation. They require energy to marginate, emigrate, phagocytize, and digest substances. Because they can function in the absence of oxygen, they are

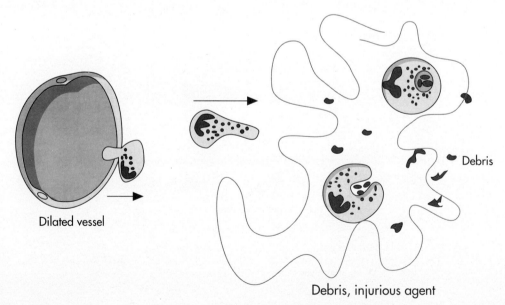

Dilated vessel

Debris

Debris, injurious agent

Fig. 3-4 Migrating neutrophils surround, engulf, and begin to digest particulate injurious agents and necrotic debris.

especially effective in areas of necrosis where oxygen availability is very low. However, they have little capacity to survive and exhaust readily in the demanding environment of inflammation. Neutrophil metabolism and cell death result in the release of neutrophilic proteins, enzymes, acids, and other products. Some of these products cause further tissue injury. However, many of these products further aid the inflammatory process. For example, neutrophilic enzymes can activate complement (alternate pathway), prostaglandin, and kinin systems yielding continuation of vasodilation and vascular permeability. In addition, metabolic acids and neutrophilic proteins can function as chemotactic agents for the next cells of inflammation, the monocytes.

The Late Cellular Stage

Monocytes are also white cells that normally circulate in the blood and are of bone marrow origin. These cells metabolize aerobically and have a longer life span. Monocytes can be activated into phagocytic cells that function to engulf and digest amounts of cellular debris and large injurious agents. Monocytes have chemotactic receptors that are sensitive to neutrophilic byproducts and other chemotactic substances. Monocytes are also attracted to a focal area by *lymphokines,* which are secretory products of activated T lymphocytes. This attraction serves as another link between inflammation and immunity and plays an important role in monocyte function in types of long-term (chronic) inflammation.

Like neutrophils, monocytes emigrate from hyperemic blood vessels and aggregate in the area of chemotactic concentration—the area of necrosis and early cellular inflammation. They engulf considerable amounts of cellular debris and markedly increase in size. Under the microscope, digestive vacuoles can be noted. These large digesting phagocytic monocytes are now termed *macrophages.* Macrophages digest primarily by lysosomal degradation, with indigestible substances being defecated into the tissue or stored within the large macrophages (Fig. 3-5). These cells have the ability to synthesize new lysosomes and to survive for long periods of time (months) at the focus of inflammation.

Lymphocytes and *plasma cells* play only a minor role in the early stages of inflammation. Lymphocytes do not readily respond to chemotaxis and therefore do not concentrate in or migrate to areas of acute inflammation. However, if the injurious agent is antigenic, lymphocytes that happen to be exposed to the antigen may be *sensitized* during the late cellular stage. This sensitization may result in antibody production by plasma cells or lymphokine production by T lymphocytes to facilitate the inflammatory process. More importantly, this exposure sensitizes lymphocytes to become memory cells that will help eliminate a similar antigen-bearing injurious agent at the next exposure or during continuous exposure (Chapter 4).

The stages of acute inflammation are characterized clinically by obvious signs and symptoms. Recognition of these signs and symptoms helps us make a correct diagnosis of inflammation and gives us information about the cause of the inflammatory reaction. Because hyperemia is the hallmark of the vascular phase, the engorged inflammatory tissues often appear *red* (rubor) and feel *warm* (calor). The capillary permeability allows for watery fluid exudation (edema) into the surrounding tissues; therefore, the tissue appears *swollen* (tumor). The edema stretches pain receptors, and activation of prostaglandin and kinins further enhances *pain* (dolor). The damaged, painful, swollen tissue frequently becomes dysfunctional; therefore, *loss of function* is an additional cardinal sign of inflammation (Fig. 3-6). The exudation associated with acute inflammation is varied in content, and the content is often characteristic of the cause of injury. Exudates leak into the tissues and onto the surfaces of inflamed tissues, where they may be recognized. Certain

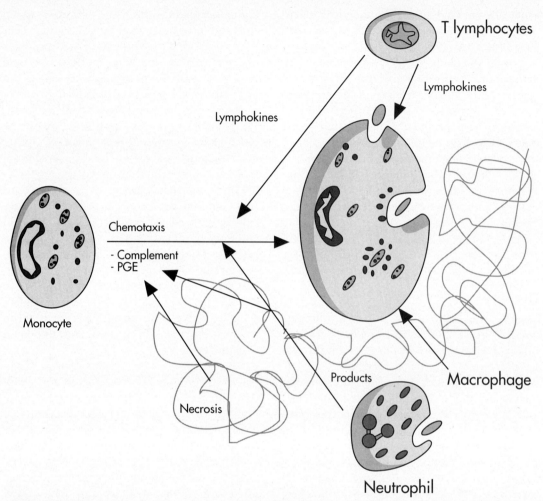

Fig. 3-5 Monocytes are attracted to the area of inflammation by neutrophil products, products of necrosis, and by lymphokines secreted by activated lymphocytes. Monocytes transform into larger phagocytic macrophages.

injuries (burn, friction) tend to cause very watery (*serous*) exudates that fill the tissues or leak into a body cavity (edema). Other injurious agents (bacteria) tend to stimulate exudates especially rich in neutrophils. This exudation is termed *purulent* or *suppurative.* The combination of live and dead neutrophils and serum is commonly termed pus. Some injuries (immune, physical) tend to stimulate an exudate that is rich in fibrin—the clotting

protein activated by the blood. This *fibrinous* exudate is sticky. When present on the skin, fibrinous exudates usually dry and crust as a scab. Within the oral cavity, fibrinous exudates appear as a white coating or pseudomembrane. Rarely, exudates contain serum and red blood cells from diapedesis or hemorrhage. This bloody exudate is termed *sanguineous.* When the respiratory tract is inflamed, the mucous glands and

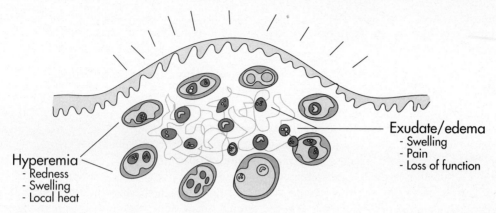

Fig. 3-6 The cardinal clinical signs and symptoms of acute inflammation result from hyperemia and exudation.

mucous cells of the system are stimulated to oversecrete, and a mucin-rich *catarrhal* exudate is formed. Mixtures of exudates (fibrinopurulent, catarrhosanguineous, sero-sanguineous) are common (Table 3-1).

Other systemic clinical features frequently accompany acute inflammation. Macrophage secretory factors, prostaglandins, and products of microorganisms frequently affect and alter the portion of the hypothalamus that regulates body temperature. The hypothalamus is stimulated by these substances, and an increased temperature or fever results. In some instances a high fever may actually cause additional illness or even death. Viruses and bacteria tend to cause fever due to elaboration of the factors listed previously. However, fever may result from nonmicrobial inflammation.

Factors released from microorganisms, neutrophils, and activated macrophages can also stimulate the bone marrow stem cell to become hyperplastic and produce more white cells (leukocytosis). These white cells are frequently released into the blood as immature forms. Some injurious agents stimulate such intense leukocytosis that the white cell count approaches that of leukemia. This is referred to as a leukemoid reaction. Other

TABLE 3-1
Inflammatory exudates

Exudate	Component	Cause
Serous	Serum H$_2$O	Burn, blister (friction)
Purulent (suppurative)	Pus Neutrophils Serum Liquefaction	Bacteria
Fibrinous	Fibrin	Injury Immune Physical Ulcerative
Sanguineous	Blood serum	Hemorrhagic
Catarrhal	Mucus	Irritation Respiratory GI
Mixed Fibrinopurulent Serosanguineous Catarrhopurulent	—	Infection of ulcer, bleeding into blister, infection of respiratory system

Inflammatory exudates may reflect the type of injurious agent responsible for the injury.

systemic reactions such as malaise and drowsiness can also result from the acute inflammatory reaction.

REPAIR

In our uncomplicated inflammatory reaction, the fluids and cells have neutralized, isolated, and destroyed the injurious agent and cleaned the necrotic tissues. The process of repair begins in coordination with the inflammatory process and is triggered by the events of necrosis and inflammation. We define *repair* as the restoration of functional or morphologic integrity to the injured tissue. Ideally, both functional and anatomic integrity will be achieved. This process, termed *regeneration,* is not always possible because (1) some tissues cannot divide and grow and (2) many tissues do not have the capacity to fill very large necrotic defects in a functional fashion. When regeneration cannot occur, the tissue is healed by an alternative form of repair termed connective tissue substitution.

Tissue Regeneration

Labile tissues are tissues in which stem cells are readily available and can divide easily, with little stimulus. The skin, oral mucosa, gut mucosa, germ cells, hematopoietic tissues, and tracheobronchial mucosa are composed of labile tissue. These tissues constantly are replaced through cell division, with new cells functionally replacing senescent ones. When necrosis occurs, mitotic rates increase and regeneration readily occurs in most circumstances. In *stable* tissues such as glands, the liver and kidneys, and most connective tissues, there is moderate or limited mitosis in response to physiologic stimulus. However, under pathologic stimulus (cell necrosis), stem cells divide and the tissue can be regenerated functionally and morphologically. Several tissues are considered *permanent.* Such tissues as cardiac muscle, neurons, and skeletal muscle have few stem or reserve cells that can mitotically divide. Therefore, these tissues cannot regenerate in response to either a physiologic or a pathologic stimulus.

Connective Tissue Substitution— Scarring

A second mechanism of repair is termed *connective tissue substitution.* As the term implies, this process substitutes strong collagenous connective tissue (scar tissue) for the original functional cells (parenchyma) of the organ. Although the tissue does not regain its function, it does regain and sometimes even increases its strength and anatomic integrity.

The process of repair, be it by regeneration or connective tissue substitution, must be stimulated and directed by localized tissue factors. In normal nondamaged tissues, cell-to-cell interactions help regulate tissue growth. Some of these subtle intercellular physical and chemical factors constantly inhibit division of other cells. When necrosis occurs, there is a void in the tissues, and *contact-inhibitory factors* are no longer released by the dead cells. In fact, necrotic cells now release factors that stimulate cell division and growth in the adjacent stem cells. In addition, products of the inflammatory process and inflammatory cells initiate cell division, cell migration, and cellular maturation. For example, macrophage-derived growth factor (MDGF) stimulates blood vessel and fibroblast formation; and platelet-derived growth factor (PDGF) (hemostasis is also occurring) stimulates proliferation of endothelial and smooth muscle cells (also see atherosclerosis in Chapter 10). Other mitogens such as epidermal growth factors (EGFs) are activated by necrosis and stimulate regeneration of skin. Indeed, biochemists can now manufacture EGF and use it to treat patients who have large surface burns to stimulate regeneration of the skin.

The process of repair occurs in close coordination with the process of inflammation. The surviving stimulated stem cells—be they parenchymal or connective tissue—divide, grow, and migrate to fill the tissue defect. Cell migration is directed and further stimulated by matrix-to-tissue interactions. The necrotic zone has become filled with a matrix of exudation and clotting components consisting of fibrin, fibronectins, platelets, and macrophages. This matrix is both mitogenic (stimulating mitosis) and chemotactic for regenerating cells such as fibroblasts. In addition, it provides a scaffold for cellular migration and growth from the periphery. Regenerating parenchymal cells, fibroblasts, and angioblasts are attracted to and migrate over this superstructure. Therefore, the new reparative tissue fills the previously voided space.

When connective tissue substitution occurs, the fibroblasts and angioblasts are the predominate cells to grow from the undamaged margins into the area of repair. After a period of days, the fibroblasts begin to secrete immature collagen and the angioblasts form capillary buds that develop into miniature blood vessels. Within a period of days—depending on the size of the damaged tissue—the space becomes filled with a combination of fibroblasts, fibrocytes, angioblasts, capillary buds, and late-stage inflammatory cells. This combination of reparative tissues is designated *granulation tissue* (Fig. 3-7). Over a subsequent period of weeks to months, the granulation tissue matures. Fibroblasts secrete more collagen, which polymerizes. Angioblasts and capillary buds mature into blood vessels. As more collagen is formed, the tissue

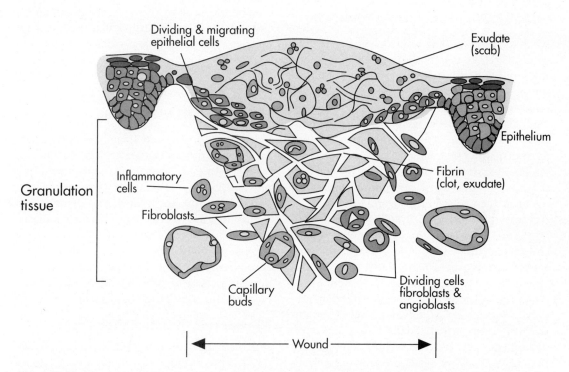

Fig. 3-7 This wound is healing by regeneration of epithelial cells and by granulation tissue that closes the defect. Fibrinous exudate and clot provide a framework for this regeneration.

becomes more dense, less cellular, less vascular, tough, and contracted. This highly collagenous tissue is termed scar tissue and is the sequela of connective tissue substitution.

With regeneration, there is a similar mitogenic stimulation of stem cells with activated factors from products of necrosis and inflammatory cells, as well as stimulation and chemotaxis of new cells by exudates and blood clots. The preservation of tissue architecture is essential for effective reestablishment of organ and tissue function. If, in labile and stable tissues, the basic tissue architecture is intact, the regenerative tissue will duplicate the form and function of the previously damaged tissue. If, however, the defect is very large and tissue architecture is disintegrated, the repair may occur in a haphazard, nonfunctional arrangement, or connective tissue substitution (scarring) may replace some of the functional tissues.

COMPLICATIONS OF INFLAMMATION

We have now outlined the basic events responsible for uncomplicated inflammation and repair. There are, however, many variables throughout this process that are readily altered. When this occurs, the process becomes complicated and prolonged. Many factors can alter, inhibit, and delay the inflammatory and reparative processes. Such factors include conditions that reduce the vascular or cellular responses, repeated or continuous injury to the area, persistent infection, and loss of integrity of the healing area. Systemic disease and nutritional deficiency may also delay repair and regeneration. In addition, some injurious agents are by their nature resistant to the inflammatory process and are persistent even when the inflammatory process is fully operational. For example, individuals with certain vascular diseases that reduce blood flow will demonstrate delayed inflammatory and reparative response. You have probably observed that a baby heals much more rapidly than a senior citizen with decreased circulation,

when a similar injury occurs. Numerous drugs can inhibit the vascular response, chemotaxis, phagocytosis, digestion, fibroblast proliferation, and mitosis of stem cells. Cortisone affects almost all of the above functions and therefore reduces and delays the inflammatory reaction and the reparative response. Patients with white cell diseases (agranulocytosis, leukemia) have a deficiency in number or function of white blood cells (WBCs). Such patients may exhibit prolonged or inadequate inflammatory reactions to uncomplicated injurious agents, or exaggerated infections from organisms that normally do not cause severe disease. Some organisms have specific characteristics that make them slippery, indigestible, or undetectable by the inflammatory response. If inflamed and repairing tissues are also infected or traumatized, if the matrix is lost, or if the cells and vessels of inflammation are damaged, the process will be prolonged. Finally, the growth of new tissues (repair) is dependent on nutritional elements for energy, cellular construction, and collagen formation. Therefore, nutritional deficiency will delay this response (Table 3-2).

CHRONIC INFLAMMATION

Long-term, complicated inflammation is known as *chronic inflammation* and is usually the result of one or several of the factors listed previously. Most chronic inflammatory reactions are nonspecific; that is, they demonstrate similar histopathologic and clinical manifestations. Some specific injuries, however, cause the microscopically distinctive granulomatous chronic inflammation. Histopathologic recognition of this type of inflammation provides many clues to the etiology of the disease.

Nonspecific Chronic Inflammation

Nonspecific chronic inflammation is characterized by a reduced vascular response and reduced early cellular response. Tissue necrosis is usually reduced because the injurious agent has been at least somewhat neutralized—or was never very destructive to begin with. Hyperemia, exudation, and neutrophilic infiltrations are not particularly notable. The low-grade injurious agent, however, is persistent and has not been completely eliminated for whatever reason (Table 3-2). Therefore, the late cellular stage—consisting of macrophages, lymphocytes and plasma cells, granulation tissue, and scar tissue—is enhanced and prolonged. The lymphocytes react to the antigens of the injurious agent by transforming into plasma cells (B lymphocytes) or by attracting, transforming, and capturing macrophages (T lymphocytes). Granulation tissue, fibroblast proliferation, and collagen formation are im-

TABLE 3-2
Prolonged inflammation and repair

Mechanism	Cause
Decreased blood to area	Vascular disease, heart disease, aging, anemia
Decreased vasoactive substances	Drugs, medications
Decreased WBC quantity	Bone marrow depression, drugs
Decreased WBC quality	Diabetes, drugs, genetic disease, leukemia
Decreased fibroblast activity, collagen	Starvation, nutritional deficiency, drugs
Increased number of microorganisms	Reinfection
Increased resistance of microorganisms	Specific organisms Indigestible Coated
Decreased fibrin	Loss or failure of clot
Reinjury	Reinjury

Interruption or interference with any of the mechanisms of inflammation and repair will prolong the process and slow healing.

portant components of the chronically inflamed tissue that is attempting to repair itself during the extended period of time.

The clinical signs and symptoms of nonspecific chronic inflammation reflect these tissue changes. The duration of the lesion is prolonged. The tissue appears normal to pale in color, depending on the degree of scarring. The tissue may be swollen and firm because of proliferation of granulation tissue, scar tissue, and accumulation of mononuclear inflammatory cells. The lesion is usually not particularly painful, red, or warm—since all these symptoms reflect the vascular and exudative phases of acute inflammation that are now absent. Nonspecific chronic inflammatory lesions may exist for years, may finally resolve and repair with scarring, may revert to a more acute phase when they become further complicated, or may actually become very proliferative and even tumor-like. Treatment usually involves identification and removal of the injurious agent.

Granulomatous Inflammation

Granulomatous inflammation is a specific type of *chronic* inflammation that is recognizable at the histopathologic level. The granulomatous pattern is a manifestation of the immune and inflammatory reactions to several very specific etiologic agents. In general, granulomatous chronic inflammation occurs in response to injurious agents that have strong T lymphocyte antigenicity and are relatively indigestible by macrophages. The antigenicity elicits T cell activation and elaboration of lymphokines. As we have already seen, lymphokines chemotactically attract monocytes and transform them into macrophages (Fig. 3-5). The result is a lesion dominated by macrophages. These macrophages engulf the injurious substance. Since digestion is difficult, the macrophages tend to accumulate the agent and change in morphology. Macrophages become elongated cells (epithelioid cells) and cluster in spherical masses or granulomas. Some macrophages coalesce with others to form giant multinucleated cells. Lymphocytes some plasma cells, granulation tissue, and scar tissue outline the periphery of each granuloma. In some diseases, the granulomas encase the regions of necrosis and injury (Fig. 3-8). In other diseases, there is little necrosis. The granulomatous reaction itself may be the lesion responsible for morbidity of the tissue—the causative agent injures the tissue by stimulation of the chronic granulomatous response. Diseases such as tuberculosis, deep fungal infections, and many inflammatory reactions to foreign bodies are classically granulomatous in nature.

NOMENCLATURE OF INFLAMMATION

Nomenclature allows us to communicate with other dental and medical personnel without lengthy explanation. In general, *acute inflammation* is of short duration and is characterized by redness, swelling, heat, pain, and loss of function. Fever and leukocytosis may or may not occur. *Chronic inflammation* is relatively nonpainful, pale, firm, swollen, and of a duration ranging from weeks to years. The suffix *-itis* is used to designate inflammation of an organ or tissue, regardless of its cause. For

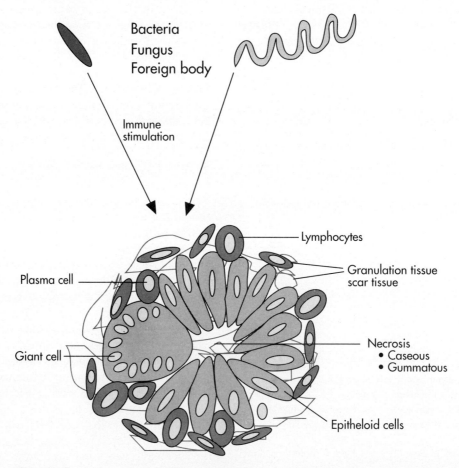

Fig. 3-8 The microscopic lesion of granulomatous inflammation is characterized by epithelioid cells, giant cells, lymphocytes, granulation tissue, and scar tissue arranged in a spherical cluster (granuloma).

example, a recent, red, swollen inflammation of the gingiva is designated as *acute gingivitis.* A proliferative, slow-growing, pale, painless inflammation of the periodontium is termed *chronic periodontitis.* We can further characterize the nature and, perhaps, cause of an inflammatory lesion by using a descriptive term to describe the exudate, associated necrosis, and/or type of inflammatory pattern. An acute suppurative gingivitis is probably caused by *pyogenic* (pus-forming) bacteria, whereas a chronic granulomatous caseous gingivitis is most likely a manifestation of tuberculosis.

Sometimes we name the inflammatory lesion by its appearance. A diffuse, swollen acute inflammation with much seropurulent exudation is termed a *cellulitis.* A focal accumulation of pus (purulent exudate) in a localized area of liquefaction is termed an *abscess.* An inflammatory break in a mucosal or epidermal surface is termed an *inflammatory ulcer.*

DISCUSSION

We have now nearly completed our discussion of the inflammatory process. Vascular and cellular changes isolate, neutralize, and destroy injurious agents and clean necrotic debris. Even the chronic inflammatory response isolates the agent and destroys the bulk of the offending organisms or substances. What happens if there are disorders of the inflammatory or immune processes? Debilitating diseases may occur as a result of either inflammatory deficiencies or inflammatory overreaction.

It should be apparent that if the inflammatory-immune processes are deficient, injuries will persist and enlarge, and offending agents might continue to spread and destroy tissues. Individuals with severe deficiencies will most likely die of infections from common, often nonvirulent organisms. Cancer patients with reduced inflammatory responses, AIDS patients, and patients with leukemia and leukopenia are all likely to develop such problems. As we have already seen, patients with minor inflammatory system problems such as aging or diabetes demonstrate chronic infections and delayed wound healing. An intact inflammatory-immune system, then, is necessary for optimal patient health.

The inflammatory system can also be responsible for patient morbidity and mortality. Because inflammation itself can cause loss of function and dysfunction, there are instances in which the injurious agents cause disease by stimulating an inflammatory reaction. We have already noted that certain microorganisms cause disease by stimulating gross exudation (pneumonia) or granuloma formation (foreign body) without causing significant direct tissue necrosis. In other instances, low-grade traumatic injury can cause an inflammatory reaction where there is marked loss of function. In hypersensitivity and allergic reactions, the inflammatory system overreacts to a perceived injurious agent that is relatively harmless. Pollens do not cause tissue necrosis; however, when one is allergic to pollen, the immune system causes the mast cells to release histamines and leukotrienes. The resultant vascular and cellular inflammatory response leaves the individual with uncomfortable manifestations. Likewise, the oils of the poison ivy plant are not very toxic for tissues. Instead, these oils stimulate a hypersensitive inflammatory-immune response that may harm the tissues. Such overreactions are therefore treated by removal of the stimulus and medication with antiinflammatory and immune suppression drugs (aspirin, cortisone, antihistamine, etc.). These drugs reduce the inflammatory response and make the patient more comfortable.

Case Studies

Case 1
M.K. is a 51-year-old man who scheduled a routine dental visit for the first time in 5 years. He was having no oral problems and sought dental

care because his company had a new dental insurance plan. Oral examination revealed calculus, moderate to severe periodontal bone loss, focal mild gingivitis, recurrent caries, and a 1-cm well-demarcated radiolucent area apical to tooth #20. M.K. remembered that a restoration had broken from #20 4 years earlier; but the tooth had never bothered him, so he did not seek treatment. The tooth was extracted because of the periapical and periodontal involvement, and the periapical lesion was submitted to an oral pathology laboratory. The laboratory reported that the lesion was composed of granulation tissue, fibrosis, plasma cells, lymphocytes, and macrophages. The socket healed without complication and M.K. began comprehensive dental treatment.

Case 2

H.G. is a 21-year-old college-football player who suffered a strained left knee during preseason practice. The torn ligament was diagnosed, and rest was the prescribed therapy. Before the day of the opening game, the knee became swollen and painful, and could not be bent to the maximal degree. One day before the game, H.G. had fluid drained from the knee and was given a cortisone shot in the joint. He caught nine passes, including the game-winning touchdown pass with 3 minutes to go.

Case 3

M.P. is an 18-year-old woman who complained of a very painful swollen red gingiva buccal to tooth #15. The pain had been present for 3 days. Oral examination revealed a swollen, reddened 0.8 cm area of the attached gingiva and alveolar mucosa buccal to tooth #15. The tooth was vital, there was no obvious lesion, and the radiograph showed no abnormality. A periodontal probe in the buccal sulcus measured a pseudopocket of 6 mm, and copious purulent drainage resulted. A foreign body resembling a popcorn shell was removed from the "pocket." M.P. recalled eating popcorn at the movies 1 week before. She was placed on antibiotics for 7 days. Ten days later, at the time of the follow-up visit, all signs and symptoms had resolved themselves, the pocket had regressed to 3 mm, and the gingiva looked healthy.

Case 1

1. What do you think accounted for the periapical lesion?
2. Why were the periapical and periodontal lesions not painful?
3. Does the histopathology help diagnose the cause of the apical lesion?
4. What kind of healing would you expect to occur after surgery?

Case 2

1. Do you think the knee was inflamed? Why?
2. Explain the presence of fluid on the knee.
3. Why was a cortisone shot given and what was its effect?
4. What risks result from such treatment?

Case 3

1. Do you think there was acute inflammation present?
2. Name the lesion.
3. What role did popcorn and bacteria play in etiology and pathogenesis of the lesion?

SUMMARY

- The inflammatory reaction is an efficient process that isolates, destroys, or removes injurious agents, and cleans the necrotic area in preparation for tissue repair.
- Uncomplicated inflammation is of short duration and consists of vascular, early cellular, and late cellular responses.
- Each stage of the inflammatory response helps trigger and facilitate subsequent stages until repair is accomplished.
- The inflammatory response shares intermediate activated substances with the parallel hemostatic and immune responses.
- Mediators of the inflammatory response are usually multifunctional.
- The inflammatory response in itself can cause harm or additional injury to tissues. The degree of injury may exceed that caused by the inciting injurious agent.

- The acute inflammatory response can be characterized clinically by the signs, symptoms, and exudates related to the pathogenesis of the inflammatory disease.
- A specific nomenclature is used to help communicate the diagnosis of inflammatory disease.
- The inflammatory response is often compromised by agents that are resistant to or interfere with the inflammatory response. Chronic inflammation is the result.
- Tissue repair results from accelerated cellular division and replacement of damaged tissues. Increased cellular division is based on loss of growth inhibitors and increase in growth factors activated from necrotic tissues and inflammatory cells.
- All tissues do not have the same capacity for cellular division. Some tissues have little or no capacity for cell regeneration and therefore must repair by connective tissue substitution.
- Granulomatous inflammation results when specific antigenic agents stimulate a T lymphocyte-mediated response. Granulomatous inflammation can further injure tissue.

Suggested readings

1. Bomalaski JS, Williamson PK, and Zurier RB: Prostaglandins and the inflammatory response, Clin Lab Med 3:695, 1983.
2. Fantone JC and Ward PA: Inflammation. In Rubin E and Farber JL, editors: Pathology, Philadelphia, 1988, JB Lippincott.
3. Finch RF, Aker F, and Miller RL: The inflammatory reaction: a programmed workbook on the sequence of inflammation and its modification, Columbus, Ind, 1981, Thompson.
4. Gross M and Dexter M: Growth factors in development, transformation and tumorigenesis, Cell 64:271, 1991.
5. Karnovsky MJ: The ultrastructural basis of capillary permeability studied with perioxidase as a tracer, J Cell Biol 35:213, 1967.
6. Kumar V, Cotran RS, and Robbins SL: Basic pathology, Philadelphia, 1992, WB Saunders, chapter 2.
7. O'Flaherty JT: Lipid mediators in inflammation and allergy, Lab Invest 47:314, 1982.
8. Samuelsson B: Leukotienes: mediators of immediate hypersensitivity reactions and inflammation, Science 220:568, 1983.
9. Snyderman R and Goetzl EJ: Molecular and cellular mechanisms of leukocyte chemotaxis, Science 213:830, 1981.
10. Taussig MJ: Processes in pathology and microbiology, ed 2, Oxford, 1984, Blackwell, section 1.
11. Wedmore CV and Williams TJ: Control of vascular permeability by polynuclear leukocytes in inflammation, Nature 289:646, 1981.

4 Immune Reaction

After studying this chapter, you should be able to meet the following objectives and define the key terms:

- Explain the role of the immune response in controlling disease.
- Explain the role of the immune response in causing disease.
- Define self-antigenicity.
- List the common cells of the immune system.
- List the functions of the common cells of the immune system.
- Define immune "memory."
- Discuss autoimmune disease and common causes.
- List the sequelae of immune deficiency states.
- List the common causes of immune deficiency.
- Define cytokines and list their functions in the immune response.
- Describe immune hypersensitivity diseases and give examples.

The immune reaction is designed to help the healthy body resist and defend against certain injurious agents. We have already seen that the immune reaction plays a helping role in the cellular stage of acute inflammation and a sustaining role in both nonspecific and granulomatous chronic inflammation. These are very important functions. The immune system also functions to prevent injurious agents such as certain microbes, toxins, parasites, and even altered cells (cancer, transplantation) from becoming established, proliferating, and causing harm. Basically, four types of diseases can result from immune system dysfunction. These are (1) immune deficiency disorders, (2) hypersensitivity disorders, (3) autoimmune disorders, and (4) immune cellular proliferative disorders (leukemia, lymphoma). We will review the normal immune process and describe the first three types of mentioned disorders in this chapter.

NORMAL IMMUNE SYSTEM FUNCTION

In review, the normal immune system functions to destroy and isolate antigen-bearing injurious agents. Remember that most body tissues are antigenic. However, the immune system learns to recognize "self" during development and therefore usually does not attack the body's own cells. The immune system is composed of two distinct classes of lymphocytes (T cells and B cells), as well as antigen-processing and antigen-presenting cells (APCs), which are most frequently macrophages. The lymphocytes are memory cells. When a lymphocyte precursor is stimulated and becomes sensitized to a specific nonself antigen—usually a protein on a microbe or cell—the sensitized lymphocyte will react to that antigen. All progeny of the sensitized lymphocyte will also develop a memory for the specific antigen and will react (attack) when the antigen (injurious agent) reappears. If you were cheated in a business relationship, you might describe the specific characteristics of the person who cheated you to your children. They in turn would pass on this description (antigen code) to their children and grandchildren. Generations later a similar-appearing cheater (silk tie, big car, Rolex watch) would be instantly recognized by your great-grandchildren, who might tar and feather him (antibodies), tear his pin-striped suit (cytolytic cells), or call the police (lymphokines). The antigen would be inhibited and the damage prevented or restricted.

B Lymphocytes

The B-lymphocyte precursor cells reside in lymph nodes and are sensitized by certain antigens. The progeny of sensitized B lymphocytes mature into sensitized plasma cells within lymph nodes and tissues. The plasma cells produce antibodies specifically directed against the antigen. Antibodies circulate in the blood and percolate through tissues until they encounter the specific antigen (the Rolex cheater). The antibody binds itself to the antigen material. Once the binding occurs, the antigen-antibody complex may be opsonized, agglutinated, or precipitated for inflammatory phagocytosis. In addition, complement may be activated for opsonization or proteolytic destruction of the antigenic agent. (See Fig. 4-1.) This classical complement fixation also can lead to chemotaxis of neutrophils and

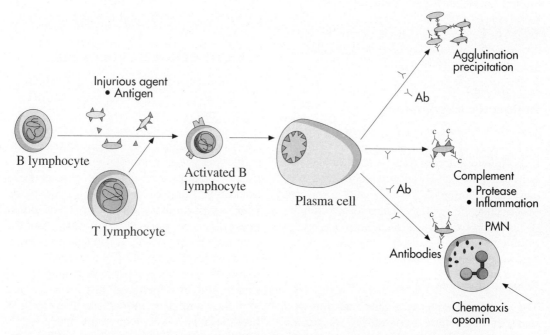

Fig. 4-1 The B lymphocyte is sensitized by contact with an antigen. With stimulation by T lymphocyte cytokines, the B lymphocyte develops a memory for the antigen. Daughter B lymphocytes from this cell will develop into plasma cells that secrete specific antibodies that help inactivate the antigen (injurious agent).

enhance the vascular inflammatory reaction. All of these functions promote inhibition and destruction of the injurious agent.

T Lymphocytes

The T-lymphocyte precursors are processed (educated) in the thymus gland and subquently reside in the lymphoid nodules that they share with B-lymphocyte precursors. These T cells also develop a memory for a single specific foreign antigen associated with an injurious agent. The antigenic memory is passed down through generations to numerous T-cell progeny. When sensitized T cells encounter the "silk tie antigen," they react by sending messages to other cells, including T cells, B cells, and macrophages. These chemical messages are termed lymphokines or cytokines, and they instruct the other cells to shred, club, punch, and generally disable the antigenic agent. Some sensitized T cells (cytolytic) can directly destroy the agent, whereas some simply call other cells to help. (See Fig. 4-2.) The net result is that the silk tie bandit is destroyed or at least inhibited. Review chronic granulomatous inflammation. This is a good example of this process.

Antigen-Processing Cells

The third series of cells to participate in the immune reaction is the antigen-processing cells. In many cases the T lymphocytes are quite farsighted and do not immediately recognize the antigenic substances. Antigen-processing cells such as macrophages initially change or process the antigen until it is recognizable to the lymphocytes. Then the lymphocytes can react and function.

Coordination of Cells

The three cell systems usually function as a team, and therefore, communications are important. In many situations a team leader functions to call and coordinate signals. The T-helper lymphocyte, also called the T_4 lymphocyte, usually serves in this role. Once the T_4 lymphocyte has been presented with the antigen by the APC, it sends chemical lymphokines, termed interleukins, to other T_4 and T_8 lymphocytes and B lymphocytes, instructing them to proliferate and function. (See Fig. 4-2.) Other lymphokines have effects on macrophages, such as initiation of macrophage chemotaxis, activation of phagocytosis, and aggregation at the area of injury (antigen). T_8 lymphocytes function to (1) directly destroy the antigenic agent and (2) send messages back to T_4 cells (again via interleukins). Some of these messages inhibit further immune response so that there is not an overreaction. Because T_8 cells function to limit the immune response, they are often referred to as suppressor cells. Activated macrophages and B cells also communicate by interleukins. Other types of lymphocytes (NK cells) and macrophages participate in the immune reaction with extensive communication and feedback by interleukins. The system therefore is very complex and precise and is easily distorted.

IMMUNE DEFICIENCY DISEASES

Immune deficiency diseases occur when the immune system does not form or mature completely (primary disease) or when the lymphocytes or APCs are suppressed or destroyed by exogenous factors (secondary disease). Regardless of cause, immune deficiency diseases usually demonstrate common clinical manifestations. Immune suppressed patients develop opportunistic infections from organisms that are normally controlled by the immune system. These organisms are ubiquitous (widespread within the everyday environment), are not very virulent, and usually cause mild or subclinical disease in normal immune competent individuals. For example, histoplasmosis is a common fungal spore found in the soil and air in the middle United States. About 80% of all young adults in the Ohio-Mississippi valley have a positive histoplasmosis skin test, indicating that they have

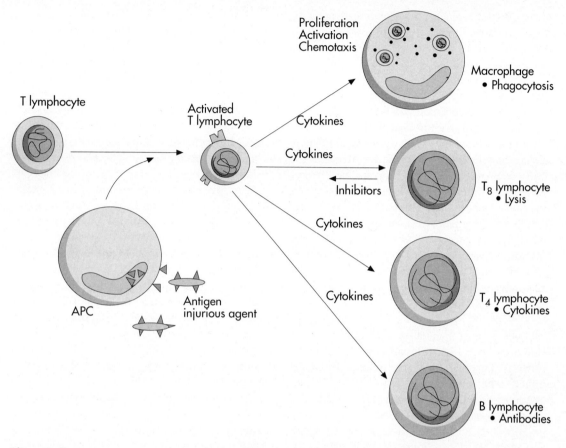

Fig. 4-2 The T lymphocyte receives the antigen from the APC. The T lymphocyte is now specifically sensitized and activated to the antigen and via cytokines initiates antigen destruction by macrophages, T lymphocytes, and B lymphocytes.

been infected by this organism. Only a few of these individuals can recall being ill from this organism (flu-like respiratory disease), and clinical lesions are rare. However, if individuals are immune suppressed, histoplasmosis can readily become a widely disseminated infection of most tissues, resulting in morbidity and mortality. In fact, the majority of patients with widespread histoplasmosis are immune suppressed. Similar morbid sequelae occur with herpes viruses, tubercu-

losis, protozoans, and common bacteria in immune compromised patients. These infections frequently involve the oral cavity. You will learn some specifics of these "opportunistic" diseases when we discuss human immunodeficiency virus (HIV) and immune suppression, and some of the commonly associated oral infections.

Since the immune cells also patrol for cancer and transplantation cells, immune suppressed patients are also more susceptible to development of certain cancers—especially those supposedly caused by microorganisms— than are normal patients. Long-term immune suppression patients have a higher incidence of cancers in general, and certain highly specific cancers (lymphoma, Kaposi's sarcoma), than do nonsuppressed patients.

Immune suppression is common. The condition most often is a result of medication such as corticosteroid drug therapy. Interestingly, corticosteroids are usually prescribed to reduce the immune and inflammatory processes in conditions where these processes are hyperactive (severe edema of inflammation) or overreactive (autoimmune disease, hypersensitivity disease). Other common diseases such as AIDS, leukemia, and lymphoma (lymph cancer) will also suppress the immune system.

Transplantation

All cells of an individual bear surface antigens called major histocompatibility complexes (MHCs). These antigens are genetically determined and therefore vary among all individuals—except perhaps identical twins. The immune system of each individual is programmed to recognize these antigens as self and therefore does not attack one's own cells. However, if tissues from another individual are transplanted into the patient, the immune system will detect, but fail to recognize, the "foreign" MHCs, and the lymphocytes and macrophages will begin the immune process and ultimately reject the transplanted tissues. Physicians attempt to match the MHCs of the transplant donor to those of the recipient (by matching family, blood type) to diminish the immune response. However, some immune rejection is inevitable. Therefore, immune suppressive drugs have been developed and are used to reduce the immune response and increase transplant survival. This therapy, however, makes transplantation patients susceptible to the opportunistic infections and cancers mentioned earlier.

Hypersensitivity disease

In hypersensitivity disorders, the immune system overreacts to an antigen that otherwise might, in itself, cause little or no harm to tissues. Both T-lymphocyte and B-lymphocyte hypersensitivity conditions exist. Some individuals seem especially prone to hypersensitivity diseases (allergy) and often have inherited this predisposition from their parents. Four basic mechanisms of hypersensitivity are noted (Fig. 4-3).

The overreaction of the immune systems can cause necrosis and dysfunction of tissue by each of these mechanisms. Therefore, management and prevention frequently involve suppression of the inflammatory and immune systems with such drugs as antihistamines, antiinflammatory drugs, and immune suppression agents. Avoidance of the antigenic substance (TB, drugs, pollen) is paramount in prevention of further disease.

Type 1: Anaphylaxis, allergy. Individuals react to harmless antigens by making IgE-class antibodies. These antibodies attach to mast cells. When the antigen is again encountered, the mast cells degranulate, histamine and leukotrienes are activated, and a severe acute inflammatory response causes clinical signs and symptoms. Example: Antibodies to harmless pollen attach to the mast cells of the nasopharynx. Hay fever results from pollen contact and inflammation of sinus and respiratory membranes.

Type 2: Cytolytic effect. "Normal cells" appear antigenic to the immune system and are regarded as foreign by B cells. Either the antigenicity of the normal cells has been altered by an exogenous agent, or the confused B cell makes antibody to "normal" antigen. Antibodies coat these normal cells, resulting in cell lysis from either complement fixation or lymphocyte cytotoxicity. Example: A drug stimulates antibodies that coat normal red blood cells (RBCs). The red cells are lysed and hemolytic anemia results.

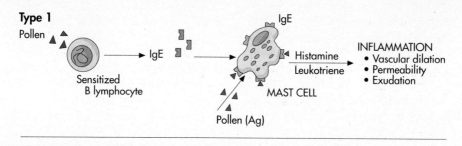

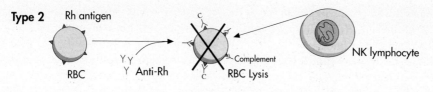

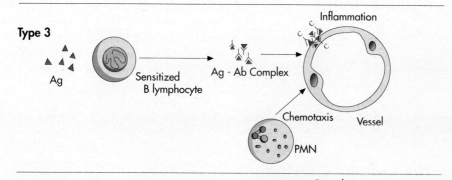

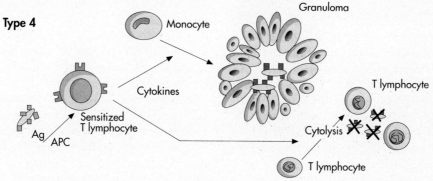

Fig. 4-3 Hypersensitivity reactions damage tissues in response to relatively harmless antigens. Damage occurs because of allergy and inflammation (Type 1), cell lysis by complement, or lymphocytes (Type 2), inflammation due to antigen-antibody complexes (Type 3), and granulomatous inflammation or T lymphocyte mediated cell lysis (Type 4).

Type 3: Immune complex disease. Numerous, relatively harmless antigens form complexes with antibodies. These complexes are entrapped in blood vessel walls where complement is activated. Complement fractions stimulate vascular and cellular stages of acute inflammation (vasculitis), which damages the tissue. Example: Antibodies and antigens from a streptococcal throat infection form complexes in the blood and settle in the vessels of the glomeruli of the kidney. Glomerulonephritis results.

Type 4: Delayed hypersensitivity. A relatively harmless antigen stimulates a T-lymphocyte sensitivity. The sensitized T cells either initiate a chronic granulomatous inflammation or initiate T-cell cytotoxicity of any cell to which the antigen attaches. Either way, normal tissue may be damaged by the immune response. Example: Tuberculosis (TB) bacillus initiates a chronic granulomatous response that destroys and occludes pulmonary tissues. Example: Hepatitis virus infects liver cells. T cells react to the viral antigens by cytolytically destroying liver cells.

AUTOIMMUNE DISEASE

In autoimmune diseases, the immune cells either become confused and attack normal cells (self), or normal cells are altered antigenically and are no longer respected as self by the immune system. Either way, the immune system is stimulated to destroy normal cells. Occasionally, antibodies are made against exogenous injurious agents (bacteria). These antibodies *crossreact* with and thereby destroy normal tissues that appear antigenically quite similar to the exogenous antigen. For example, antibodies against the M protein of β-streptococcus (strep throat) may destroy normal heart tissues that have somewhat similar self antigens (rheumatic heart disease). In some cases, confusion is due to mutations within cells and tissues that result in *new antigenicity* based on the mutation or changes. We will see later that such an immune reaction is helpful when these new antigens are found on cancer cells. However, such mutations may trigger immune destruction of otherwise normal tissues. This is comparable to the nervous spouse who doesn't recognize her drunken (mutated) husband stumbling through the window at 2 AM. She shoots the "burglar" without recognition or realization of who it is. Another mechanism for autoimmune reaction involves changes or mutations within the immune cells. These immune cells may change so that they no longer recognize self antigens. They will then begin to react to normal tissues and destroy them. This reminds one of the frightened policeman who shoots the store owner instead of the robber because, in his fright, he fails to recognize the uniform of the store owner. Exogenous agents like drugs, viruses, or chemicals frequently contribute to such changes or mutations.

We have superficially reviewed the immune system and noted many complex interactions that stimulate and depress immune function. Remember that interleukins carry messages that stimulate or repress other immune cells. When the interleukins are altered or modified, feedback can be inhibited or stimulation can be exaggerated. The net result might be overreaction of the system, to attack self tissues. Tissue destruction will follow. In this instance, the immune reaction shoots everything that moves and asks questions later. Again, exogenous substances can contribute to this autoimmune defect. Finally, during development of the immune system, there is a period of time when self-tolerance recognition is developed. If exogenous antigens are introduced during this time, they might be tolerated as self. For example, a prenatal transplant might never be rejected—even without immune suppression. But the opposite also occurs. Some normal antigenic tissues and substances might be hidden (sequestered) from the immune system during natal development. These antigens will not be tolerated as self in the future.

If events occur that later expose this antigen to the immune system, the cells will attack and destroy "normal cells" demonstrating the sequestered antigen. (See Fig. 4-4) Orphaned siblings may be separated from each other. Lacking knowledge of their relationship, they may fall in love and marry. Legal and genetic dysfunction results. Numerous fairly common diseases—including rheumatoid arthritis, lupus erythematosus, Hashimoto's thyroiditis, scleroderma, Sjögren's syndrome, atrophic gastritis, and many others—are morbid diseases with an autoimmune component. In all of these conditions, antibodies and/or activated T lymphocytes are responsible for de-

struction of normal tissues. Once again, treatment consists of administration of immune suppressive agents. Immune deficiency may be secondary to the therapy.

You will later study controlled and uncontrolled proliferations (cancer) of cells and tissues. Both situations commonly involve the immune system. The etiology and pathogenesis of cancer will also be explained later. Primary cancer of the immune system can involve solid tissues (cancer of the lymph nodes and bone marrow) and circulating cells (leukemia). Because cancer cells are dysfunctional, cancerous immune disorders generally result in immune suppression.

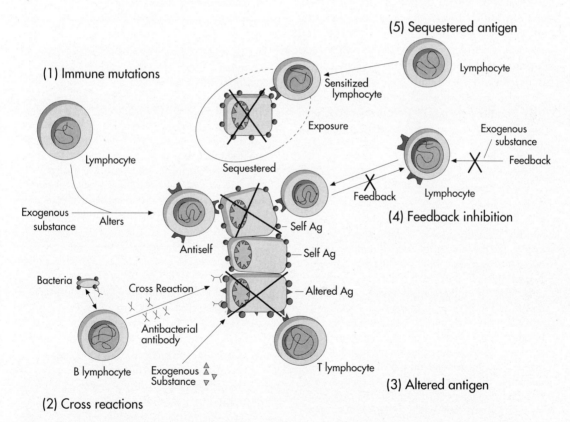

Fig. 4-4 The immune system can injure self tissues through (1) immune mutations that allow lymphocytes to attack self, (2) cross reactions where antibacterial antibody also attacks self antigen, (3) alteration of self cells that makes them antigenically susceptible to immune cells, (4) loss of feedback inhibition of antiself cells, or (5) recognizing and attacking formerly hidden antigenic tissues.

DISCUSSION

In summary, the immune reaction is necessary and responsible for policing potentially harmful exogenous and endogenous intruders and preventing them from causing tissue injury. In addition, the immune police are expected to respect the integrity and appearance of the normal cell citizenry. When the immune system is depressed, either by exogenous or endogenous agents, morbidity will occur secondary to proliferation of infections or neoplastic intruders. In some instances, however, the immune system may overreact, as in hypersensitivity to a relatively harmless agent, and thus further injure the tissues by virtue of the immune reaction itself. In autoimmune diseases, the immune cells become either confused or disoriented and injure the normal tissues they are supposed to respect. Immune system cancer often leads to crowding and destruction of adjacent normal tissues as well as deficiencies of the immune system. Therefore, balance of the immune system is vital to maintenance of patient health.

Case Studies

Case 1
B. J. is a 48-year-old woman who developed heart failure secondary to a medication she was taking. She received a cadaveric heart transplant and recovered well from the surgery. She was placed on daily doses of prednisone, cyclosporine, and azathioprine, immune suppression drugs used to prevent rejection of the heart. The transplant did well, and B. J. became active and resumed employment without limitation. She, however, developed frequent yeast (candida) infections on the tongue and oral mucosa, and pulmonary histoplasmosis. Both conditions were cleared by antifungal medications. Her oral treatment plan was adjusted by her dentist, after consultation with her physician, to include prophylactic use of an antifungal mouthwash.

Case 2
D. S. is a 28-year-old woman who developed chronic oral ulcers, painful arthritis, kidney disease, and a skin rash across the bridge of the nose. All lesions were diagnosed as stemming from systemic lupus erythematosus based on biopsy and blood tests that demonstrated immune B- and T-cell reaction to her own deoxyribonucleic acid (DNA), kidney, skin, and mucous membranes. She was placed on antilupus therapy, including immunosuppression medication. Constant adjustment of her medications controlled her disease and reduced her symptoms for 5 years. Three years after diagnosis, she developed primary herpetic gingivostomatitis, which was controlled by her dentist with an antiviral medication. Subsequently her physician altered her immune suppression medication.

Case 3
D. L. is a 40-year-old man who bought a book on natural foods. He then pulled "sassafras" roots from the woods and prepared a tasty natural tea. Two days later he developed blisters of his entire oral mucosa that rapidly ulcerated. He also developed diarrhea, cramping, and bloody stools. Tests revealed that D. L. had ulcerative gastroenteritis secondary to type IV hypersensitivity to a contact substance—probably, poison ivy root. He was hospitalized for 2 weeks for nutritional and fluid support and subsequently recovered. D. L. had a history of skin sensitivity to poison ivy leaves.

Case 1

1. Why did B. J. need to take immune suppression drugs?
2. What are the consequences of taking long-term immune suppressive drugs?
3. Do you think the fungal infections were related to the immune suppression? How?
4. Will she always be susceptible to opportunistic infection?

Case 2

1. Is the clinical presentation consistent with that of systemic lupus erythematosus?
2. Do you think there might be a relationship between her medications and the severity of her herpes infection?
3. How can B and T cells react to her own tissues and organs (kidney, skin, etc.)?

Case 3

1. Explain the pathogenesis of the oral and gastrointestinal disease.
2. Do you think D. L. had a previous contact with poison ivy?
3. What do his gastrointestinal symptoms indicate?
4. What other treatment might shorten the disease duration?

SUMMARY

- The immune reaction helps prevent injury by nonself antigen-bearing agents such as microorganisms and cancer cells. Upon initial exposure, immune cells develop a memory for a specific antigen. The progeny of these sensitized cells respond with a cellular, humoral, or combined response to destroy the challenging antigenic agent.
- The immune response can cause tissue injury through normal activity, hypersensitive reactions, or confused autoimmune reaction. In these conditions, the immune response may need to be depressed.
- Immune cells function as a team and communicate with each other with interleukins to repress or stimulate activity of other cells.
- Immune deficiency diseases can lead to opportunistic infections from common organisms of low virulence and increased incidence of cancer formation. An intact immune system would normally control the growth and spread of these organisms or tumors.
- The function of immune cells is determined by genetic MHCs. MHCs are also transplantation markers that can lead to immune rejection after transplantation of an organ to a nonmatched recipient.
- Immune hypersensitivity disease may be caused by one of four basic mechanisms termed type 1 to type 4. Each type has its own pathogenesis.
- Autoimmune disease results when immune cells attack "self" tissues. This occurs because of alterations of the immune cells, changes in the antigenicity of self tissues, sequestered antigenic tissues, or hypersensitivity reactions.
- Immune proliferative disorders often result in immune deficiency.

Suggested readings

1. Cohen S: The role of cell-mediated immunity in the induction of inflammatory responses, Am J Pathol 88:502, 1977.
2. Dinarello CA and Mier JW: Current concepts: lymphokines, N Engl J Med 317:940, 1987.
3. Jawetz E, Melnik JL, and Adelberg EA: Review of microbiology, ed 7, East Norwalk, Conn, 1987, Appleton & Lange, chapters 12, 15.
4. Kumar V, Cotran RS, and Robbins SL: Basic pathology, Philadelphia, 1992, WB Saunders Co, pp 122-134.
5. Reinherz EL and Schlossmann SF: The differentiation and formation of human T lymphocytes, Cell 19:821, 1980.
6. Roitt IM: Essential immunology, ed 7, Oxford, 1991, Blackwell Scientific Publications, Inc.
7. Taussig MJ: Processes in pathology and microbiology, ed 2, Oxford, 1984, Blackwell Scientific Publications, Inc, section 2.

5

Infectious Diseases and Specific Infections

IN THIS CHAPTER

1. Virulence
2. Host defenses
   - External barriers
   - Inflammation
   - Internal barriers
   - Other defenses
3. Specific infections
   Viral diseases
   - Herpes simplex type 1
   - Varicella-zoster virus
   - Coxsackie virus
   - Mumps
   - Measles
   - Epstein-Barr virus
   - Hepatitis
4. Bacterial diseases
   - Recurrent aphthous stomatitis
   - Chronic periodontitis
   - Streptococcal pharyngitis
   - Tuberculosis
   - Syphilis
5. Fungal diseases
   - Candidiasis
   - Deep fungal infections
6. Human immune deficiency virus
7. Case studies

After studying this chapter, you should be able to meet the following objectives and define the key terms:

- Identify factors that contribute to virulence of organisms.
- List common host defense factors that inhibit virulence and infectivity of organisms.
- Explain the pathogenesis of viral diseases by examining the mode of cellular injury.

- Distinguish the lesions of herpes simplex type 1 virus by clinical features.
- Recognize clinical tests used to differentiate herpes family infections.
- Differentiate herpes simplex infections from recurrent aphthous ulcers and other viral stomatitis.
- Relate the pathogenesis of varicella-zoster virus to shingles.
- Discuss the relevance of measles and mumps to dentistry.
- Recognize the symptoms of mononucleosis.
- Relate Burkitt's lymphoma to Epstein-Barr virus.
- List diseases caused by Epstein-Barr virus.
- Differentiate hepatitis A, B, and C by mode of infection, carrier state, and chronic disease state.
- Discuss the prevention of hepatitis B and C by vaccination.
- Interpret the common serologic (antibody) tests for hepatitis A, B, and C and comment on the significance of these tests.
- Explain the suspected etiology and pathogenesis of recurrent aphthous stomatitis.
- Differentiate the subtypes of recurrent aphthous stomatitis by clinical presentation.
- Discuss the management of chronic periodontitis based on its pathogenesis.
- Explain poststreptococcal autoimmune disease.
- Explain the pathogenesis of tuberculosis.
- Discuss reasons for the increasing incidence of tuberculosis in the United States.

- List and differentiate the clinical stages of syphilis and their manifestations.
- Discuss the environmental interactions that normally control the growth of *Candida albicans*.
- List factors that commonly lead to candidiasis.
- Recognize clinical types of candidiasis and tests that help in diagnosis of these types.
- List the risk practices and behaviors that contribute to HIV infection.
- Name opportunistic oral diseases that occur in association with HIV infection.
- Define AIDS.

- Follow special care and treatment-planning procedures necessary to better treat HIV and AIDS patients.
- Recognize the degree of risk of HIV transfer in a dental setting.

An infection is caused by the invasion of microorganisms into body tissues and their replication there, frequently resulting in tissue injury and necrosis. The injury may be caused by products of the organisms, competitive metabolism, intracellular replication and cell lysis or stimulation of the immune and inflammatory processes (Figs. 5-1 and 5-2). The resultant degenerative and necrotic products

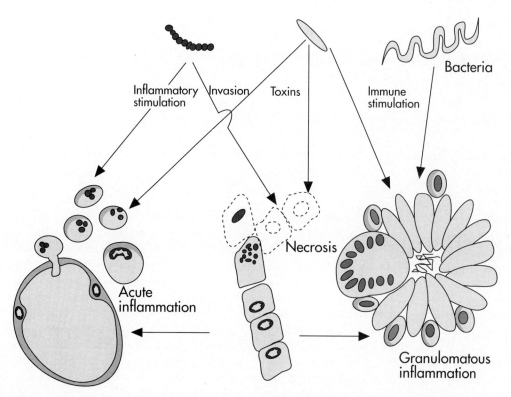

Fig. 5-1 Bacterial infection can damage tissues by direct tissue invasion, toxin production, or inflammatory and immune stimulation. The resultant lesions include tissue necrosis, acute inflammation or granulomatous inflammation, or a combination.

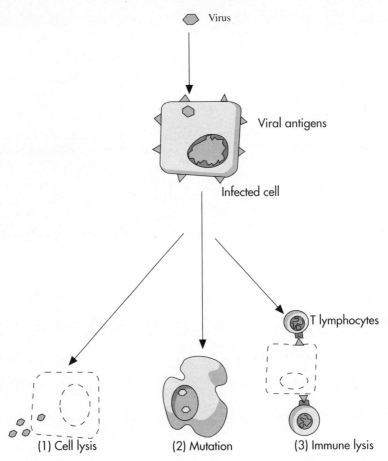

Fig. 5-2 Viral infections can damage tissues (1) by direct cell lysis, (2) by mutating the tissues to nonfunctional cells, and (3) by changing the antigenicity of tissues to make them susceptible to immune lysis.

frequently initiate an inflammatory response. This response may be subclinical (not apparent), acute, or chronic, depending on host factors and the virulence (ability to damage tissue) of the microorganism. The virulence of the microorganism is dependent on the ability of the organism to enter and grow in tissue (invasiveness), the toxins and tissue-damaging byproducts produced by the microorganism (toxicity), and the ability of the microorganism to stimulate a cell-mediated immune response (immune reaction). For example, some organisms (syphilis) are highly invasive, pen-etrate intact skin, and actively destroy tissue without significant toxin production. Other bacteria (clostridia) can produce fatal disease by virtue of their toxin production, with only limited invasion of tissue. Certain fungi and bacteria can produce illness and even death by virtue of stimulation of the granulomatous inflammatory response or acute inflammatory response, with superficial tissue invasion or minimal toxin production. Species of microorganisms vary in their virulence. The α-streptococci seldom cause serious disease and live in a commensal (sharing) or even symbiotic (helping) relationship with human oral mucous membranes. These organisms may cause mild infections when they penetrate through wounds into the submucosa or tissue cavities. The β-streptococci, on the other hand, are much more virulent; they infect intact mucous membranes and produce ulcers, abscesses, and purulent exudates as indications of the tissue necrosis and acute inflammation.

The pathogenicity (ability to cause disease) of microorganisms is dependent on the offensive characteristics of the microorganism and the defensive characteristics of the host. The body and the environment form a constant battlefield, with offensive thrusts and defensive fortification and counterattacks. In order for microorganisms to survive and thrive, they must develop relationships with host tissues. Many microorganisms must become parasites of host tissues, using host metabolites and tissue components for their own survival. Such organisms are invariably pathogenic. Other organisms produce poisons as metabolic byproducts (exotoxins) or as products of their own cellular degeneration (endotoxins). These toxins damage the host tissues. Some organisms compete with the host tissues for food or fluids. These competitive microorganisms capture needed substances at the expense of the host tissues, thereby causing disease.

Many microorganisms live in commensal or even symbiotic relationships with the host, on the skin, in the mouth, and throughout the intestines. Bacteria of the intestine help us process and digest certain foodstuffs and absorb certain nutrients. Nonpathogenic symbiotic organisms of the oral mucosa compete with and destroy more pathogenic organisms. Therefore, an ecologic situation occurs in many areas. The host supports the microorganisms and the microorganisms aid the host. When the ecology system is disturbed (as by antibiotic therapy for a nonrelated infection), symbiosis is reduced and disturbances such as malnutrition and superinfection can result.

VIRULENCE

Microorganisms have evolved and adapted offensive mechanisms in certain ways to allow them to cause disease. These offensive mechanisms include toxin production and excretion or secretion of certain enzymes. A microorganism that produces a neurotoxin (as in botulism) will have a profound effect on the nervous system, where it might cause paralysis. A microorganism that produces a hepatotoxin will most likely cause liver necrosis and its sequelae—unless the host defense mechanism is adequate to prevent it (Fig. 5-1). Some microorganisms (such as virulent streptococci) excrete enzymes that dissolve cell connections, destroy collagen, dissolve blood clots, and dissolve cell membranes. These microorganisms will therefore be quite invasive because they can penetrate tissue by virtue of the enzymes produced. Other microorganisms are highly mobile and can infiltrate and squeeze between cells and fibers. They are therefore invasive through intact skin or mucous membranes.

Many viruses parasitize cells and force the cells to reproduce thousands of viruses. The result of this viral replication is usually cellular death, with new viruses infecting and destroying other cells (HIV). Other viruses mutate and change cells without killing them. The mutated cells may become dysfunctional or even begin to grow, divide, and act in uncontrolled fashion (cancer). We will explain this more in Chapter 7. Finally, some viruses change the antigens of the cell in such a way that the immune system attacks the virally infected cell. The result may be destruction of both the virus and the cell, with resultant disease (Fig. 5-2). Several forms of viral hepatitis occur because of this type of pathogenesis.

Certain microbes learn to hide from the host defensive factors which we will discuss next. Bacteria with capsules may escape inflammatory phagocytosis; organisms that produce peroxidase may be indigestible by neutrophils; and organisms that produce dry spore forms may be resistant to phagocytosis, digestion, immune response, or antiseptic agents. Some viruses actually have the ability to combine with cells and survive through generations of cell division without being detected by the immune response. (This state of being "hidden" is known as latency.) These viruses can ultimately be activated and again become infectious. Many other mechanisms of microbial virulence are known. These mechanisms dictate the type of disease caused by the organism, and knowledge of the mechanisms helps us develop defensive agents.

HOST DEFENSES

The host is not defenseless before microbial attack. Host defenses can be stimulated or fortified to prevent or reduce infection. Natural host defense mechanisms can be classified as first-, second-, or third-line mechanisms. Further, internal (immune) and external (vaccine, antibiotic) acquired mechanisms can further strengthen host defense and help prevent or diminish future infections.

External Barriers

First-line defense includes barriers to invasion or toxin absorption, such as keratinized, thick, impervious skin and mucous membranes. Most microorganisms—except the most invasive—cannot penetrate this barrier; therefore, infection only occurs when there is a break or cut present. Secretory products such as sweat, semen, saliva, tears, and gastrointestinal (GI) secretions contain numerous antimicrobial substances. A patient with dry eyes may develop a corneal infection; a patient with dry mouth may develop caries. Such enzymes as lysozyme in tears and saliva, ferritin in sweat and saliva, amylase in saliva and intestinal secretions, and acids in gastric secretions—as well as antibodies in many secretory substances—afford important primary protection from microorganisms. The mucous secretions of the respiratory and gastrointestinal cavities entrap microorganisms and allow them to be expectorated or swallowed for digestion in the stomach. Respiratory cilia lining the bronchial mucosa push mucus and its microorganisms from the vulnerable lung tissue toward the mouth for expectoration or digestion. Fluid secretion—including saliva, sweat, bile, and urine—washes microorganisms away from vulnerable glandular tissues. Any obstruction or decrease in flow will allow for glandular infections (such as postsurgical parotitis). Finally, as we have previously mentioned, symbiotic microorganisms of the skin, mouth, mucous membranes, and respiratory and GI tracts help protect us from infection by pathogenic intruders (Fig. 5-3).

Inflammation

The second line of defense involves the inflammatory process that we have already studied in detail. In overview, the inflammatory process can dilute, detoxify, and destroy toxic substances, and the cells help phagocytize, digest, immobilize, entrap, and inhibit invasive microorganisms. In patients where the inflammatory process is reduced in quantity or quality (by AIDS, leukopenia, leukemia), infection with common microorganisms (herpes, candida, oral streptococcus) is frequent and quite marked, whereas in normal patients the same infections would be mild or subclinical.

Internal Barriers

A third line of defense involves establishment of barriers to prevent spread of infectious microorganisms once infection is established. The density of connective tissues provides such a barrier. An infection within a body cavity or loose connective tissue can spread

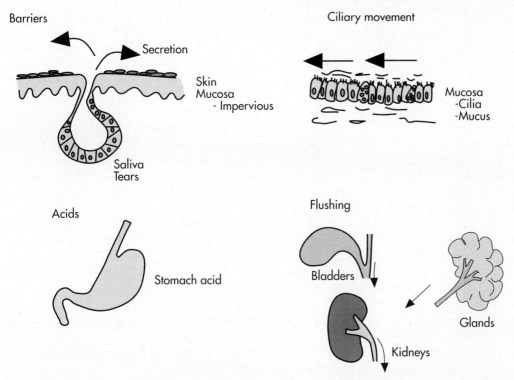

Fig. 5-3 Barriers and natural defense mechanisms, such as impermeable skin, antimicrobial secretions, acids that destroy microbes, flushing of secretory organs, and mucus and ciliary movement, protect the organism from infection. Loss or diminishment of any of these barriers predisposes a system to infection.

quite readily. Once the infection spreads to dense tissues (bone, muscle, capsules), the spread will be slowed or arrested. Of course, some microorganisms secrete enzymes that can dissolve and overcome these barriers. By understanding the anatomy of these barriers, we can often predict the pathways of the spread of infection. The lymphatic system also serves as a filtration barrier to infection. Lymph vessels drain most tissues, and lymphatic drainage of infected tissues is increased by the edema of inflammation. The draining fluid carries microorganisms away from the tissue into the filtration system of the lymph node. The microorganisms are there entrapped, phagocytized, and digested by the histiocytes contained within lymph nodes.

Toxins are further diluted. Finally, most organs contain tissue macrophages, and most blood vessels are lined with reticuloendothelial cells. The reticuloendothelial system (RES) functions in a manner similar to the inflammatory macrophages and lymphatic histiocytes. That is, the RES cells entrap, phagocytize, and digest microorganisms that may be spread to the blood vessels, spleen, liver, or other tissues. When the RES and lymphoid histiocytes become dysfunctional, clinical infections will increase in number and severity.

OTHER DEFENSES

We have previously discussed the immune system, and you are aware that this system enhances and supports the inflammatory process and functions to prepare the body to recognize antigen-bearing substances—like microorganisms—upon reinfection. Both the humoral and cellular immune systems can be stimulated to help protect (acquired resistance) against infection by microorganisms. Many microorganisms are antigenic and activate natural immune response. The procedure of vaccination takes advantage of the immune protective mechanisms. In vaccination, nonvirulent antigenic substances are supplied (orally, by injection) to the host. The host mounts an immune reaction to the antigen, which remains ready for years. Upon challenge by the offending microorganism, the humoral or cellular immune response will quickly destroy the infectious agent before significant infectious disease can occur.

Numerous other forms of prophylactic resistance and treatment can be used to support host defense. Antibiotics, antifungal agents, and antiviral substances interfere with microbe replication or metabolism and thereby limit infection. Other substances may (1) stimulate nonspecific immune reactions (thymosin), (2) stimulate cells to inhibit viral replication (interferon), or (3) cause immune cells to react more readily and aggressively. Infections of the oral cavity are very frequent in occurrence, can cause considerable illness, and are potentially contagious. Therefore, these diseases are of major interest to the dental team.

SPECIFIC INFECTIONS

Viral Diseases

Herpes Simplex Type 1. The herpes simplex virus is extremely common and ubiquitous. The herpes simplex type 1 virus (HSV-1) survives best in an oral environment and usually causes perioral and oral lesions. Approximately 85% of the population demonstrates antibodies to herpes simplex type 1. Antibody

formation serves as evidence of infection by this virus. Antibodies only give the infected patient partial protection from the virus. The formation of antibodies limits the severity and spread of the herpes infection, but the antibodies do not always prevent recurrence of infection. Only about 35% of the population ever develop clinical herpetic lesions. This means that more than half of the population infected by this virus never develop disease, or have developed the disease with such minor symptoms (subclinical) that they are not aware of the infection. Three clinical forms of the disease may occur in the 35% who do develop lesions. The clinical forms are primary herpetic gingivostomatitis, recurrent herpes labialis (cold sores, fever blisters), and recurrent intraoral herpes.

The herpes simplex type 1 infection is usually acquired by direct contact with an infected patient (through kissing, dental procedure) or by contact through instruments, utensils, dishes, or other contaminated *fomites*. In the days before dental personnel used barrier techniques such as gloves and eyewear, occasional instances of herpetic lesions of the fingers and eyes acquired by these personnel from patient contact were reported. The use of gloves and eyewear has decreased this incidence markedly.

Once HSV-1 has infected the tissues, the virus migrates up the trigeminal nerve and hides itself in the cells of the trigeminal ganglion. In most cases, no clinical disease accompanies this primary infection. The immune system reacts to this subclinical infection by forming antiherpetic antibodies. These antibodies partially control any viral proliferation; however, they do not usually destroy all the virus—especially not the viral particles sequestered in the trigeminal ganglion. Uncommonly, the immune reaction does not control the viral proliferation. This occurs because the patient is immune suppressed (by HIV, drugs) because the immune system has not fully developed (as in infants), or because the viral inoculum is enormous. In such cases where resistance is low, the patient may develop a severe primary oral infection and viremia. We will describe the clinical features of this primary disease subsequently. In those patients with an adequate immune response, the virus may survive in an inactive form within the ganglion. There are several predisposing factors that tend to activate the virus at a later date. The factors include the common cold, fever, localized trauma, the menstrual cycle, and ultraviolet light (from sun and other sources). Once reactivated, many viruses will migrate down the trigeminal nerve and infect the epithelial cells of either the skin and lip, or the palate and gingiva. Some viruses remain hidden in the ganglion; therefore, reinfection may be recurrent and may occur whenever the susceptible patient encounters the predisposing factor.

Recurrent herpes labialis is by far the most common clinical form affecting 30% to 35% of the population. The lesions occur near the vermilion border and on the skin of the lips, and occasionally about the nose and face. Lesions usually occur within the middle two thirds of the upper or lower lips. Typically the lesions occur in phases. The first phase consists of a prodromal burning or tingling without a visually apparent change. After 12 to 24 hours of prodromal burning, multiple crops of clear liquid-filled blisters (vesicles) form at the infected site. These vesicles range from 1 to 5 mm in size and from 1 to 100 in number (Fig. 5-4). The vesicles remain for 1 to 2 days and subsequently dry and crust to yellow-brown ulcers. The irritating crust stage lasts for 3 to 6 days and heals—usually without scarring. Occasionally, crops of lesions occur simultaneously at multiple locations, even involving both upper and lower lips. It is also not uncommon for new lesions to form on a patient with lesions of several days' duration (Fig. 5-5). The frequency of recurrence varies among individual patients from weeks to years. Predisposing factors play an important role in initiating recurrence.

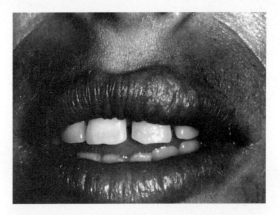

Fig. 5-4 Herpes labialis vesicle stage of 1-day duration. There is a history of cold sores.

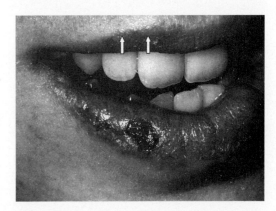

Fig. 5-5 Herpes labialis, ulcer crust stage of 5-day duration. Note vesicles of upper lip (*arrows*). There is a history of fever blisters.

Recurrent intraoral herpes occurs in less than 1% of the population. Trauma, fever, and stress seem to be important predisposing and activating factors. These lesions occur only on the mucous membranes that are tightly bound to bone and are void of salivary tissues. The lesions are usually located on the hard palate and the maxillary palatal and buccal gingiva. Rarely, the mandibular gingiva is involved. These lesions follow a course similar to that of herpes labialis—that is, lesions begin in prodrome and progress to vesicular and ulcerative stages. The vesicular stage is short-lived (hours) because mastication easily ruptures the vesicles. Crops of multiple small ulcers with red margins result. These ulcers give the examiner the impression that the palate and gingiva have been perforated with an instrument such as an ice pick (Fig. 5-6). The ulcerative stage is usually quite painful because of masticating pressure on the lesions. These lesions are usually recognizable clinically by the history of recurrence, the location, and the multiple small ulcers that irritate the patient.

Primary herpetic gingivostomatitis is the most severe oral form of herpes simplex and occurs in less than 1% of the population. As the name implies, the lesions usually occur after the initial contact with the herpes simplex virus. Children are most frequently affected, although this manifestation can occur in adults. Oral lesions include numerous vesicles and small (1 to 3 mm) ulcers of the lips and any or all of the oral mucosa. These ulcers can coalesce or expand to form large, ragged ulcers that may be very painful. Usually ulcers appear with an intense red margin and yellow-white central exudate. The gingiva is classically edematous and demonstrates nu-

merous vesicles and ulcers. The gingivitis is very red and painful and bleeds readily from simple pressure (Fig. 5-7). The oral lesions are accompanied by fever, malaise, and irritability (Table 5-1). Oral and systemic symptoms frequently make the patient vulnerable to dehydration and malnourishment because of the pain associated with eating and drinking. Children must be monitored closely and sometimes hospitalized to correct dehydration with intravenous fluid support. The course of the disease usually lasts approximately two weeks. Individuals with persistent primary herpes may have an underlying immune deficiency. The pathogenesis of primary herpes involves an initial infection with a significant number of viruses in the absence of any previously established immune protection. Mode of viral transfer is the same as with recurrent herpes—through contact with a lesion or contaminated utensil or instrument. Remember, the majority of primary-contact infections result in subclinical disease; only 1% result in primary gingivostomatitis. Once the primary disease resolves, recurrent herpes labialis or recurrent intraoral herpes may develop at a later date, or there may be no further lesions. When an individual with a

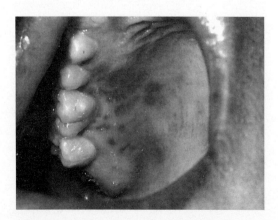

Fig. 5-6 Recurrent intraoral herpes. Painful crops of ulcers of the gingiva and palate. There is a history of similar lesions forming.

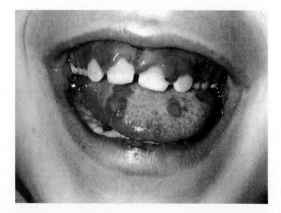

Fig. 5-7 Primary herpetic gingivostomatitis. Note swollen ulcerated gingiva and mucosal ulcers in this child.

TABLE 5-1

Oral ulcerative lesions

Disease	Recurrent history	Vesicles	Location	Ulcer characteristics	Related factors
Recurrent herpes labialis	+ + + +	Multiple crops	Vermilion	Multiple, dry, crusting	Sun, URI, fever
Recurrent intraoral herpes	+ + + +	Multiple crops	Hard palate, maxillary gingiva	Small (1-3 mm), punctate, multiple	Trauma, stress
Recurrent aphthous stomatitis	+ + + +	—	Lips, buccal mucosa, floor of mouth, soft palate, ventral surface of tongue, alveolar mucosa	Singular, volcanic, 0.5-1 cm, raised, round	Trauma, stress
Major aphthous ulcers	+ + + +	—	Lips, buccal mucosa, floor of mouth, soft palate, tongue, alveolar mucosa	1-2 cm, healed by scarring	Trauma, stress
Herpetiform aphthae	+ + + +	—	Lips, buccal mucosa, floor of mouth, soft palate, ventral surface of tongue, alveolar mucosa	Multiple, 1-3 mm, red, painful	Stress, menstrual cycle
Coxsackie virus	—	Multiple	Herpangina—pharynx, HFM (hand foot and mouth disease)—all oral mucosa	Multiple, 1-3 mm, red, painful	Contagion
Primary herpetic gingivostomatitis	—	±	All mucosal surfaces and lips	Multiple, 1-3 mm, red, punctate	Contagion
Measles	—	—	Buccal mucosa	White-coated, Koplik's spots	Precedes rash

††††Usually present.
—Absent.

reliable history of recurrent herpes suddenly develops primary lesions or chronic lesions, immune suppression should be suspected.

Other diseases (Coxsackie virus, herpetiform aphthous ulcers, allergic gingivostomatitis, necrotizing gingivitis) can mimic the symptoms of primary herpes. Cytologic study of vesicles or fresh ulcers becomes a useful tool in making the distinction, along with history and physical examination. Virally infected epithelial cells can be removed by scraping a vesicle or fresh ulcer from any of the clinical forms of herpes simplex. These cells can be recognized on a cytology (smear) slide by an oral pathologist, and specific therapy can be initiated. In most situations involving recurrent herpes labialis or recurrent intraoral herpes, the lesions can be diagnosed based on location, recurrence, and appearance of stages. Treatment for all forms includes antiviral substances (acyclovir), and occasionally, antibiotics against secondary bacterial infection. Prevention may include avoidance of predisposing factors, antiviral substances, and diet supplement (lysine). Rare cases result in severe viremia and widespread herpes of the brain and internal organs, with morbid or fatal result.

Varicella-Zoster Virus. The varicella-zoster virus (VZV) is a member of the herpes family. Like herpes simplex, this virus infects a majority of the general population, stimulates a partially protective antibody response, and is often hidden from the immune system in the dorsal root and trigeminal ganglia. Whereas primary herpes gingivostomatitis occurs in only 1% of infected individuals, the varicella-zoster virus almost always causes a generalized primary infection (chickenpox). Chickenpox is a varicella infection of skin and mucous membranes that is very common as a contagion in children. These children develop disseminated vesicles and pustules of the skin and of the gingiva and oral mucous membranes. Since the pustules of the skin are common and easily recognized and since oral

lesions are less common, the disease is seldom presented to the dental office environment.

Shingles (herpes zoster) occurs rarely, and only among those already infected with VZV when varicella-zoster virus is activated from the dorsal ganglion or the trigeminal ganglion where it was sequestered. Usually a predisposing factor (stress, debilitating disease, immune suppression) can be identified. The previously hidden virus migrates down the peripheral nerve and infects the skin and mucous membranes supplied by the nerve. Lesions begin as prodromal paresthesia or pain, followed shortly by multiple crops of vesicles and subsequent ulcers and crusts. The total lesion duration is usually less than 1 month. Since the virus cannot migrate far beyond the area of skin or mucous membrane supplied by the infected nerve, the lesions usually do not cross the midline but conform to the anatomic pattern of the branches of the affected nerve (Fig. 5-8). Severe pain is a common accompanying feature. It is not uncommon for pain to persist (post-herpetic neuralgia) in the area for months after resolution of lesions. This painful sequela may mimic tic douloureux, toothache, or other pain syndromes. Shingles is

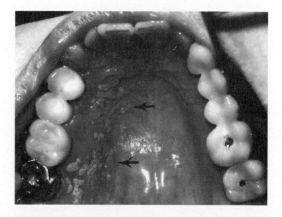

Fig. 5-8 Herpes zoster. Crops of vesicles are confined to one side of palate (*arrows*). The corresponding side of the face also exhibits vesicles and ulcers.

best treated with antiviral drugs (acyclovir). Patients who have recurrent shingles or chronic shingles should be suspect for immune suppression (HIV or medication induced).

Coxsackie Virus. A number of Coxsackie viruses are quite contagious and cause oral infections, most commonly in children. Contagion and epidemics are common in nursery school or elementary school settings. These viruses are passed by saliva or eating implements, toys, hands, and coughing or sneezing. The infected children usually develop fever, malaise, and mouth sores. The Coxsackie lesions begin as small vesicles that readily ulcerate. The ulcers are herpetiform—that is, they are multiple and small (1 to 2 mm), and appear as punctures of the mucosa. Ulcers may enlarge and become secondarily infected and confluent. In the Coxsackie disease *herpangina,* the vesiculoulcerative lesions are confined to the soft palate and oropharynx. In *hand-foot-and-mouth disease* the vesiculoulcerative lesions resemble those of primary herpetic stomatitis. Ulcers can occur on any oral mucosal surface, and gingivitis may accompany the condition. Skin vesicles and ulcers, especially of the palms and soles, are a diagnostically important component of the disease (Fig. 5-9). Diagnosis of Coxsackie infection is usually made by clinical presentation, although viral culture is possible. Treatment consists of bed rest and nutritional-liquid support. The diseases limit themselves to 2 weeks, and immunity is conferred. Again, severe cases and recurrent infections may accompany immune deficiency disease.

Mumps. Mumps (epidemic parotiditis), a viral infection of glandular tissue, was formerly one of the most common contagious children's diseases in the United States. Public immunization has decreased the incidence considerably; however, occasional outbreaks occur in nonimmunized groups. The virus is shed in saliva and spread via utensils, hands, kissing, coughing, and sneezing. Infection involves fever, malaise, and acute parotitis, usually bilateral in nature. The parotid glands become markedly swollen and painful, especially in the region of the neck (Fig. 5-10). Xerostomia (dry mouth) may result, and the parotid papillae may be inflamed. Acute pancreatitis and orchitis in males are somewhat less common components of the infection. Occasionally sterility in young adult males can be the sequela of orchitis. Spread of the virus in the blood (viremia) can result in meningoencephalitis. The disease usually lasts for 2

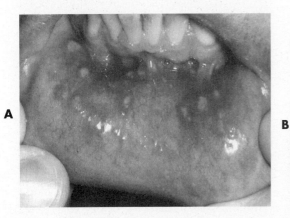
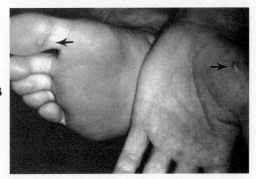

Fig. 5-9 Hand-foot-and-mouth disease. **A,** Typical viral vesicles and ulcers of several days' duration. **B,** The hands and feet exhibit vesicle formation.

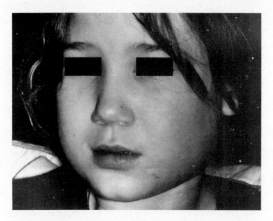

Fig. 5-10 Mumps. Bilateral painful parotid swelling of 3 days' duration. The patient's sister has similar lesions.

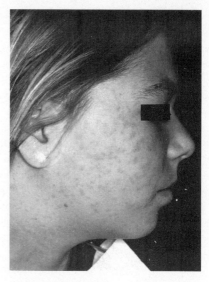

Fig. 5-11 Measles. Exanthematous rash of face, torso, arms and legs.

to 3 weeks and is self-limiting. Vaccination is highly effective in prevention of epidemic parotiditis.

Measles. The infection known as measles (rubella) is another that formerly caused widespread epidemics in children but has recently been controlled by vaccination. The virus is transferred by saliva and is highly infectious. After a short incubation period, the patient develops fever, malaise, photophobia (intolerance to sunlight), and an exanthem (itching rash) of the face, arms, legs, and trunk (Fig. 5-11). Respiratory symptoms such as cough and sore throat are common. Occasionally, patients will develop accompanying herpetiform mouth ulcers and gingivitis. Small, multiple, white ulcerative lesions on a red base occur on the buccal mucosa bilaterally and are termed *Koplik's spots*. Koplik's spots are frequently prodromal and therefore precede development of the more characteristic exanthem of the skin. Secondary bacterial infections of the rash and meningitis can be morbid sequelae. Although the virus has been well controlled by vaccination, several recent epidemics among college students, with re-

sultant quarantine, have emphasized the need for booster vaccinations.

Epstein-Barr Virus. The Epstein-Barr virus (EBV) is a ubiquitous pathogen that seems to have an affinity for immune system cells (lymphocytes, antigen-processing cells). Because this virus is so common and causes known diseases in laboratory animals, it has been implicated as the cause of numerous systemic and oral conditions. *Infectious mononucleosis* involves infection of the immune system by the EBV, resulting in T-lymphocyte hyperplasia. Patients may develop swollen lymph nodes, spleen, and liver; marked malaise and fatigue; pharyngitis; skin rash; and other less specific symptoms. Lymphocytes appear abnormal when examined with a microscope, and the white cell count usually increases to a level above normal. Specific blood tests help confirm the diagnosis. The symptoms usually last for a week to a month, but both chronic and recurrent forms have been reported. Patients also exhibit intraoral lesions, including pinpoint palatal bleeding spots (petechiae) and exudative acute pharyngitis. The lymphadenopathy frequently involves the posterior cervical nodes of the neck. Treatment includes bed rest and nutritional support.

Burkitt's lymphoma is a malignant neoplasm of solid lymphoid tissues that usually occurs in children of central Africa. The tumors grow in abdominal lymphoid tissue and the jaws. The significance of two features of these tumors has been studied and debated for years: (1) Tumor incidence is almost exclusive to African geographic areas of great rainfall and high average temperature, leading one to speculate on an insect vector; and (2) Epstein-Barr virus is found in most Burkitt's lymphomas—the implication being that EBV causes this cancer. Although these tumors initially respond well to chemical therapy, the long-term mortality rate is fairly high. Both the etiology and pathogenesis of this tumor continue to be debated.

Oral hairy leukoplakia (OHL) is a benign hyperplastic growth of the oral mucosa appearing as white, ridged, rough lesions of the oral mucosa—usually bilateral, on the lateral surfaces of the tongue (Fig. 5-12). These lesions are almost exclusively secondary to immune suppression, with the majority diag-

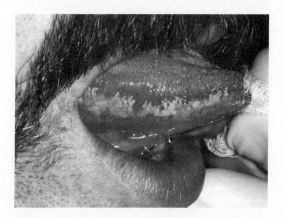

Fig. 5-12 Oral hairy leukoplakia. The white lesion is bilateral and present in an HIV-positive patient.

nosed in patients with HIV infection. EBV is frequently demonstrable within these epithelial lesions and is considered by many to be the opportunistic causative organism. OHL is considered important because it serves as an indicator in diagnosis and predicting prognosis of immune suppression and AIDS. The recognition of these lesions helps us diagnose HIV infection and predict that the patient is becoming severely immune suppressed. The lesions respond well to antiviral medications but frequently recur. Oral hairy leukoplakia has no major sequelae and should be considered in itself a benign, nonharmful condition that usually does not require treatment.

Hepatitis. *Hepatitis A virus* (HAV) is caused by a common RNA virus that is transferred by fecal contamination of water or food. Outbreaks and even epidemics result, usually because of a breach in public health protocol. Recent epidemics in Kentucky involved a contaminated water system (causing 250 cases in one county) and contaminated food material (tomatoes, lettuce) at Louisville restaurants (causing 300 cases). Other epidemics have involved ingestion of contaminated shellfish and spreading among male homosexuals. There is a relatively short incubation period after ingestion of the virus of 2 to 6 weeks. Most infections show early flulike symptoms of malaise, fever, and anorexia. Jaundice occurs in the majority of cases and lasts up to 6 weeks. The condition tends to be self-limiting. There is no significant chronic disease state and no carrier disease state. Sequelae such as cirrhosis are rare, and natural immunity is life-long. Rarely, patients develop severe fulminant acute disease with resultant morbidity or cirrhosis. Antibodies (anti-HAV) can be detected in the infected patient's blood, usually after development of symptoms, and are therefore useful in diagnosis and determination of the type of hepatitis the patient has, or has had. Hepatitis A is best controlled by sound public health measures.

Hepatitis B virus (HBV) is caused by a DNA virus that is sometimes referred to as Dane particles. This virus can be transmitted via contaminated blood, urine, semen, feces, or even saliva, and is most often transferred by parenteral (puncturing) or sexual activity. Therefore, sexually active individuals, male homosexuals, intravenous (IV) drug abusers, dialysis patients, and health care workers are at greatest risk. Epidemics associated with medical and dental contagion have been reported secondary to poor sterilization and disinfection practices (for surgery, hygiene procedures) in the health care setting.

The organism is highly virulent and most often infects adults. A 45- to 120-day incubation period is usual. The majority of infected individuals develop subclinical or mild flulike symptoms. Those who develop acute hepatitis demonstrate malaise, weakness, anorexia, fatigue, and frequently, jaundice. The absence of jaundice, however, certainly does not exclude the diagnosis of hepatitis B. A small number of patients (2%) develop acute fulminant disease resulting in death. The majority of clinically affected patients are ill for 3 to 8 weeks with subsequent resolution. About 12% of patients infected develop chronic forms of the disease and become carriers who can spread the virus via contact with others through the transmission factors previously listed. The majority of carriers are asymptomatic or only exhibit very mild symptoms of hepatitis. This condition, known as chronic persistent hepatitis B, is frequently unknown to the carriers, or to the physician or dentist treating them. Therefore, infection-control precautions are necessary for all patients. After years, long-term immunity can occur in patients with the chronic persistent form (Fig. 5-13).

A small percentage (3%) of HBV-infected individuals develop chronic active hepatitis. In this condition, fatigue, anorexia, and jaundice are severe and persistent, lasting for years. These patients are infectious and are frequently bedridden or unable to function socially. After years of disease, death can result from liver failure, cirrhosis, or liver cancer—all sequelae of the HBV infection. Recent reports have indicated an increased risk of liver cancer from all clinical forms of hepatitis B.

Certain antigens and antibodies of HBV can be detected in the blood and aid in diagnosis of the disease and carrier states of hepatitis B. The most important antigen for carrier state detection is hepatitis B surface antigen (HB$_s$Ag), sometimes called the Australian antigen. The presence of this surface antigen in blood indicates the presence of infectious HBV. The body responds with natural immunity to HB$_s$Ag by making anti-HB$_s$ antibodies that are protective against the virus. Therefore, presence of anti-HB$_s$ antibody implies a previous infection, with subsequent immunity. Vaccinations with HB$_s$Ag preparations (Heptavax, Recombivax) are readily available and highly effective. It is recommended that all health care workers attain anti-HB$_s$ antibody status—usually by vaccination. Public and private blood supplies should be thoroughly screened.

Hepatitis C is sometimes referred to as a non-A, non-B hepatitis. This RNA virus is the most common cause of blood-transmitted hepatitis. Its incidence should decrease now that blood-screening tests have been developed to reduce the possibility of tainted blood. The pathogenesis of the disease(s) seems similar to that of HBV. The majority of cases occur from parenteral or sexual spread. Chronic active states and carrier states can develop, resulting in cirrhosis, liver failure, or liver cancer. Since the virus can be transferred parenterally, since blood testing is new and not widespread, and since vaccinations are not yet available, hepatitis C continues to be a risk in the health care setting—even to the hepatitis B–vaccinated individual. Contagion can be controlled by sound sterilization, barrier techniques, and sharp instrument hygiene.

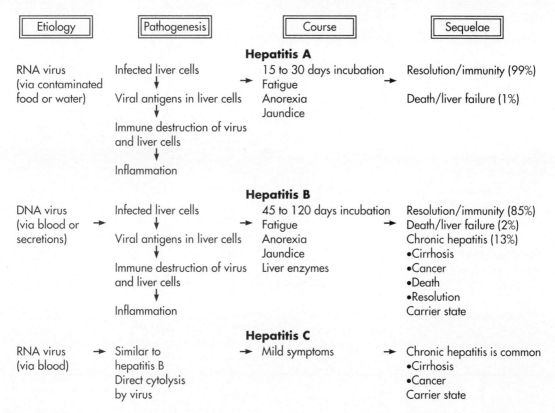

Etiology	Pathogenesis	Course	Sequelae

Hepatitis A

| RNA virus (via contaminated food or water) | Infected liver cells ↓ Viral antigens in liver cells ↓ Immune destruction of virus and liver cells ↓ Inflammation | 15 to 30 days incubation Fatigue Anorexia Jaundice | Resolution/immunity (99%) Death/liver failure (1%) |

Hepatitis B

| DNA virus (via blood or secretions) | Infected liver cells ↓ Viral antigens in liver cells ↓ Immune destruction of virus and liver cells ↓ Inflammation | 45 to 120 days incubation Fatigue Anorexia Jaundice Liver enzymes | Resolution/immunity (85%) Death/liver failure (2%) Chronic hepatitis (13%) •Cirrhosis •Cancer •Death •Resolution Carrier state |

Hepatitis C

| RNA virus (via blood) | Similar to hepatitis B Direct cytolysis by virus | Mild symptoms | Chronic hepatitis is common •Cirrhosis •Cancer Carrier state |

Fig. 5-13 The etiology, pathogenesis, course, and sequelae of hepatitis A, B, and C are compared in this chart.

Bacterial Diseases

Recurrent Aphthous Stomatitis. Recurrent aphthous ulcers—also called recurrent aphthous stomatitis (RAS)—are common causes of mouth sores (canker sores, stomach ulcers) and affect up to 20% of the population. It is thought that these ulcers represent an immune hypersensitivity reaction to oral mucosa and perhaps to common endemic streptococci of the oral cavity; therefore, we are including this discussion in the category of infectious diseases. The condition tends to occur in families, with an expected history of lesions in parents and siblings. The lesions do not seem to be contagious. Since the α-streptococci implicated are found in most mouths, whether affected or not, and since patients who develop lesions show increased antibody titers to both

α-streptococci, and oral mucosa, an autoimmune or hypersensitivity mechanism seems most acceptable. Although some clinical forms of aphthous stomatitis resemble viral ulcers (herpetiform), no viral cause can be established despite numerous attempts and projects intended to do so. Recurrent aphthous ulcers are frequently confused by physicians, patients, and even dental practitioners with intraoral herpes lesions. In most instances, this should not happen, because the two are easily distinguished clinically (Table 5-2).

Aphthous ulcers usually occur as single lesions located on oral mucous membranes that contain minor salivary glands. These locations include all oral mucosa except the gingiva, and the anterior and lateral surfaces of the hard palate. Predisposing factors play a

TABLE 5-2

Comparison of oral herpes and aphthous stomatitis

Lesion	Location	Clinical characteristics	Course
Oral herpes (caused by herpes simplex type 1)			
Gingivostomatitis	Gingiva, all mucous membranes	Multiple vesicles; multiple ulcers; fever; malaise	7-14 days
Herpes labialis	Lips—vermilion	Prodrome; multiple small vesicles; crust(s)	7-14 days; recurrent; with predisposing factors
Intraoral recurrent	Gingiva, palate	Prodrome; multiple small vesicles; multiple small ulcers	7-14 days; recurrent; with predisposing factors
Aphthous stomatitis			
Recurrent aphthous ulcers	Salivary-bearing mucous membranes	Singular, enlarging ulcers	7-14 days; recurrent; with predisposing factors
Major aphthous ulcers	Salivary-bearing mucous membranes	Singular, very large ulcers; scarring	14-28 days; frequent
Herpetiform ulcers	Salivary-bearing mucous membranes	Multiple, small, herpetiform ulcers	7-14 days; frequent

significant role in lesion development and include low-grade trauma (toothbrush abrasion, lip biting), stress, certain foods (nuts, tomatoes), menstrual cycle, and other factors. Patients frequently recognize these factors and try to avoid them if they can. The lesions start as a red edematous area that rapidly ulcerates. No prodromal paresthesia or vesicle stage occurs. The ulcer rapidly expands to up to 1 cm in diameter. The ulcer margins are red and edematous, and the ulcer surface is usually coated with a yellow-white fibrinopurulent exudate. The lesion is usually round and has the appearance of a volcano with a central crater (Fig. 5-14). The ulcers are exquisitely painful. Patients may have difficulty talking or eating when lesions are either large or multiple. Associated cervical lymphadenitis is common. Some patients even report low-

grade fever and malaise at times of recurrence. The painful lesions often stimulate increased salivation. The ulcers usually last from 7 to 14 days and heal without scarring. Patients frequently use topical over-the-counter medications to relieve the pain. Some of these medications can actually enlarge the ulcers and should be avoided.

Uncommonly, other more severe forms of aphthous stomatitis occur. *Major aphthous ulcers* occur as very large ulcers (1 to 3 cm) that persist for weeks and heal by scarring (Fig. 5-15). Patients who suffer with major aphthae are quite uncomfortable and may exhibit malnutrition because they are unable to eat properly. *Herpetiform oral ulcers* are another uncommon form of RAS. These lesions are usually multiple, and the ulcers are frequently quite small (1 to 3 mm) and very painful.

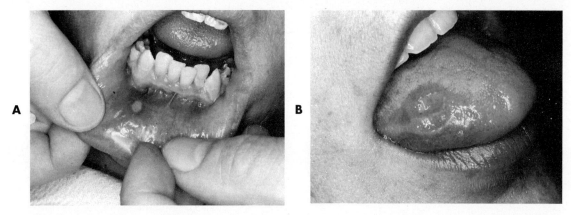

Fig. 5-14   Recurrent aphthous ulcer. **A,** This cratered ulcer of 3 days' duration is in a typical location. **B,** This painful edematous tongue ulcer occurred in a patient with recurrent aphthous lesions of other mucosa.

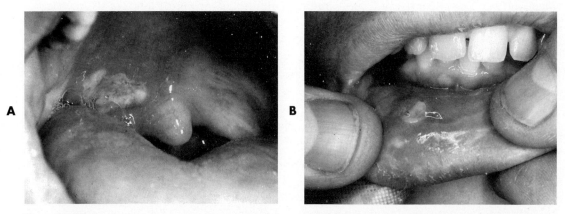

Fig. 5-15   Major aphthous ulceration. **A,** The patient has a long history of similar scarring lesions. **B,** A smaller ulcer and scars from previous ulcers.

These lesions are far more common in young women and may be clinically confused with primary herpes (Fig. 5-16). The recurrent history and lack of gingival involvement helps make the distinction between this and primary herpes.

In addition, there is an increased incidence of RAS associated with such systemic conditions as Crohn's disease, ulcerative colitis, pernicious anemia, and iron and vitamin defi-ciency. Several rare ulcerative conditions of the skin, eyes, and genital mucosa (Behçet's disease, Reiter's syndrome) have been associated with aphthous oral ulcerations. Therefore, these conditions should be considered in the patients with RAS.

Diagnosis of RAS is usually based on recurrence, location, appearance of ulcers, and history of predisposing factors. There is no definitive test for the disease, and biopsy will

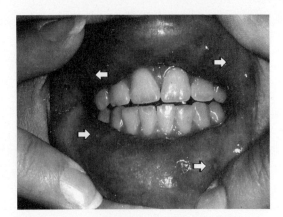

Fig. 5-16 Herpetiform aphthous ulcers. Recurrent ulcers (*arrows*) are multiple and painful.

not be helpful in a definitive diagnosis. Treatment and prevention consist of topical antibiotics for streptococci and secondary bacteria, and corticosteroids (topical or systemic) to suppress the hypersensitivity response. Over-the-counter medicines usually have an anesthetic effect.

Chronic Periodontitis. Chronic inflammatory destruction of the periodontal structures is one of the most common diseases of adults. It is estimated that after age 30, more teeth are lost to chronic periodontitis than to any other condition. The etiology of chronic periodontitis is complex and not fully understood, even though many millions of dollars have been spent on research. For purposes of this discussion, the following interrelated factors play important roles in a patient's susceptibility or resistance to chronic periodontitis. These factors include bacterial causative agents, plaque, calculus and dental accretions, immunologic factors, inflammatory mediators, nutrition, hygiene and prophylaxis, saliva, local factors (alignment, occlusion), and systemic factors. In addition, hereditary factors play a part because they influence such elements as composition of saliva, occlusion, immune competence, calculus formation, and inflammatory

modulation. It is accepted knowledge that endemic microorganisms grow in crevicular plaque and secrete numerous byproducts that either directly damage periodontal structures or indirectly stimulate immunologic and inflammatory mediators (PGE, leukotrienes) that in turn initiate collagen breakdown, cellular and bony degeneration, and destruction. The growth of these low-grade pathogens can be inhibited by plaque control, salivary factors, and bacterial immunity, or stimulated by systemic diseases (diabetes), immune suppression (AIDS), inflammatory suppression (agranulocytosis), nutritional deficiency, hereditary and racial predisposition, and local factors. You will spend your career in continued study of this disease.

The pathogenesis involves the slow, chronic, nonpainful, subclinical degeneration and destruction of all the periodontal structures, including the periodontal connective tissues, cementum, alveolar bone, epithelial attachment apparatus, and gingival fibers. As the periodontium degenerates, crevicular deepening (pockets) occurs, which facilitates local accretions and bacterial accumulation. The progression of the disease becomes a vicious cycle, with more inflammatory disease leading to deeper pockets leading to more destruction. Immune and inflammatory cells and mediators help control the infectious microorganisms, but they also contribute to further destruction of bone, cementum, and periodontal membrane. Treatment involves meticulous hygiene in susceptible individuals, pocket reduction, removal of accretions and local factors, and sometimes antibiotic therapy.

Streptococcal Pharyngitis. Streptococcal pharyngitis is a common acute suppurative pharyngitis that is caused by β-hemolytic streptococci. These highly contagious microorganisms are easily transferred by droplet or utensils. Infected patients usually develop very painful pharyngitis and tonsillitis that may extend to the palate and the tongue (Fig. 5-17). Purulent exudates, ulcerations, and even abscesses may occur, and lymphadenitis (swollen, painful nodes) of the neck is common. Some specific strains of β-streptococci elaborate erythrotoxins that cause a skin rash and red, painful strawberry tongue, as well as acute suppurative pharyngitis. This symptom complex is termed *scarlet fever.* Occasionally, streptococcal pharyngitis has reduced symptoms and is then easily confused with viral pharyngitis or other bacterial forms of pharyngitis. Patients with acute pharyngitis are best referred to their physician, who can usually control streptococci with antibiotics. The use of culture is debatable since some cases give false negative cultures.

Streptococcal pharyngitis can cause disease in ways other than through direct bacterial tissue destruction and inflammation as just described. Streptococcal organisms may evoke an immune response mediated by formation of anti-streptococcal antibodies. Although these antibodies help control the streptococcal infection, they also may cause serious sequelae because of type 3 and type 2 immune hypersensitivity reactions (see the discussion of the immune system in Chapter 4).

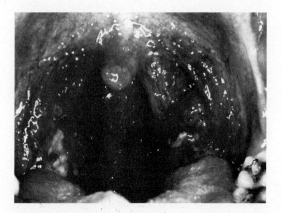

Fig. 5-17 Streptococcal pharyngitis. Intensely red tonsils and oropharynx with inflammatory exudates on surface.

These autoimmune reactions can result in aseptic immune damage to the heart, joints, and brain (rheumatic fever, rheumatic heart disease). We will discuss this later. In addition, type 2 and type 3 hypersensitivity can also cause acute and chronic kidney diseases (glomerulonephritis) (Fig.5-18). Therefore, the control and prevention of streptococcal pharyngitis is essential since its autoimmune sequelae can result in significant illness or death.

Tuberculosis. Tuberculosis is a common and significant worldwide infection that is caused by the bacterial organism *Mycobacterium tuberculosis.* The organisms are spread in droplets (cough, spray) and in sputum on utensils and instruments. This organism typically causes a chronic granulomatous inflammatory response in tissues (review Chapter 3). *Primary* infection usually occurs in the lungs after TB organisms are inhaled. The organisms lodge in the lung periphery. After a brief acute inflammatory response, granulomas form at the lung periphery. These peripheral granulomas are termed the *Ghon focus.* Commonly, the organisms from the Ghon focus spread by way of lymphatics to a lymph node in the hilar (central) area of the lungs. More granulomas form in these nodes, and the combination of peripheral and central granulomas is termed the *Ghon complex.* Usually, this inflammatory response is sufficient to isolate or neutralize the infection, and the disease is prevented from spreading further. Commonly, the persistent Ghon complex becomes scarred and calcified and is therefore easily detected on a chest radiograph. Although the primary Ghon complex arrests spread of TB, the organisms may survive within the granulomas for years. The granulomatous response is a type 4 hypersensitivity involving activated T lymphocytes and macrophages reacting to TB antigens. Formation of the Ghon complex is usually without significant symptoms.

Secondary tuberculosis occurs after primary exposure and sensitized T-lymphocyte

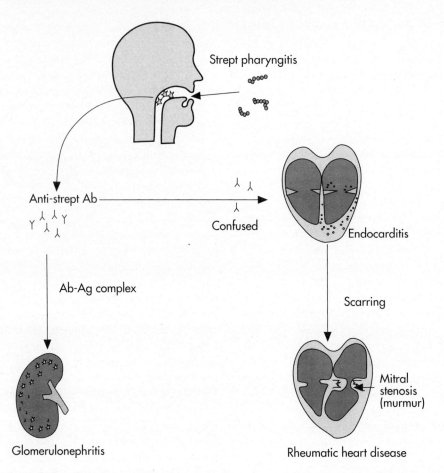

Fig. 5-18 Streptococcal infections can lead to rheumatic heart disease following anti-strep antibody cross-reaction with heart antigens (endocarditis). Also, immune complexes to strep antigens may cause inflammation of kidney glomeruli (glomerulonephritis).

formation has occurred. Either new tubercular bacteria are inhaled, or bacteria escape the primary Ghon lesions. There is an enhanced type 4 hypersensitivity response, and granulomas are formed within the lung alveoli—usually at the apices of the lungs. Caseous necrosis frequently occurs with the proliferating granulomatous response. Multiple large granulomas form and cause symptoms such as productive cough and night sweating. The granulomas may either arrest the further spread of the disease or cavitate (form cavities) and spread organisms throughout the lungs. Some granulomas may erode vessels and seed organisms throughout the bloodstream to other organs, where more caseous granulomas form. This spread is termed miliary tuberculosis. Severe secondary pulmonary tuberculosis and miliary tuberculosis are life-threatening diseases (Fig. 5-19).

Oral manifestations of tuberculosis are rare and usually occur as a result of implantation of bacteria in sputum from a cavitating pulmonary lesion into an oral cut or ulcer, or as a result of miliary spread. Oral lesions occur as chronic granular ulcers, most frequently in-

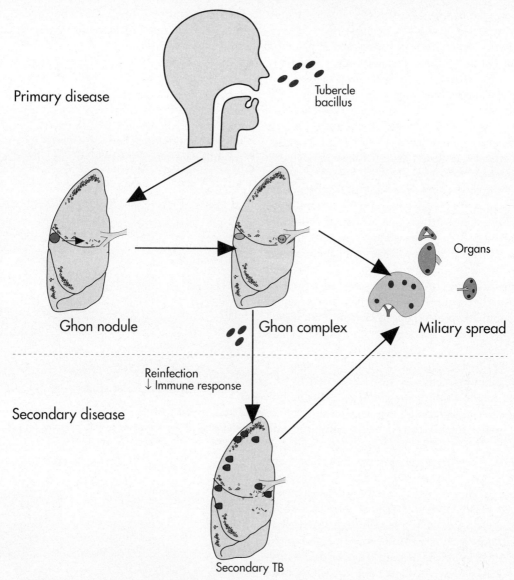

Primary disease

Tubercle bacillus

Ghon nodule

Ghon complex

Organs

Miliary spread

Reinfection
↓ Immune response

Secondary disease

Secondary TB

Fig. 5-19 Initial tuberculosis frequently results in formation of the Ghon nodule or Ghon complex. Reinfection or reduced immunity can result in secondary pulmonary tuberculosis or miliary spread.

volving the gingiva, tongue, and buccal mucosa. Diagnosis requires identification of granulomas and TB organisms through biopsy and culture.

In the United States, tuberculosis has been controlled, but not eradicated, by using public health testing and antitubercular drug therapy. The TB skin test is widely used and is based on the presence of cellular immunity to the organism. Once an individual has been infected, sensitized T lymphocytes circulate and monitor for further infection. When killed TB antigen is applied to the skin, the previously infected individual will show a positive delayed type 4 hypersensitivity response at the application site on the skin. A positive skin test simply denotes that an individual has been previously infected by the TB organisms. That individual has immune hypersensitivity but may also have active tuberculosis. Chest radiography and other tests help detect those positive–skin tested patients that have active disease.

Recently, there has been a resurgence in numbers of cases of tuberculosis in the United States. Many of these new cases are caused by organisms that are resistant to the antituberculosis drugs. Also, since the cellular immunity response limits spread of the organisms, the infection rate of tuberculosis is high in HIV and AIDS patients because of the impaired immune response. These new and additional cases provide a reservoir for spread of the disease to the general population.

Syphilis. Syphilis is usually a venereal (sexually transmitted) disease caused by the spirochete *Treponema pallidum*. This mobile species of bacteria is very invasive and is able to penetrate intact mucous membranes and skin. Once infection occurs, three stages of clinical lesions may develop. The first stage develops at the site of contact or invasion—usually the genitalia. The lesion is a raised, firm, relatively painless ulcer termed a *chancre* (Fig.5-20). The chancre usually appears within several weeks after infection and lasts 2 to 4 weeks before healing. The regional lymph nodes become swollen, and the spirochetal organisms are spread through the blood to other tissues.

Secondary syphilis occurs on the skin and mucous membranes and develops in most of the untreated cases. The skin lesions, termed mucocutaneous rash, are often red and cause itching. Lymphadenopathy is very common. Oral mucosal lesions are common and consist of red, superficial plaques and ulcers that are often coated with a white mucuslike inflam-

matory exudate (Fig. 5-21). They are therefore termed *mucous patches*. These lesions are easily confused with other oral ulcers and white lesions (as in candidiasis); and therefore, history, associated rashlike skin lesions, lymphadenopathy, and laboratory tests provide necessary data for diagnosis. Other mucosal and skin lesions of secondary syphilis, termed condyloma lata, are warty or mushroomlike growths that may become persistent

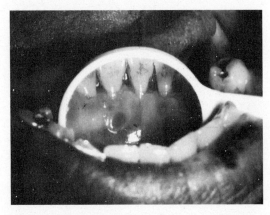

Fig. 5-20 Chancre. Edematous ulcer of the lingual alveolar mucosa is seen reflected in the mirror.

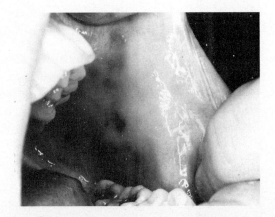

Fig. 5-21 Secondary syphilis. Rashlike lesions and mucous patches of the buccal mucosa. This patient has a corresponding skin rash.

or regress with treatment. They may occur on oral and genital skin and mucosa. All primary and secondary lesions of syphilis are teeming with numerous spirochetes and are therefore highly contagious to contact—including non-venereal contact in a health care setting. Therefore, proper diagnosis and adequate protective procedures are mandatory. Both primary and secondary syphilitic lesions show nonspecific plasmacytic chronic inflammation under the microscope. Although some clues exist microscopically, the diagnosis of the lesions is better verified by examination of clinical appearance and history, and serologic testing for antitreponema antibodies. A minority of untreated cases progress to tertiary syphilis. These lesions are characterized by perivascular chronic infection and granulomatous inflammation with gummatous necrosis. Classic lesions include necrotic gummas of bone (including palate), aneurysms of the ascending aorta, and permanent damage to the spinal cord and brain. Tertiary lesions are usually not very infective. The majority of cases demonstrate cardiovascular or central neurologic disease.

The spirochetal organisms are very sensitive to numerous antibiotics, including penicillin, and transmission can be prevented using barrier techniques and antiseptic procedures. Paradoxically, in this age of sexual disease–awareness, the incidence of primary syphilis is again on the increase.

Congenital syphilis occurs when an infected mother transfers the organism via the placenta to the fetus. Numerous developmental defects of the heart, bones, teeth, and nervous system can occur. Much less commonly, *Hutchinson's triad*—notched central incisors, interstitial keratitis (blindness), and eighth-nerve deafness—is a sequela of the rare congenital syphilis. Mulberry-shaped permanent molars may also be seen (Fig. 5-22). The newborn with congenital syphilis may also develop other classic secondary or tertiary lesions and may be infective.

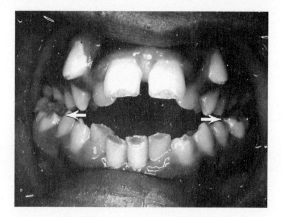

Fig. 5-22   Congenital syphilis. Notched incisors and mulberry molars (*arrows*).

Fungal Diseases

Candidiasis. The species *Candida albicans* is a common fungus that is found as normal commensal flora in oral and genital mucous membranes and that survives under moist environmental conditions. As you are aware, the oral cavity is an ecologic system involving numerous bacterial and fungal interactions. The growth of *Candida albicans* within this system is controlled and inhibited by the flora, by secretory antibodies and anticandidal lymphocytes, by antifungal factors found in saliva, and by hereditary, endocrine, and hygienic influences. If any of these factors are altered, the system is changed and the candidal organisms may have the opportunity to grow and flourish. For example, patients who take specific antibiotics may frequently develop intraoral candidiasis. Competing bacteria are reduced by the antibiotic, and the fungal organisms therefore have an opportunity to proliferate. Patients who are immune suppressed (by AIDS, cortisone therapy) frequently have intraoral candidiasis. Patients with dry mouths (drug induced), poor denture hygiene, endocrine diseases (diabetes, hypoparathyroidism), or hereditary predisposition to fungal infections have a greater incidence of intraoral candidiasis. The organism grows well on superficial mucosa, where it causes a mild irritative mucositis. Commonly the organisms themselves can be scraped from the infected mucosa and seen with a microscope. Several clinical forms of intraoral candidiasis exist. The most common are the pseudomembranous, atrophic, and hyperplastic forms.

Pseudomembranous candidiasis is one of the most common clinical forms of the disease. It frequently is acute and immediately follows antibiotic or corticosteroid therapy. Colonies of candidal organisms proliferate on all oral mucosal surfaces (Fig. 5-23). These colonies resemble white milk curds that easily wipe off with a tongue depressor. The mucosa beneath the pseudomembrane appears red and may bleed slightly. The patient complains of mild irritation, burning, and perceived swelling or dryness of the affected areas.

Atrophic candidiasis is also a common form of the disease. The mucosa appears red and atrophic, is nonpainful or slightly irritated, and is therefore easily confused with other red mucosal diseases. The condition is usually long-standing (chronic atrophic candidiasis) and most often occurs beneath a nonhygienic ill-fitting denture. When a denture is involved, the atrophic mucositis follows the outline of the denture that covers it (Fig. 5-24). Sometimes pseudomembranous areas are also present. Occasionally, atrophic candidiasis is acute in presentation. These acute lesions may be burning or painful and are frequently associated with antibiotic or corticosteroid therapy or delivery of a new denture. Chronic atrophic candidiasis of the commissures of the lips is termed *perlèche* (Fig. 5-25) and that of the posterior dorsal surface of the tongue is termed *median rhomboid glossitis* (Fig. 5-26).

Hyperplastic (hypertrophic) candidiasis is a far less common clinical presentation than the pseudomembranous or atrophic forms. This chronic candidiasis is most often associated with genetic or endocrine-induced disease. The lesions appear clinically as white hyperkeratotic plaques that do not scrape off with a dental instrument. The white areas are often somewhat raised and must be differentiated from other white lesions we will describe later (hyperkeratosis, dysplasia, carcinoma).

The association of candidiasis with oral cancer and precancerous lesions has been discussed and debated in the scientific literature. Clinically, there is an increased incidence of candidal growth in precancerous and cancerous oral diseases. Since *Candida albicans* grows in an altered environment with reduced

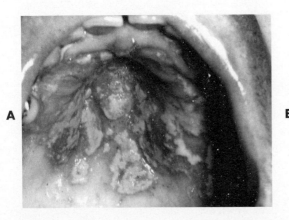
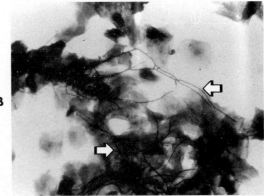

Fig. 5-23 Pseudomembranous candidiasis. **A,** White areas of the palate scrape off in a patient taking antibiotics. **B,** A smear of the palate shows fungal organisms (*arrows*).

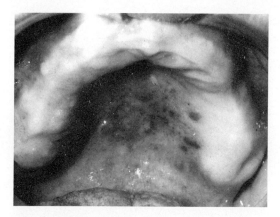

Fig. 5-24 Chronic atrophic candidiasis. Red painless areas of palate beneath a denture.

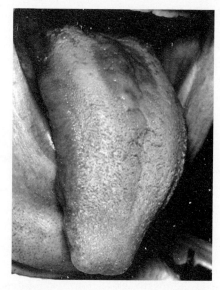

Fig. 5-26 Median rhomboid glossitis. Red painless area is positive for candidal organisms.

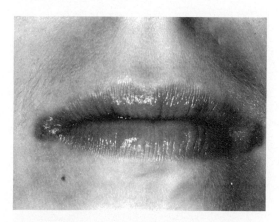

Fig. 5-25 Perlèche. Candidiasis and angular cheilitis.

protective mechanisms, the presence of *Candida* in these lesions probably is secondary to the cancerous growth rather than causative of the malignancy.

Candidiasis is controlled by a number of antifungal medications that are administered either topically or systemically. However, since these organisms usually grow in an altered ecologic environment, it is important that the contributory factors be identified and eliminated if possible. Otherwise, the infection will soon return, or not resolve with medication. Since

the organisms grow in the superficial layers of the mucosa, cytologic tests are useful in verifying the clinical diagnosis.

Deep Fungal Infections. Infections such as histoplasmosis, coccidioidomycosis, blastomycosis, and cryptococcosis are termed deep fungal infections because they usually occur in internal organs and submucosal connective tissue. The infecting organisms are common in nature and are found as spores in soil, dust, and circulating air. Some are concentrated in geographic areas such as the Ohio valley (histoplasmosis) or the Western desert (coccidioidomycosis). These organisms, like TB, are usually inhaled and evoke a chronic granulomatous response. Primary and secondary infections frequently mimic the stages of tuberculosis. Since these organisms are controlled by cellular immunity, individuals who are immune suppressed are especially susceptible to more severe secondary and disseminated infections. Oral lesions may result either from direct implantation of preexisting lacerations or from miliary spread. Oral lesions usually appear as chronic granular ulcers that must be differentiated from tuberculosis and some oral cancers (Fig. 5-27). Treatment consists of antifungal drugs and removal of the cause of immune suppression.

HUMAN IMMUNE DEFICIENCY VIRUS

The HIV virus is an RNA virus that infects susceptible cells such as T_4 lymphocytes, antigen-processing cells (macrophages), and nerve cells of the central nervous system. The infection causes cytolysis with resultant immune deficiency and central nervous system degeneration (psychosis). Immune and inflammatory responses to the HIV virus do not provide significant protection. Once infection occurs, the condition becomes chronic and progressive. A subclinical carrier state may exist for years before any symptoms arise. Therefore, infected individuals are frequently unaware of the infection and frequently cannot recall the source of the inoculum. Acquired immune deficiency syndrome (AIDS) occurs as the advanced stage of HIV infection, when the immune system is severely depressed and opportunistic infections and ma-

lignant tumors begin to overwhelm the patient (Fig. 5-28). AIDS invariably leads to patient death.

The virus is predominantly transmitted between individuals in three ways: (1) through sexual activity, (2) parenterally (as by injection of blood products), and (3) transplacentally from mother to fetus. Male homosexual activity, intravenous drug abuse, and promiscuous heterosexual activity account for the majority of cases in the United States. However, blood transfusions, injected blood products, and placental transfer to the fetus account for a small but significant number of cases of HIV infection. The HIV virus has been detected in most secretions from infected individuals, including blood and saliva. Therefore, dental care personnel must be diligent in infection control to avoid transfer of the infection to patients or to themselves.

Because the virus specifically targets the immune system (T lymphocytes, antigen-processing cells), the disease is primarily that of

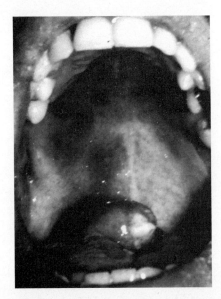

Fig. 5-28 Oral manifestations of AIDS. This HIV-infected patient has Kaposi's sarcoma of the tongue, herpes ulcers, candidiasis, and acute progressive periodontitis.

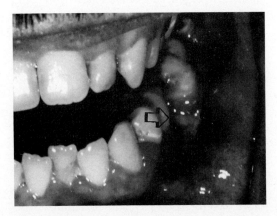

Fig. 5-27 Histoplasmosis. Chronic gingival ulcer and granular-appearing tissue in an HIV patient.

non-specific immune deficiency. As the number of T lymphocytes decreases from viral cytolysis, patients begin to develop opportunistic infections such as tuberculosis, disseminated deep fungal infections, primary herpetic gingivostomatitis, shingles, candidiasis, Epstein-Barr virus lesions, and pneumocystic (protozoan) pneumonia. The opportunistic organisms that produce these diseases produce mild, subclinical, or no disease when they infect immune competent individuals. However, since the HIV patient is immune deficient, this patient develops more frequent, more long-lasting, and more serious infections, as well as multiple infections. The result is an additional stress of infections on the patient that overwhelms the immune system with resultant illness and death. For example, pneumocystic carinii, a ubiquitous protozoa, seldom cause disease in normal individuals. Pneumocystis pneumonia, however, is the single most important cause of death in AIDS patients to date.

We have previously discussed the role of T lymphocytes in rejecting forming cancer cells. In general, immune deficient individuals have increased rates of morbidity and mortality from cancer because of depression of this immune-monitoring function. In HIV infection, several opportunistic cancers such as Kaposi's sarcoma and non-Hodgkin's lymphoma are markedly increased in incidence and contribute to high rates of patient morbidity. In fact, the majority of the cases of Kaposi's sarcoma occur in AIDS patients. Some investigators speculate that cancers associated with HIV infection may be caused by opportunistic viruses (e.g., EBV) that are allowed to infect and mutate tissues. The newly formed opportunistic cancers, in turn, can proliferate unchecked because of the immune deficiency.

You can expect several categories of special dental problems in patients with HIV infection and AIDS. These problems include those associated with (1) care of oral lesions caused by the opportunistic infections and tumors; (2)

diagnosis of HIV infection based on oral disease; (3) proper dental care in immune compromised and medically compromised patients; and (4) infection control and fear of contagion.

We have previously described the oral presentation of candidiasis as pseudomembranous, atrophic, or hyperplastic. Approximately 60% of HIV-infected individuals will develop upper aerodigestive candidiasis—including that of the oral cavity. These infections will respond to antifungal medication; however, recurrence, reduced sensitivity to antifungal agents, and increased severity of lesions should be expected. Therefore, HIV-infected patients often must be prophylactically treated and closely monitored to reduce candidiasis, or they may become debilitated from the disease.

Herpes simplex virus is frequently manifest as primary gingivostomatitis or as severe chronic recurrent herpes labialis. The incidence and duration of shingles (secondary herpes zoster) is also markedly increased with HIV infection. Oral hairy leukoplakia (caused by EBV) is found almost exclusively in HIV-infected patients and frequently signals progression toward more severe immune suppression (AIDS). These opportunistic viruses can be controlled to some extent with antiviral prophylaxis and therapy; however, some lesions can cause severe illness.

Bacterial oral infections associated with HIV immune suppression are also very common. HIV-gingivitis (HIV-G), HIV periodontitis (HIV-P), and acute necrotizing ulcerative gingivitis (ANUG) occur frequently and acutely in HIV-infected patients. These bacterial infections are caused by resident microorganisms of the gingival and crevicular tissues. These bacteria produce disease by virtue of pathogenic overgrowth of fusospirochetal organisms (in ANUG) and Gram-negative anaerobic organisms (in HIV-G and HIV-P). Patients have acute, reddened, painful gingivitis (HIV-G), necrotizing ulcerative pseudomembranous gingivitis

(ANUG), destructive acute periodontitis with bleeding, pain, and rapid bone loss (HIV-P), and combinations of all of these (Fig. 5-29).

Tooth loss is inevitable unless these conditions are controlled. Occasionally, these infections spread to adjacent mucosa and bone as necrotizing ulcerations and erosions (noma) that can be life threatening. Systemically and topically administered antibiotic and antibacterial medications are useful in control and prevention of these lesions.

HIV-infected patients may have a myriad of deep fungal, bacterial, protozoan, and tuberculosis-like granulomatous infections. The oral lesions usually appear as chronic ulcerative lesions and frequently represent life-threatening disseminated spread of the organisms. Needless to say, intervention and referral at an early stage are mandatory.

Kaposi's sarcoma associated with HIV infection commonly involves the oral cavity and is particularly common on facial skin. This blood vessel cancer causes red to blue growths of the submucosa—most frequently in the palate and gingiva (Fig. 5-30). These lesions may be flat but usually become raised with growth. They must be distinguished—usually by biopsy—from other inflammatory

and reactive red and blue tumors. As with all cancer, early diagnosis and treatment gives the optimal result. Another cancer, non-Hodgkin's lymphoma, may appear in the oral cavity as a firm, rubbery swelling, usually located in the tonsil area or palate. However, any mucous membrane or even bone may be involved. The diagnosis is made with biopsy. Both lymphomas and Kaposi's sarcomas can be treated and, at times, cured.

Since HIV infection is frequently subclinical for several years, the dental patient will often be unaware of the infection. The health history may or may not give clues to the patient status. Since the opportunistic diseases associated with HIV infection (candidiasis, herpes, HIV-P) are both commonly oral and occur early in the course of the disease, the initial suspicion of HIV infection may arise in a dental setting. Detection of these oral conditions, associated systemic conditions, risk factors (by history), and other laboratory abnormalities should warrant referral for counseling and testing. As we will see, it is important that the dental team know if the patient is HIV infected, so that the dental treatment plan can be designed to minimize the development of complications for the patient.

HIV-infected dental patients may have many other HIV- or immune suppression–related problems. These include hemorrhage because of reduced platelet quantity, susceptibility to infections after minor dental procedures, failure to heal properly, intolerance to medications because of systemic disease, as well as many others. In addition, these patients may be taking anti-HIV drugs, as well as multiple drugs to control opportunistic infections and cancers. Many of these medications are newly developed or experimental, and most will have some impact on routine dental care. Therefore, very careful, updated patient assessment is necessary. This assessment should involve physician consultation, treatment plan adjustment, and anticipation of prognosis. For example, would it be justified to electively

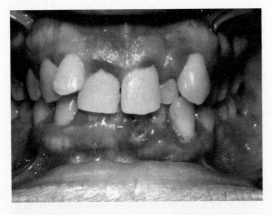

Fig. 5-29 Early HIV-related gingivitis and periodontitis. Note the marginal erythema and ulceration.

extract bony impacted third molars from an AIDS patient with a 6-month prognosis for survival and a 10% platelet count? Should we draw up a treatment plan for an HIV patient for implants and expensive fixed prostheses when that patient has a history of pneumonia and psychosis? These questions illustrate extreme situations but make a medical and ethical point for consideration. By definition, persons with AIDS (PWAs) have major medical problems and diseases. They should therefore receive dental treatment in a setting that readily permits intervention or emergency medical care. Many routine dental procedures might better be performed on PWAs in a hospital setting than in the dental office. In the hospital, emergency personnel and experts are readily available when severe complications arise.

Infection control is mandatory in any health care setting to avoid spread of organisms. Although HIV is not a particularly contagious organism, the spread of this virus in a health care setting is of great concern to our patients because of (1) reported spread of the virus in a single dental practice, and (2) the decidedly negative prognosis associated with HIV infection. Certain guidelines of infection control should be established. These include (1) stringent sterilization of reusable equipment that may be used in invasive procedures; (2) use of barrier procedures (gloves, eyewear) and coverage or disinfection of surfaces contaminated by blood or saliva; (3) use of disinfectants in preparing noninvasive equipment for use; (4) cleanliness, and (5) stringent handling and disposal procedures for sharp instruments (needles, blades, cutting instruments). Furthermore, these guidelines should be used for all patients (universal precautions), since it is impossible to determine absolutely which patient is HIV infected and which patient is not infected, and since asymptomatic carrier states are common.

Case Studies

Case 1

F. G. is a 29-year-old man who came to the dentist with severe acute painful gingivitis. Oral examination revealed bilateral oral hairy leukoplakia, candidiasis, and acute hemorrhagic gingivitis. The dentist commenced treatment for the gingivitis (chlorhexidine, cleaning) and candidiasis (antifungal therapy) and referred F. G. for HIV testing. F. G. identified known risk factors and tested HIV positive. He was scheduled for quarterly dental visits consisting of oral assessment and cleaning. His gingivitis and candidiasis were both controlled for 3 years, and the hairy

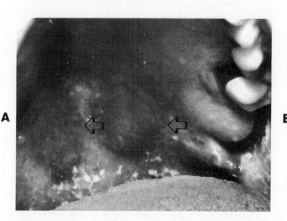
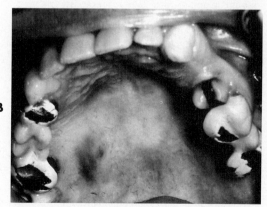

Fig. 5-30 Kaposi's sarcoma. **A**, These are flat purple lesions of the palate (*arrows*) in an AIDS patient. Note the pseudomembranous candidiasis. **B**, A singular flat sarcoma of the palate.

leukoplakia persisted. He subsequently developed primary herpetic gingivostomatitis involving gingiva, tongue, palate, and labial mucosa. He was placed on antiviral medication (acyclovir). The herpes was resolved, and F. G. is taking prophylactic doses of acyclovir without apparent lesions.

Case 2

C. V. is a 14-year-old girl who developed acute blisters and crusts on the upper and lower vermilion borders following a sunburn. She gave no history of cold sores or fever blisters and admitted to a prodromal "swelling sensation" one day previously. The clinical impression was that of herpes labialis, and a cytologic smear test was performed that confirmed the diagnosis. The lesions healed without treatment and have recurred 4 times when C. V. has sunburned her lips. She has had no lesions for the past 2 years and is using sunscreen preparations and occasional antiviral prophylaxis.

Case 3

P. D. is a 50-year-old woman who developed burning beneath her upper partial dentures subsequent to antibiotic treatment of a throat infection by her physician. Examination revealed a red burning palatal mucosa beneath the denture and occasional white milky plaques of the dorsal surface of the tongue and buccal mucosa. Cytologic tests on both sites were positive for overgrowth of *Candida*. P. D. was given antifungal mouth lozenges and told to soak her denture nightly in diluted hypochlorite solution. Her antibiotic prescription expired. Burning stopped in 2 days and the redness disappeared in one week's time. Follow-up cytologic tests after two weeks were negative for fungus.

Case 4

R. W. is a 38-year-old man who gave a history of chronic active hepatitis B. He noted that he had related liver cirrhosis, was occasionally jaundiced, and suffered from extreme fatigue. Oral examination revealed submucosal bleeding of the palatal mucosa and spontaneous bleeding of the gingiva. R. W. was weak and had lost 35 lbs in

the past year. The dentist chose to schedule extractions of 9 periodontally involved teeth to be done in a hospital-based dental unit. Blood-clotting tests were performed prior to extraction. Because clotting was prolonged, the teeth were extracted singularly in separate sessions.

Case 1

1. Why did the dentist refer F. G. for HIV testing? Would the referral have been proper if the patient history for HIV infection had been negative?
2. What is the significance of oral hairy leukoplakia? Should it have been treated also?
3. Is there any association between primary herpes and HIV infection? Can herpes be prevented with prophylactic acyclovir?
4. What special problems does this patient pose when seeking dental care?
5. Should special infection control precautions be initiated specifically for this patient?

Case 2

1. Is there any association between herpes labialis and sunburn?
2. How did cytologic testing help the dentist diagnose the lesion?
3. Is the course of the lesion recurrence consistent with herpes labialis?
4. What do you think was the primary lesion in this case?

Case 3

1. What caused the red burning of the palate?
2. Why was the denture soaked in hypochlorite solution?
3. What do you think triggered the candidiasis? Explain how this can occur.
4. What do you expect might occur if the patient takes the antibiotic again?

Case 4

1. What is chronic active hepatitis?
2. How do you think R. W. contracted the hepatitis B virus?
3. Do you think there is a relationship between hepatitis B, cirrhosis, and bleeding problems?
4. Why was dental surgery done in a hospital?
5. How can it be determined whether the patient has hepatitis B in an active state?

SUMMARY

- The virulence of microorganisms is determined by their ability to invade and grow within tissues, produce toxins, and elicit an injurious inflammatory and immune response.
- Microorganisms can produce both toxins and virulence factors that facilitate pathogenesis.
- Viruses damage cells by causing cell lysis, by inducing mutations, or by stimulating an immune response that subsequently injures the infected cell.
- Both external and internal defense mechanisms help defend against infection. Loss of these barriers and mechanisms enhances infectivity.
- Herpes simplex virus causes common vesiculoulcerative recurrent lesions of the lips and uncommon ulcers of the palate and gingiva. These lesions are readily distinguished clinically.
- Primary herpetic gingivostomatitis is a severe oral condition usually occurring in children or immune suppressed individuals. Other conditions can demonstrate similar clinical characteristics.
- Shingles represents recurrent infection from the latent chickenpox virus.
- Other viruses such as Coxsackie virus, measles, and varicella-zoster virus cause oral herpetiform lesions.
- Epidemic parotiditis is well controlled by vaccination, although sporadic outbreaks continue to occur.

- Epstein-Barr virus has been implicated in causing mononucleosis, Burkitt's lymphoma, and oral hairy leukoplakia. All have oral manifestations.
- Hepatitis A virus causes acute hepatitis and is contracted from fecally contaminated food or water. No chronic disease state or carrier state exists.
- Hepatitis B virus is usually transmitted parenterally or sexually. Acute fulminant and chronic states can be morbid or fatal. Carrier states exist. Vaccinations and infection control procedures are useful and necessary in the dental setting.
- Hepatitis C can be spread through dental procedures and can result in chronic disease and carrier states. Infection control is mandatory.
- The etiology and pathogenesis of aphthous ulcers reflect hereditary hypersensitivity. These recurrent ulcers are usually easily diagnosed by clinical features and behavior. Several unusual subtypes can cause diagnostic problems.
- Streptococcal pharyngitis can cause local purulent acute infection and morbid autoimmune sequelae such as rheumatic heart disease.
- Tuberculosis is highly contagious in sputum and can cause disease in otherwise healthy individuals. Previously infected individuals are at risk for reinfection. The prevalence of infection is increasing because of drug-resistant strains and HIV patient susceptibility.
- Syphilis occurs in primary, secondary, tertiary, and congenital forms. All forms occasionally demonstrate oral lesions.
- Candidiasis is usually caused by interference with the oral ecosystem that controls growth of the fungus. Acute and chronic infections can cause different recognizable clinical forms of the disease. Testing is simple and inexpensive. Treatment is dependent on antifungal therapy and removal of the predisposing factor.
- HIV infection is spread in a manner similar to that of hepatitis B. The virus causes immune suppression. The disease is usually slow in progression but is relentless, with no known immunity or cure.

- Proper infection control procedures eliminate any risk of HIV transfer within the dental practice setting.
- Patients with AIDS have a very low T_4-lymphocyte count and therefore are very susceptible to oral and systemic infections and tumors. Many of these oral conditions can be anticipated, prevented, and treated in a normal dental setting.

Suggested readings

1. Abrutyn E: Diseases caused by mycobacteria. In Rose LF and Kaye D, editors: Internal medicine for dentistry, ed 2, St Louis, 1990, Mosby, pp 221-227.
2. Antoon JW and Miller RL: Aphthous ulcers: a review of the literature on etiology, pathogenesis, diagnosis and treatment, JADA 101:803, 1980.
3. Carranza FA: Glickman's clinical periodontology, ed 7, Philadelphia, 1992, WB Saunders Co, chapter 11.
4. Cawson RA and others: Pathology: the mechanisms of disease, ed 2, St Louis, 1989, Mosby, chapter 6.
5. Finlay BB and Falkow S: Common themes in microbiol pathogenicity, Microbiol Rev, 53:210, 1989.
6. Jawetz E, Melnick JL, and Adelberg EA: Review of medical microbiology, ed 7, East Norwalk, Conn, 1987, Appleton & Lange, chapters 30, 44, 46.
7. Klein RS and others: Low occupational risk of human immunodeficiency virus infection among dental professionals, N Engl J Med 318:86, 1988.
8. Lehner T: Oral candidosis, Dent Pract 17:209, 1967.
9. Robertson PB and Greenspan JS: Perspectives on oral manifestations of AIDS, Littleton, Mass, 1988, PSG Publishing Co.
10. Scuibba J and others: Hairy leukoplakia: an AIDS-associated opportunistic infection, Oral Surg Oral Med Oral Pathol 67:404, 1989.
11. Scully C: Orofacial herpes simplex virus infections: current concepts in epidemiology, pathogenesis and treatment, and disorders in which the virus may be implicated, Oral Surg Oral Med Oral Pathol 68:701, 1989.
12. Shafer WG, Hine MK, and Levy BM: A textbook of oral pathology, ed 4, Philadelphia, 1983, WB Saunders Co, chapter 6.
13. Shearer BG: MDR-TB: another challenge from the microbial world, JADA 125:43, 1994.
14. Spruance SL and others: The natural history of herpes simplex labialis, N Engl J Med 297:69, 1977.
15. Vincent SD and Lilly GE: Clinical, historic and therapeutic features of aphthous stomatitis: literature review and open clinical trail employing steroids, Oral Surg Oral Med Oral Pathol 74:79, 1992.

6

Disturbances of Cell Growth

After studying this chapter, you should be able to meet the following objectives and define the key terms:

- Explain why some tissues can divide and other tissues cannot.
- List common causes of hypertrophy and hyperplasia.
- Explain why connective tissue hyperplasia is often persistent after the stimulus is removed.
- Define metaplasia and give several examples of the process.
- Differentiate hyperplasia and metaplasia.
- Define hamartoma and choristoma and give several common examples.
- Develop a rationale to explain the presence of teeth, hair, bone, and gut in a teratoma.

All cells have the genetic apparatus necessary to allow for regulation of cell division. The series of events necessary for tissue growth and cell division is complex and is genetically regulated. In normal tissues, cell division is regulated by both the inherent activated genetic material within the cells and the environmental stimuli for cellular growth. In studying regeneration and repair, we discovered that certain (labile) tissues have a controlled rapid rate of cell division under normal physiologic stimuli while other (stable) tissues have a slower rate of cell division that occurs only after stimulants are released by injury. Some (permanent) tissues have little or no ability to divide, no matter what the degree or intensity of the stimulus. Tissues that have the capacity to divide and regenerate contain immature, less differentiated cells termed *reserve cells,* which can be stimulated to mitotically "divide and produce" new cells to replace lost ones. In labile tissues, reserve cells maintain genetic machinery that can be easily switched on by growth factors, loss of cell-to-cell contact, and exogenous factors released by necrosis, inflammation, or the reparative processes. In stable tissues, fewer reserve cells are present, and stimulation must be significant and concentrated. Permanent tissues lack reserve cells. All the genes for division within permanent tissue cells are repressed. In embryonic, labile, and stable tissues, cell division yields a new reserve cell and a maturing (differentiating) cell. As these differentiating cells mature, they lose the potential to divide.

CELL REGULATION

The normal cell division in labile and stable tissues can be regulated by several factors. These factors include systemic and local hormones. Many trophic hormones (adrenocorticotropic hormone, thyroid-stimulating hormone) induce cell division. We will study the function and pathology of these in Chapter 19.

Local hormones, including macrophage-derived growth factors and epidermal growth factor hormones, also induce cell division. Exogenous factors can also stimulate cellular division. Such factors as physical forces (friction, heat, pressure) and chemical substances frequently stimulate cell division. Certain microorganisms and their products can also stimulate cell division.

The genetic regulation of cell division is important. Although all cells have the same genetic components, only the labile and stable tissue stem cell populations have genetic material available for stimulation of cell division. In permanent tissues, the genetic materials for cell division are repressed and permanently locked. In certain pathologic conditions, the regulation of cell division is diminished or lost, resulting in more rapid and frequent cell division and subsequent overgrowth of cells. Finally, in order for tissues to divide and grow, there must be available nutrients for cell construction and metabolism. In tissues where vascular or nutritional deficiency exists, there will most likely be atrophy because of cellular shrinkage and decreased mitotic rates. Less commonly, in tissues where there is increased nutrition there may be an actual stimulation of cell division.

CHANGES IN CELL GROWTH

Hypertrophy

An increase in cell size caused by an external stimulus (hormone, increased nutrients, physical force) is termed *hypertrophy*. For example, a weight lifter's muscle mass increases because of the external physical forces of constant physiologic stimulation and increased nutrition. Likewise, heart muscle cells will become hypertrophic and the heart will enlarge greatly when it must work harder to push blood against increased peripheral resistance such as high blood pressure (Fig. 6-1). The thyroid gland will become hypertrophic if the pituitary gland releases increased thyroid-stimulating hormones on a sustained basis.

Hypertrophy is a reversible process. Thus, when the stimulus is removed, the cell and tissue size should revert to normal.

Hyperplasia

Hyperplasia denotes an increase in number of cells caused by increased cellular division. A stimulus is involved. Naturally, only reserve cells of labile and, occasionally, stable tissues are affected. When the stimulus is removed, the division rate will return to normal and the tissue mass will shrink over time to reflect this (Fig. 6-1). In some cases of hyperplasia, however, products of increased cell numbers may remain after the stimulus is removed, and therefore the tissue will remain enlarged. This is common in connective tissue hyperplasias where collagen fibers, bone, or cartilage are formed and the matrix remains following removal of the stimulus. Hyperplasia of fibrous connective tissue is frequently termed *desmoplasia*, and a growth of collagenous tissues (fibroma) can result from it. Other common examples of hyperplasia include the callus—a hyperplasia of parakeratinized skin cells in response to friction—and the analogous white hyperkeratosis that may occur on the oral mucosa in response to cheek biting, irritation by the teeth, or irritation from a denture clasp or denture. Hyperplasias are common. Upon clinical examination, they often resemble other more serious or morbid lesions and therefore must be distinguished from these lesions. If the suspected cause can be determined, the hyperplasia will regress when the cause is removed. If, however, the cause cannot be detected or desmoplasia persists after the cause is removed, it might be necessary to surgically remove the lesion to ensure it is not a more serious condition. We will discuss the most common types of oral hyperplastic conditions in Chapter 13.

Metaplasia

Metaplasia is a term used to denote change from one mature tissue type to another tissue

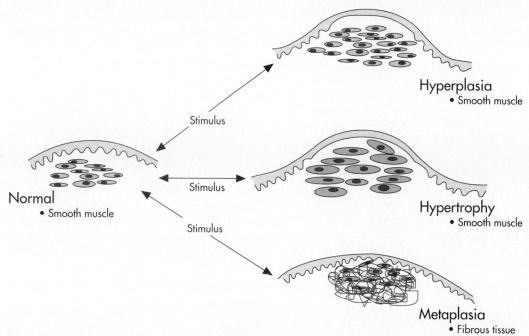

Fig. 6-1   When stimulated, smooth muscle cells may increase in number (hyperplasia), increase in size (hypertrophy), or change to fibrous connective tissue (metaplasia).

type in response to a stimulus. The reserve cells respond to the stimulus by dividing. The daughter cells, however, are induced by the stimulus to form cells that are dissimilar in form and function to the native cells of the tissue (Fig 6-1). For example, respiratory mucous membrane is normally composed of pseudostratified ciliated columnar epithelium with mucus-secreting goblet cells. This mucosa functions to entrap microbes within the mucus and remove the contaminants from the respiratory tract by ciliary action. We have seen that this is a form of defense by the body against infection. When cigarette smokers inhale, they irritate this mucous membrane with the chemical irritants (tars) of the smoke, as well as with the heat and drying associated with inhalation. Over a period of time, depending on the degree of smoking, the epithelial reserve cells will divide at an increased rate, and the new cells will mature as kerati-

nized squamous cells without cilia or goblet cell formation. What was previously pseudostratified ciliated mucosa becomes metaplastic keratinized stratified squamous mucosa. Although the keratin better protects the submucosa from tars and heat, the antimicrobial function is now diminished. Therefore, the heavy smoker develops chronic bronchitis and chronic cough resulting from the unrestricted passage of microorganisms into the bronchi and lungs. If the individual stops cigarette smoking, the metaplasia will be reversible over a period of time. Therefore, the squamous metaplastic tissues just described will revert to ciliated cells and goblet cells after the patient ceases smoking cigarettes, and function should return to normal.

An example of connective tissue metaplasia occasionally occurs within the oral cavity. A loose lower denture may pinch the connective tissue of the supportive mucosa. Fibrous connective tissue hyperplasia and cartilaginous metaplasia (cartilaginous rest) may result in response to the chronic irritation. When the irritation is corrected, the growth will stop. However, cartilage and collagen may remain as clinical swellings that should be surgically removed. Although metaplasia is a benign, reversible process, the stimuli for metaplasia may also stimulate cancer. Therefore, every effort should be made to identify and eliminate the stimulus in order to prevent more serious disease.

DEVELOPMENTAL DISORDERS OF CELL GROWTH

Hamartoma and Choristoma

Several types of disturbances causing exaggerated cell growth may be present at birth (congenital) or develop in conjunction with normal growth and development. These disturbances are very common and are termed *hamartoma* and *choristoma.* They represent developmental overgrowths (too much tissue) that grow in coordination with normal tissues. When normal somatic growth ceases (age 16 to 20), so does the growth of these lesions. For example, the *hemangioma* is a common overgrowth of localized blood vessels that occurs at birth or during development of connective tissues. A mass of normal blood vessels grows beneath the skin or mucous membranes and causes a soft red-blue swelling (birthmark). Instead of the normal four to five vessels within a unit of the tissue, this hamartomatous growth might lead to hundreds of vessels in a tissue mass (Fig. 6-2). The hemangioma is benign and will stop growing when the patient stops growing. It is not uncommon, however, for such lesions to be removed for diagnostic and esthetic reasons.

The choristoma represents similar overgrowth of normal tissues but in an abnormal location. Melanocyte-like cells may be developmentally entrapped beneath the skin or mucous membranes. The common mole *(intradermal nevus)* results from overgrowth of these entrapped cells and is representative of a choristoma (Fig. 6-3). (See the discussion of nevi in Chapter 8.) This is coordinated growth that usually ceases as the patient's growth diminishes.

Teratoma

The *teratoma* is a growth of embryonic cells that were implanted in a tissue during tissue development and became proliferative during a subsequent time. The ovaries and testes are the organs in which teratomas most frequently occur. The entrapped tissue begins to grow and differentiate because of an unknown stimulus. The teratoma may develop mature derivations of any of the embryonic precursor layers. Therefore, the tumor may contain hair, teeth, brain cells, skin (ectodermal cells), bone, cartilage, loose connective tissue (meso-

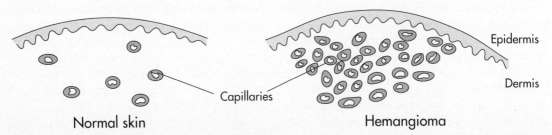

Fig. 6-2 This hemangioma represents a developmental overgrowth of capillaries within the dermis. Note the capillaries located in the normal location.

dermal cells), and gut, glands, and ducts (endodermal cells). Epithelial proliferation frequently becomes cystic, and the resultant cystic teratoma is common. Teeth are commonly formed within teratomas, and this is a noteworthy feature since this tumor seldom occurs in the jaws. Teratomas can have the growth attributes of both a malformation and a neoplasm. Occasionally, teratomas become malignant and can kill the patient.

Case Studies

Case 1

M. O. is a 58-year-old man who noted a rough area on his right buccal mucosa that lasted for 4 months. The 1 cm white lesion is at an area where he keeps his pipe stem about 12 hours a day. Biopsy revealed increased keratin and hyperplasia of the epithelium. The remaining lesion disappeared 8 weeks after M. O. stopped smoking his pipe.

Case 2

J. D. is a 43-year-old woman who noticed a very slow-growing submucosal knot on her lower lip opposite tooth No. 23. The lesion was raised, pink, and slightly firm. Tooth No. 23 had a broken incisal edge that constantly irritated the area. Removal of the labial mucosal lesion revealed fibroblast hyperplasia and associated collagenization (fibroma). The lesion did not recur subsequent to its removal and restoration of tooth No. 23.

Case 3

R. J. is a 73-year-old woman who has worn the same mandibular free-end partial denture for 23 years. One clasp was broken and one of the guiding teeth had been extracted. The denture was very loose and moved freely. There was a 2.5 × 0.8 cm soft, raised, pink tissue mass growing from her buccal vestibule in the area of the denture flange. The tissue had been growing for at least 2 years. The tissue was removed and diagnosed as fibrous hyperplasia (epulis fissuratum). One year following excision, a smaller lesion recurred. There had been no denture correction performed. Biopsy of the new lesion also was diagnosed as fibrous hyperplasia. A new denture was constructed, and no new lesions formed in 3 years. (See Chapter 14.)

Case 1

1. Do you think there was a relationship between the pipe smoking and the keratosis of the buccal mucosa?
2. Why did the lesion regress after discontinuance of pipe smoking?
3. Why was a biopsy performed on the lesion?

Case 2

1. If tooth No. 23 had been repaired before surgery, do you think the fibroma would have disappeared on its own? Why?
2. If tooth No. 23 had not been repaired, do you think the fibroma might have recurred?

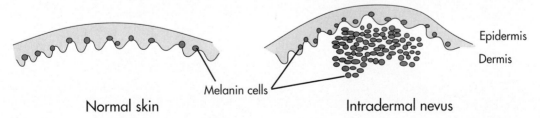

Normal skin   Intradermal nevus

Epidermis
Dermis
Melanin cells

Fig. 6-3 This intradermal nevus represents a developmental overgrowth of melanin cells within the dermis. Note the melanin cells located in an abnormal location compared with their location in normal skin.

3. Is the clinical appearance of the lesion consistent with the diagnosis of fibroma?

Case 3

1. What caused the epulis fissuratum to form and reform?
2. Why were these lesions removed for biopsy?

SUMMARY

- Labile and stable tissues have reserve cells that can be stimulated to divide by hormones, local growth factors, and exogenous physical and chemical substances.
- Hypertrophy of cells exists when cell size increases in response to a stimulus.
- Hyperplasia of cells occurs when the number of cells increases in response to a stimulus.
- Metaplasia of a tissue occurs when a stimulus induces a change in tissue type resulting from cell division that produces cells dissimilar to the native cells.
- Hypertrophy, hyperplasia, and metaplasia are reversible processes in which tissues normally revert to original type and size when the stimulus is discontinued.

- Hamartomas and choristomas are common growths in which normal tissues grow in excessive amounts. Both cause tumors that grow in coordination with the normal growth process.
- Teratomas are tumor malformations derived from entrapped embryonic elements that begin to grow and differentiate into a mixture of tissue types.

Suggested readings

1. Baserga R: The biology of cell reproduction, Cambridge, Mass, 1985, Harvard University Press, pp 117-133.
2. Gardner DG and Paterson JC: Chondroma or metaplastic chondrosis of soft palate, Oral Surg Oral Med Oral Pathol 26:601, 1968.
3. Krolls SO, Jacoway JR, and Alexander WN: Osseous choristomas (osteomas) in intraoral soft tissues, Oral Surg Oral Med Oral Pathol 32:588, 1971.
4. McGinnis JP and Parham DM: Mandible-like structure with teeth in an ovarian cystic teratoma, Oral Surg Oral Med Oral Pathol 45:104, 1978.
5. Rubin E and Farber JL: Pathology, Philadelphia, 1988, JB Lippincott Co, pp 9-13.
6. Waldron CA and Shafer WG: Leukoplakia revisited: a clinicopathologic study of 3256 oral leukoplakias, Cancer 36:1386, 1975.

7

Neoplastic Cell Growth

After studying this chapter, you should be able to meet the following objectives and define the key terms:

- Explain the role of repressors and accelerators in regulating cell growth.
- Distinguish neoplasia, carcinoma, sarcoma, cancer, adenoma, and tumor.
- Differentiate benign neoplasia from malignant neoplasia by behavior of tissues.
- Differentiate malignant neoplasia from nonmalignant tumor growth by common clinical characteristics.
- Differentiate malignant neoplasia from nonmalignant tumor growth by microscopic characteristics.
- List common benign and malignant neoplasms by tissue type.
- Discuss the role of viruses, chemicals, hormones, radiation, genetics, and the immune system in cancer etiology. Give examples of each.
- Define oncogenes and explain their role in the pathogenesis of neoplasia.
- Explain several theories of the pathogenesis of neoplasia and malignant neoplasia.
- List cellular changes that allow malignant cells to invade and metastasize.
- Discuss the prognosis of cancer based on stage, histologic features, and tissue of origin.
- List the rationale behind therapy for malignancy.
- Discuss the common routes of metastasis for cancers.

REGULATION OF CELL GROWTH

As considered in the chapter on repair and healing (Chapter 3), certain labile tissues such as skin and bone marrow have the ability to mitotically produce millions of new cells every day, while other tissues like heart muscle and neurons have only slight ability to produce new cells or replace tissues—even after severe tissue loss or damage. Why do cells of tissues with exactly the same genetic makeup have such different capacities to reproduce themselves? To answer this question, we must look at mechanisms of cellular division. All cells of one individual have essentially the same genetic material arranged in a similar manner—the DNA sequence of the cardiac muscle cell of an individual is genetically identical to that of an epithelial cell of the dorsal surface of the tongue. It is the genetic material within these cells that regulates cell division. However, much of this genetic material has been covered or repressed by nuclear and cytoplasmic substances. Consider the genetic material within each cell as having the potential for cell division, a situation analogous to a running truck at the top of an incline. Without some kind of environmental regulation, the loaded truck will accelerate down the hill. Likewise, without a braking effect (repression), a cell will divide at an accelerated rate. All cells, then, must be somewhat repressed, or there could be uncontrolled accelerated growth. Those tissues that are permanent, such as muscle and nerves, have their repressor brakes locked tightly, while those tissues with labile capacity for regeneration have many reserve cells with their repressor brakes pushed only halfway down. This repressor mechanism is not completely understood, but the following characteristics seem to hold true:

1. The braking mechanism may be influenced by extracellular and environmental substances such as hormones, chemicals, viruses, ionizing radiation, and heat. The usual result of stimulation from such substances is inhibition of the repressor mechanism—that is, the cell lets up on the brakes and the velocity of cell division increases.
2. Repression is determined environmentally during embryologic tissue development. For example, neurons have tightly locked brakes that are extremely difficult to disengage once the cells are formed (differentiated). In bone marrow, the tissue is only slightly repressed for cell division, and this repression can be easily altered by environmental stimuli.
3. As cells (not tissues) mature and begin to function, they lose their ability to divide. Immature (undifferentiated) cells divide readily, whereas mature cells (such as neurons and PMNs) cannot divide—even if stimulated. Therefore, labile tissues have numerous immature reserve or stem cells that have the capacity to divide on the slightest stimulus, whereas permanent tissues have no reserve cells and cannot regenerate.
4. Certain genetic defects in themselves can override repression and cause cell division. This is like the cell keeping one foot on the brake but nevertheless accelerating because the other foot is pressing on the accelerator.

In the previous chapter, we saw how cell division could be altered by environmental factors, resulting in controlled increased cell division or hyperplasia. When the hyperplastic stimulus was withdrawn, the rate of cell division was again repressed and returned to normal. In some instances, however, the stimulus, be it environmental or internal, can cause a permanent alteration in the rate of cell activity (mitotic regulation) either by mutating the DNA of the affected cell, or by permanently altering the cellular substance that represses cell division (Figure 7-1). Once again using our truck analogy, such an alteration is consistent with the truck traveling on a downgrade with either a jammed accelerator or a broken brake line. In either instance, accelerated cell division will continue, even after the foot (DNA mutation) has been removed from the accelerator or pressure is applied to the brake pedal (altered repressor).

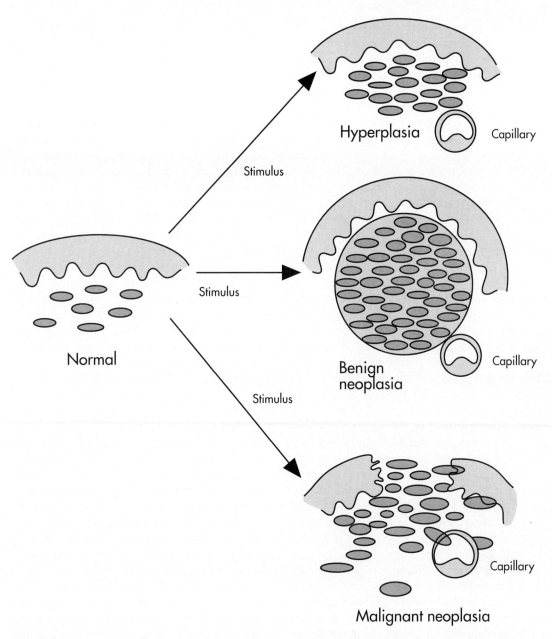

Fig. 7-1 Cells within normal tissues may be stimulated to grow in a controlled fashion (hyperplasia). Cell growth ceases when the stimulus is withdrawn. In neoplasia, cell division controls are diminished and cells grow uncontrollably. In benign neoplasia, the growth is localized and expansile. In malignant neoplasia, the growth is infiltrative to adjacent tissues and vessels.

NEOPLASIA

Such new autonomous unregulated cell growth is termed neoplasia (neo: new; plasia: formation). A neoplasm is an uncontrolled cellular growth. It is not necessarily a reckless growth, although it may be. The stimulus may not be readily apparent—in fact, it usually is not noticeable. Because the neoplastic growth is uncoordinated with normal growth, and because the neoplastic growth does not obey the laws of tissue growth, it often grows at the expense of other normal tissues (Fig. 7-1). In almost every case, the neoplastic cells arise from the undifferentiated reserve cells we discussed previously. In permanent tissues, the neoplasm may arise from embryologically entrapped reserve cells. The neoplastic cells may differentiate and acquire the function and form of the tissues from which they originate. As an example, a thyroid gland neoplasm may look like thyroid gland, and may make thyroxin. On the other hand, some neoplastic cells may show other characteristics of genetic mutation or repressor blockade, and may therefore fail to mature or function. They might even function in an aberrant fashion. Remember that the genetic focus of cell division is influenced by environmental substances. It is possible that the genetic foci of cell maturation and cell function might also be influenced by the same substances. As an example, the neoplasm of the thyroid gland might not resemble thyroid tissue or make any thyroxin at all.

For purposes of communication, a specific nomenclature is used to define and describe specific attributes of neoplastic growth. As a member of a health profession, you should acquaint yourself with this terminology. A *benign* neoplasm is a new growth that grows slowly, remains localized, and does little harm to the patient. A *malignant* neoplasm, on the other hand, is a growth that usually grows rapidly, invades and destroys tissue, spreads to distant sites, and invariably results in fatal termination if left untreated. *Cancer* is a term that denotes malignancy, regardless of the tissue of origin. A *tumor* is a swelling and may be the result of neoplasia, hyperplasia, hemorrhage, or inflammation. Remember that in our discussion of inflammation, tumor was considered one of the cardinal signs of inflammation. Nevertheless, the term tumor usually implies neoplasia and even cancer to the layman, and therefore, the term must be used cautiously.

Neoplastic growth can be named and classified according to several systems. Unfortunately, we lack a single universal system of classification; therefore, you must familiarize yourself with multiple systems and specific names. Most tumors are classified by behavior. The name of a neoplasm usually ends with the suffix -*oma*. Malignant tumors of epithelial origin are called *carcinomas,* whereas malignant tumors of connective tissue origin are designated *sarcomas*. Most neoplasms are further classified according to their tissue of origin, using the Greek designation of the tissue. Using a combination of these classifications, a benign neoplasm of fat tissue is a *lipoma,* whereas a malignant growth of the same tissue is a *liposarcoma*. Likewise, a benign neoplasm of the thyroid gland is termed a thyroid *adenoma,* and a malignant thyroid neoplasm is termed a thyroid *adenocarcinoma*. You notice the prefix *adeno-* has been inserted into our nomenclature. Many neoplasms are further classified according to their gross or microscopic appearance. An epithelial neoplasm that appears microscopically as glandular tissue is usually designated with the prefix adeno-; hence the designations such as pancreatic adenoma or pancreatic adenocarcinoma. Some tissues are even further subclassified according to their microscopic appearance. For example, follicular thyroid adenocarcinoma appears as microscopic follicles and is different from papillary thyroid adenocarcinoma. Other neoplasms are classified or subclassified according to their clinical appearance. This gives terminology such as *squamous papilloma,* for a fingerlike (papilla) benign neoplasm of squamous (scaley) epithelium, and *verrucous carcinoma,* for a warty (verruca) cancer of squamous epithelium.

To complicate things further, the system just discussed is not used in all cases. There are a number of special classifications and exceptions. Some neoplasms are classified by the name of the physician or patient who first recognized the disease. Therefore, terms (eponyms) like Hodgkin's disease, Ewing's sarcoma, and Pindborg tumor denote specific tumors and make no attempt at systematic classification. These terms and their meanings must be memorized. In addition, other terminology breaks the laws of nomenclature previously described. Such neoplasms as lymphomas, hepatomas, myelomas, and melanomas are deadly malignant and should not be considered benign—even though terms like carcinoma and sarcoma are not used.

Why do we bother with classification and subclassification of neoplasms? The treatment and prognosis of the neoplasm is often contingent on the specific qualities of the tumor as designated in the name, and numerous health personnel (hygienists, dentists, pathologists, physicians) must diagnose, treat, and react to the disease. You should examine and familiarize yourself with the nomenclature of common neoplasms (Table 7-1).

PROPERTIES OF BENIGN AND MALIGNANT NEOPLASMS

Malignant neoplastic cells are dissimilar to normal cells by virtue of their increased rate of cellular growth and their aberrant social behavior. As previously mentioned, the cellular DNA of a neoplastic cell is either derepressed, stimulated, or mutated. Therefore, both growth rate and cell maturation are affected. Because of either derepression or mutation, these cells may acquire the ability to grow uncontrollably, become mobile, physically or chemically destroy neighboring cells, travel and establish themselves at remote sites (metastasis), favorably compete with normal cells for nutrients and oxygen, survive in an environment where normal cells cannot live, and secrete chemicals and hormones that their normal analog cells are unable to produce (see box on page 94). These malignant cells have a different appearance, structure, and antigenicity than their normal cell counterparts. These differences allow both the clinician and the pathologist to recognize them diagnostically. These differences will be discussed later. The aberrant social behavior of cancer cells might be analogous to your neighbor's behavior after acquiring a motorcycle. As long as the neighbor is quiet, does not disturb your property, and controls his friends, there is no problem—even if a number of other cyclists congregate on the neighbor's property. But if the number of cyclists next door begins to uncontrollably multiply, if they begin to drive through your flower gardens, if they make noise at 3 AM, if they break your car windows, burn your house, and beat up your sister—then their social behavior becomes unacceptable and even life threatening. Such is the behavior of cancer cells. A group of cyclists next door may be an irritating but benign condition, but aberrant (invasive) cyclists manifest very malignant tendencies. Upon crowding, this gang may travel to another neighborhood or community and threaten its inhabitants. Malignant cells may acquire any one or all of these characteristics, and the threat of disaster is dependent on the number and intensity of these mutations. Cancers that show all these invasive and metastatic tendencies will rapidly contribute to the demise of the host. *Invasion* denotes the ability of cancer cells to successfully infiltrate and destroy neighboring normal tissues. *Metastasis* denotes the ability of cancer cells to travel to remote sites, where they establish themselves and proliferate (Fig. 7-2).

TABLE 7-1

Nomenclature of common neoplasms

Tissue of origin	Benign	Malignant
Epithelium		
Squamous	Papilloma	Squamous cell carcinoma
Glandular	Adenoma	Adenocarcinoma
Transitional cell	Papilloma	Transitional cell carcinoma
Liver cells	—	Hepatoma*
Respiratory	Polyp	Bronchogenic carcinoma
Connective tissue		
Fibrous	Fibroma	Fibrosarcoma
Bone	Osteoma	Osteosarcoma
Cartilage	Chondroma	Chondrosarcoma
Adipose	Lipoma	Liposarcoma
Muscle		
Smooth muscle	Leiomyoma	Leiomyosarcoma
Striated muscle	Rhabdomyoma	Rhabdomyosarcoma
Endothelium		
Blood vessel	Hemangioma	Hemangiosarcoma, Kaposi's sarcoma†
Lymph vessel	Lymphangioma	Lymphangiosarcoma
Bone marrow and lymphoid tissue		
Hematopoietic	—	Myelocytic leukemia
Lymphoid	—	Lymphocytic leukemia, lymphoma,* myeloma* Hodgkin's disease†
Reticuloendothelial	—	Lymphoma,* Hodgkin's disease,† Ewing's sarcoma†
Nerve tissue		
Nerve sheath	Neurofibroma	Neurofibrosarcoma
	Neurilemoma	Neurofibrosarcoma
Melanocyte	Nevus	Melanoma*

*Notes a misnomer
†Eponym

Both metastasis and invasion are examples of aberrant cellular behavior, and either phenomenon can lead to patient destruction.

Clinical Manifestations of Benign and Malignant Neoplasms

The clinical signs and symptoms of benign and malignant neoplastic growths reflect the features of growth and social behavior we have just discussed. Since benign neoplasms show a defect in growth rate only and not in social behavior, the clinical manifestations of benignity include the following (Fig. 7-1):

1. Benign neoplasms grow more rapidly than normal tissue—therefore, an expansive tumor appears.
2. Benign neoplasms are well demarcated, encapsulated, or isolated from the

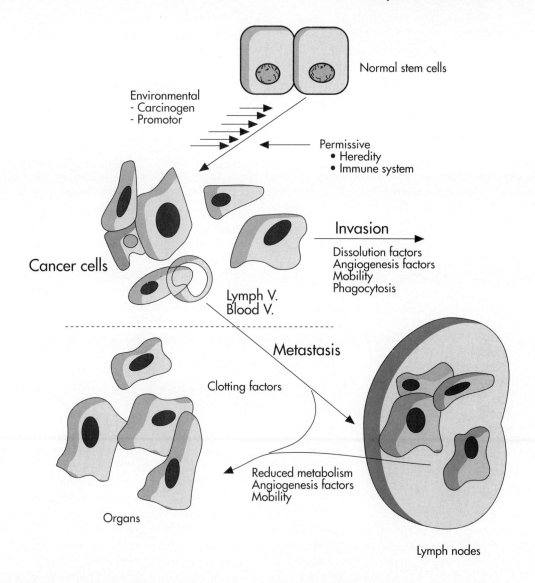

Fig. 7-2 Malignant cells are altered by environmental factors and endogenous permissiveness. The growth becomes uncontrolled, and the cells invade local tissues. Some metastasize to remote sites. Invasion and metastasis depends on acquisition of altered functions.

adjacent tissue and do not invade these tissues. Usually, this can be demonstrated clinically by movability of the tumor in relation to the normal tissue.

3. Benign tumors resemble normal tissue in color, consistency, and texture. This may be somewhat misleading when the normal tissue is mixed, because the neoplasm is usually pure and resembles only one element of the mixed tissue.

4. Benign tumors usually function as normal tissue. Because there is

---

Common behavioral characteristics of malignant cells that contribute to disease

Lose growth restraints, allowing them to overgrow normal cells
Secrete enzymes that enable them to do the following:
  Dissolve adjacent tissues
  Kill adjacent cells
  Invade other cells and spread
Undergo metabolic changes that allow them to do the following:
  Survive in poor environments
  Steal materials from adjacent normal cells
  Live for very long periods
Acquire new antigens that make it easy for the immune system to recognize and attack
Secrete angiogenesis factors that stimulate formation of a sustaining blood supply
Acquire new (embryonic) features allowing spread and metastasis:
  Mobility
  Phagocytosis
  Growth factors
  Anticoagulation and procoagulation
Undergo uncontrolled mitosis, division of cells
Lose function and ability to mature

---

excessive or uncontrolled cellular growth, this may lead to hyperfunction. For instance, our thyroid adenoma may cause the patient to exhibit a hyperthyroid state and to be clinically ill because of the neoplastic growth.

5. Benign neoplasms can sometimes cause damage or be life threatening because of physical bulk. If the tumor bulk occludes an airway, lumen, or blood vessel or compresses adjacent structures in an enclosed space (such as the cranium), it can cause obstructive disease or pressure necrosis of adjacent normal tissues.

Malignant neoplasms usually grow at a more rapid rate than benign tumors and therefore can cause exaggerated obstructive or pressure problems. The growth rate of malignant tumors is extremely variable and often unpredictable. Some malignancies grow at an extremely rapid rate, whereas others take years to develop, invade, or metastasize. The tumor classification, clinical appearance, microscopic appearance, and tumor site allow medical personnel the opportunity to predict growth rate and deleterious effects that will be caused by a malignancy. Such predictions are only educated guesses based on previous experience.

Malignant tumors exhibit other clinical features besides rapid growth that reflect the aberrant social behavior of the cells. These features include the following (Fig. 7-2):

1. Tissue fixation results because the malignant cells invade between and among adjacent tissues. The malignant tumor frequently is "fixed" to the normal tissue, meaning that it cannot be easily demarcated from or moved away from the adjacent tissue.

2. Malignant tumors cause necrosis, destruction, and ulceration of adjacent tissues, resulting from cellular invasion and the destructive influences of malignant cells. Such destruction causes dysfunction or hemorrhage of normal tissue. For example, a small malignant tumor in the brain stem might destroy the respiratory center and cause fatal respiratory failure.

3. Malignant neoplasms frequently do not resemble normal tissues clinically—at least not to the extent that benign tissues do. Since malignant tumors can acquire functional features different from those of normal tissues, they likewise acquire dissimilar morphologic features. Some very immature malignancies may not resemble the tissue of origin at all, whereas other, more mature tumors may look very much like benign growths or normal tissues.

4. Malignant neoplasms frequently lose the ability to function as normal tissues. Because these cells have altered function, they have very likely lost their ability to function normally. Hypofunction of an organ or tissue may signal malignancy. Occasionally, malignant cells will function normally or excessively; therefore, hyperfunction of organs may also signal malignancy.
5. Malignant neoplasms often metastasize. This process allows for dissemination of cells to remote tissues. The metastatic cells establish themselves and perform their aberrant acts. An adenocarcinoma of the colon might metastasize to the liver and cause death from liver failure. Routes of metastasis are somewhat predictable and will be discussed later.
6. Malignant tumors, if left untreated, will ultimately lead to death of the host. When treated, malignant neoplasms frequently recur, either because the poor demarcation of the lesion did not allow for total discovery and eradication, or because cancer cells metastasized to noncontiguous sites.

Malignant tumors seldom exhibit all of the above clinical characteristics. They may exhibit only a few characteristics. For example, a lesion should be considered malignant if it is expansile and movable, closely resembles the normal tissue morphologically and functionally, and does not cause signs or symptoms of necrosis, ulceration, or host dysfunction at the primary site, but does metastasize. On the other hand, some malignancies never metastasize, but nevertheless cause death secondary to local tissue invasion and destruction. For a comparison of clinical characteristics of benign and malignant neoplasms, see Table 7-2.

Histopathologic Changes of Malignant Tissues

The alteration of functional, morphologic, and antigenic features of malignant cells from

TABLE 7-2

Clinical characteristics of neoplasms

	Benign	Malignant
Rate of growth	Slow (years)	Rapid (months)
Demarcation	Encapsulated	Nonencapsulated
Movability	Freely movable	Fixed
Growth in bone	Expansile	Perforating
Surface changes	Stretched	Ulcerated
Neural changes	None	Pain, paralysis
Area(s) of growth	Localized	Metastatic
Color	Normal	Changed
Effects in host	None or hyperfunction	Hypofunction, cachexia

those of benign neoplasms and normal cells can be diagnosed by recognition of microscopic, radiographic, biochemical, immunologic, or other specific changes. Tests for these changes are usually performed under special conditions. The most common test used is biopsy—where the lesion or a portion of the lesion is removed and examined microscopically. Microscopic changes such as increased nuclear DNA (hyperchromatism), increased and abnormal mitotic activity, loss of morphologic evidence of maturation (anaplasia), invasion of neoplastic cells into adjacent tissues, necrosis, variations in cell and nuclear size (pleomorphism) and shape, and evidence of metastasis are all morphologic features of the malignant behavior we have previously described. Again, all these features usually do not occur at once, and the pathologist must make a diagnosis based on an ability to recognize these features gained from experience and from training and reading the literature. Because problems in diagnosis exist, a smart diagnostician uses multiple modes of diagnosis such as clinical findings, radiographic features, lesion history, histopathology, and special tests to arrive at the best diagnosis. Histopathology and special tests also give the pathologist and clinician a rough idea of the expected behavior of a malignancy, since the features they reveal reflect functional changes.

If your neighbor and his motorcycle-riding friends are unshaven and unhygienic, wear Nazi helmets and old dirty clothes, and smell of alcohol and tobacco, you can predict rather accurately that there is trouble ahead for you (a poor prognosis). Likewise, an ulcerated, anaplastic, invasive, abnormally mitotic, pleomorphic tumor probably also has a poor prognosis. Again, this is only a generalization, and exceptions exist. Howard Hughes dressed like a bum, but he was a millionaire.

Significance of Clinical and Histopathologic Changes

Prognosis involves predicting the outcome of a specific lesion. The treatment is often dependent on the prognosis. Malignant tumor prognosis is based on tumor size, tissue of origin, evidence of metastasis, histopathologic features, and specific classification of the malignancy. For example, the chance for survival of early Hodgkin's disease that is manifest as a small isolated lesion exceeds 90%, whereas the chance of surviving a tumor that is the same histopathologically but that is very large and has metastasized is less than 50%. In comparison, an anaplastic carcinoma of a lung causes death in 95% of all patients—whereas a very large basal cell carcinoma of skin causes a mortality rate lower than 5%. The prognosis in the case of benign neoplasia is usually excellent, unless the neoplasia involves an area easily obstructed or compressed, or an organ (such as the brain) characterized by vital areas that do not allow for removal of the tumor mass.

ETIOLOGY OF NEOPLASIA

The etiology of cancer is only partially understood, even after billions of dollars have been spent on research and study. We know of numerous specific agents, most of which are environmental, that cause specific cancers.

These agents are called carcinogens (carcino: cancer; genesis: formation). Chemicals, ionizing radiation, viruses, heredity, immune incompetence, hormones, aging changes, and nutritional disturbances all cause or contribute to cancer. These agents may act individually, in combination with other carcinogens (cocarcinogens), or in combination with other agents that do not in themselves cause cancer (promoters), but that help the carcinogens to mutate or derepress cells. In addition, many carcinogens are altered by normal body reactions to become different chemical forms that are more carcinogenic (ultimate carcinogens). Tracing the specific cause of cancer can be extremely complicated. Knowledge of human carcinogenesis is based primarily on data collected from population comparison studies and from production of the cancer in animals after treating them with the suspected carcinogen. It has often been stated that we live in a "sea of carcinogens" and that we eat, drink, breathe, and bathe in cancer-forming agents. It is known that certain conditions are necessary in order for cancers to form. These conditions are (1) exposure to an adequate concentration of carcinogen, (2) susceptible host or permissive host tissue, and (3) a significant period of exposure time for induction, mutation, and growth of the tumor. All these conditions must exist for cancer to form; however, there are degrees of variation depending on the carcinogen. For example, Carcinogen A might have a very long induction period, whereas Carcinogen B might induce cancer after a short period. In like fashion, Carcinogen A might induce cancer in 99% of the general population exposed for a significant period, whereas Carcinogen B might induce cancer in only one in ten thousand exposed for a similar time period.

Chemicals

Historically, the first carcinogens to be recognized were chemicals. Two hundred years ago, Sir Percivall Pott (1713-1788) noticed an association between soot and scrotal cancer in the chimney sweeps of England. Polycyclic hydrocarbons have since been isolated from coal tar, soot, and cigarette smoke, and their carcinogenic nature has been proven in laboratory animals. The surgeon general warns that smoking may cause cancer. Indeed, epidemiologic studies statistically implicate smoking in several types of cancer of the lung, mouth, larynx, esophagus, and lip.

Numerous other chemicals have been implicated statistically in human cancers. Nitrates, nitrites, and nitrosamines—all components of or additives to foods—have been implicated in cancers of the intestines. For example, aflatoxin, a product of peanut mold, is a potent carcinogen. Dye substances and vinyl chloride, chemicals used respectively in the textile and plastics industries, are known carcinogens. At last count, there were more than 400 chemicals listed as carcinogens, and the count grows daily. Components of insecticides, saccharine, and food dye have all been reported and implicated as specific carcinogens or promoters. Asbestos—a common particulate substance used in automobile brakes, fire-protective equipment, and insulation—is a known carcinogen that causes a peculiar cancer of the lungs called mesothelioma.

Viruses

Oncogenic (onco: cancer; genic: forming) viruses have been discovered and documented in animal cancers and have been implicated in human neoplasia. As discussed in the chapter on infection, both DNA and RNA viruses can contribute viral DNA that combines with host cell DNA. In some cells, specific viruses either combine or partially combine their DNA with the host DNA, thus mutating the cell. In other cases, viruses somehow derepress host cell genetic information (DNA). Either way, neoplastic genetic information (oncogenes) is now exposed and expressed. Animal sarcomas, leukemias, and breast carcinomas have been induced by

transmission of viruses in chickens, mice, and monkeys. In humans, the oncogenic potential of viruses is less clear; however, epidemiologic studies indicate that certain papilloma viruses can contribute to specific types of human cancer. The Epstein-Barr virus is a type of herpes virus that has a very high incidence in human Burkitt's tumor—a jaw cancer—and in nasopharyngeal carcinoma. Human papilloma virus is demonstrable in high levels in female patients with cervical cancer, as well as in male patients with condyloma (warts) of the penis. The implicated virus is transferred by sexual activity. Indeed, cervical cancer is practically unknown in women of little sexual experience (such as nuns) and of highest incidence in women with frequent multipartner experience (such as prostitutes). The incidence of demonstrable herpes virus antibodies in cervical cancer patients is also well documented. Several studies have reported an increased cervical cancer rate among second wives of husbands whose previous wives had cervical cancer. It can be postulated that cocarcinogenic viruses (human papilloma virus, herpes) might be transferred venereally. The recent excitement about interferon—an antiviral cellular protein—as an anticancer agent attests to the importance that investigators and clinicians attribute to viruses as oncogenic agents. Some virologists speculate that all cancers are caused by viruses (albeit hidden ones), and that other carcinogens simply allow host cells to become more permissive for viral mutation.

Radiation

Radiation injury to cells can cause DNA splitting, mutation, and recombination. Cancer incidence was shown to be markedly increased among individuals, including dental personnel, who worked with diagnostic and therapeutic radiation and did not take adequate precautions. The high rate of skin cancer among early dental personnel who held radiographs during patient exposure is well documented. The high incidence of lung cancer in uranium miners, of thyroid cancer in patients irradiated about the neck, and of leukemia in individuals exposed to nuclear explosion all attest to the carcinogenic effects of radiation. Numerous experiments in carcinogenesis in laboratory animals have proven this fact. In humans, actinic radiation received from chronic exposure to the sun has been implicated as an etiologic factor in skin cancers (squamous cell carcinoma, basal cell carcinoma, some types of melanoma) and lip cancer. Individuals with light complexion have less protection from actinic rays and a much increased risk of skin cancer as compared to individuals with dark complexion. Melanin, the primary skin pigment, absorbs actinic rays before they can alter basal (reserve) skin cells. Likewise, the incidence of skin cancer in a sunbelt area like Florida is 5 to 10 times greater than the incidence in a northern state like Michigan.

Other Environmental Factors

Additional factors affect cancer incidence, either as carcinogens or as promoters. Chronic physical injury, burns, certain nutritional deficiency states, and socioeconomic status all seem to cause or contribute to cancer incidence, although their direct or indirect role has not been precisely established.

Genetic Predisposition

Up until now, we have mentioned only exogenous or environmental agents and noted a number of them that cause or contribute to cancer. It is amazing that we do not all develop cancer when we consider the numerous carcinogens encountered daily. The fact that only about 25% of the population develops cancer indicates that there might be certain internal mechanisms that either afford protection to humans, or make them susceptible. One of these internal mechanisms may be genetic susceptibility or resistance. There are several

rare cancer syndromes that are passed down in families with an autosomal dominant pattern—no matter what the environment. For example, multiple endocrine neoplasia syndrome is a hereditary disease that causes thyroid and adrenal cancers, as well as benign tumors of the oral mucosa. In addition, genetic states seem to increase susceptibility to certain cancers. In adenocarcinoma of the breast, some familial tendencies exist, with the sibling of a breast cancer patient having tenfold the chance of the average woman of developing breast cancer. Incidentally, some evidence indicates that viruses may also have a role in breast adenocarcinoma. It is tempting to speculate, then, that the genetic defect might allow for a permissive state that makes the cell susceptible to oncogenic viral infection. It might further be theorized that a certain genetic cellular constitution might prohibit chemical carcinogen penetration, viral infection, hormonal stimulation, or radiation damage necessary for cell mutation; therefore, the individual affected would not be cancer prone.

Hormonal Factors

Hormones also seem to play a role in carcinogenesis, perhaps as promoters or permissive agents. Certain breast cancers demonstrate hormonal receptors to estrogens and are stimulated by these hormones. Tumor growth slows considerably, but does not stop, when the estrogen levels are reduced. Some prostate cancers are similarly excited by testosterone. Tumor growth is reduced considerably by either orchiectomy or testosterone antagonist therapy, or both. Although hormones have not in themselves been shown to cause cancer, evidence of the association of diethylstilbestrol (DES), an estrogen precursor taken by pregnant women, to the striking incidence of vaginal cancer in the resultant female offspring again emphasizes the linkage of hormones and cancer.

Immune System Factors

There is an increased incidence of cancer in patients with immune system problems. It has been proven that most cancer cells have an altered antigenicity, probably due to oncogene expression. These new tumor antigens should be recognized by the immune system as foreign, and the growing tumor should then be rejected in the same manner as a transplant. Specific lymphocytes recognize the neoplastic cells and initiate rejection, by way of the cell-mediated or humoral responses we covered in our discussion of the immune reaction in Chapter 4. It has been proposed that such immunologic response constantly monitors for antigenic tumor cells, and destroys these cells as they form. Again, any permissive situation caused by genetic defects, aging, drugs, viral infection, or chronic immune overload will allow tumor cells to sneak by this surveillance mechanism and prosper. Likewise, tumor cells with unrecognizable or hidden antigens will also elude such defense mechanisms. Evidence such as the increase in cancer incidence in immune suppressed transplant patients, AIDS patients, and genetic immune deficient patients lends some credence to this theory. The high incidence of cancers in the population, however, indicates that if such a surveillance system exists, it is not very effective. Research continues on the role of immune surveillance and the use of immune stimulation as a cancer-preventing or therapeutic measure.

Nutritional Factors

Nutritional deficiencies and excesses have been associated with carcinogenesis. It is not certain whether nutritional changes cause cancer, promote cancer, or result from hidden cancer. It is probable that all three situations occur. For example, obese individuals have a higher cancer rate than nonobese people. Populations with low-fiber diets have a higher colon cancer rate than do comparable populations with high-fiber diets. Certain patients with iron deficiency anemias (such as Plummer-Vinson syndrome) have a marked predisposition to oral and esophageal cancer. Other rather controversial reports have linked increased cancer incidence to deficiencies in vitamin C, vitamin A, or any of numerous trace elements. Still more reports suggest that minimal nutritional standards are inadequate for cancer protection and advocate high-dosage nutritional preventive measures.

Aging

The incidence of cancer increases dramatically with aging; however, all cancers do not occur in senior citizens or adults. Many leukemias and sarcomas are far more common in children than in adults. Other tumors show peak incidence in young adults. The majority of cancers, however, occur in adult and elderly individuals. This incidence leads one to speculate on the role of long-term exposure to carcinogens as a requisite for some cancers. The highest percentage of cancers occurs in the over-70 age group, even though the peak incidence of known environmentally induced cancers occurs at a somewhat earlier age. An extremely high incidence of prostate cancer has been noted at autopsy in men over 70 years of age, even though no clinical signs or symptoms of prostate cancer were present at the time of death.

PATHOGENESIS OF NEOPLASIA

Neoplastic disease is not a single disease, but rather a group of diseases with the common denominator of new uncontrolled cell growth. Neoplasia is caused by numerous agents, individually or in concert with others. Several mechanisms have been proposed to explain the process of cell change that results in neoplastic growth and cancerous behavior. The *mutation theory* is based on the evidence of direct cellular DNA mutations caused by a single carcinogen, multiple hits with a carcinogen, or exposure to multiple carcinogens. Certain carcinogens can mutate cultured bacteria directly and are therefore hypothesized to mutate human cells in similar fashion. *In vitro* mutation tests are considered diagnostic for carcinogenicity when used to test suspect agents. The hereditary nature of cancers resulting from rare mutations also serves as a basis of proof for the mutation theory.

The *derepression theory* is based on evidence that genetic information (oncogenes) is uncovered and activated by a carcinogen or series of carcinogenic events. This theory best explains the ability of cancer cells to function in aberrant ways. Although the aberrant social behavior of cancer cells is unusual for a specific cell from a particular tissue, that same behavior may be normal for a different tissue that has expressed the genetic information during maturation. An individual does not behave the same way in church as he or she does at a football game. An individual certainly has the capability to cheer, shout, jump, and applaud; however, this capability is suppressed in church. Likewise, a highly malignant lung cancer may produce parathormone—certainly abnormal behavior for the lung—by activation of resident genetic material that codes for this hormone. On the other hand, cells of the parathyroid gland produce this hormone "normally" due to activation of the same genetic material. Some experiments suggest that even viruses may derepress genetic material, rather than mutate the cellular DNA.

Once the cell is either mutated, derepressed, or both, carcinogens and/or promoters may play a further significant role in tumor growth and survival. Neoplastic cells may be selected for growth by certain stimulants. For example, promoters such as hormones, growth factors, chronic trauma, and certain chemicals that cause tissue hyperplasia are known to stimulate cell division. Since the only cells that can be mutated or derepressed

are cells that are dividing, agents that cause cell division create a fertile soil for cell mutation and derepression. If a tissue typically mutates at a rate of one in a million dividing cells, and cell division occurs only twice a day, there is little chance of that tissue ever mutating. If, however, that same tissue is stimulated (promoted) by a hormone to divide at a new rate of 1 million divisions per day, there is a chance that the tissue will mutate today.

Several experiments have shown that once a cell has been mutated or derepressed, it may become resistant to the toxic effects of certain carcinogens or promoters. This creates a mechanism for cancer cell selection. Let us suppose that a cell has spontaneously been derepressed and that genetic information also has been uncovered that makes this cell more resistant to Carcinogen B—a usual toxin for this tissue. Exposure to Carcinogen B will now allow for preferential growth of all derepressed cells by destroying all other, normal cells and eliminating the competition. This may explain why many carcinogens are also frequently cellular toxins or injurious agents to normal cells (such as radiation).

Lastly, we must reemphasize the role of immune surveillance in carcinogenesis. Once cancer cells are mutated, derepressed, or selected, they may express potent transplantation types of antigens and should be rejected. Probably some cancer mutation occurs spontaneously in almost everyone. Clinical cancer, then, might occur when the immune system is genetically insufficient, depressed by carcinogens or promoters, or overwhelmed by rapid tumor growth. Some evidence suggests that certain cancers can in themselves contribute to suppression of the immune system—the ultimate in self-serving aberrant behavior.

With uncommon exception, carcinogenesis appears to be multifactorial—that is, cancer development requires the influence of numerous cocarcinogens and promoters. A first event might render a cell permissive; a second agent would allow access to the carcinogen, activation of the carcinogen, and mutation or derepression; a third event might allow for cell selection; and a fourth might produce immune incompetence. In fact, each event may be part of a series or sequence of events involving multiple carcinogens and promoters. This multifactorial theory helps to explain the prolonged time interval between carcinogen exposure and appearance of cancer. It also may explain individual variability in cancer formation. Not all heavy smokers get lung cancer; in fact, the majority of them do not get it. Perhaps this is because of the absence of other agents or events necessary for the multifactorial formation.

COURSE OF MALIGNANCY

Again, malignant tumors in general act in a socially aggressive manner. This behavior is usually predictable when based on tumor histogenesis, tumor type, degree of cellular maturation or anaplasia, and other measurable factors that have been reported as predictive. Therefore, we will discuss the course of malignancies in such general terms. Malignant tumors usually metastasize: they spread to remote noncontiguous sites. Carcinomas usually metastasize by way of the lymphatic drainage system, and metastatic tumor cells are therefore initially trapped in lymph nodes. Remember, malignant cells often have the capacity to grow in a foreign environment such as a lymph node; therefore, tumor growth continues at that remote site. Sarcomas, in general, metastasize by way of bloodstream rather than lymphatics. Therefore, a sarcoma can be expected to initially metastasize to the tissue or organ in the direct line of venous drainage. For example, a sarcoma of the abdomen might metastasize to the liver, and a sarcoma of the leg might metastasize to the lungs. In addition, sarcomas and carcinomas can metastasize through cavities and tissue spaces. A cancer of the peritoneum could metastasize to another area of the peritoneum

by dropping off of cells into the cavity, whereas a tumor of the cerebellum might spread to the spinal cord by dropping cells into the cerebrospinal fluid. Occasionally, manipulation or surgical incision will spread or produce tumor metastasis, seeding cells into adjacent tissues or along the surgical site.

Cancer leads to patient deterioration in a number of ways. Malignant tumor cells may destroy the organ of origin and metastasize to and destroy remote organs, thereby causing patient illness or death through functional organ failure. An adenocarcinoma of the breast that metastasizes to the respiratory center of the medulla can cause death from respiratory failure, whereas a primary pituitary cancer can destroy the gland, and lead to severe endocrine deficiency and resultant death.

Malignant tumor cells can erode blood vessels or obstruct blood vessels, leading to hemorrhage in the former situation, and to inadequate blood supply to the organ or tissue in the latter instance. Malignant tumors of the large intestine often erode blood vessels, produce hemorrhage, and render the patient anemic. Thus, the clinical signs and symptoms of anemia frequently may be the features presented by this cancer. In addition, whole areas of the liver or brain can become necrotic because a malignant tumor has obstructed the arterial blood supply (causing infarction) to that tissue. Some malignancies obstruct a viscus or lumen and thus impede air exchange, fluid secretion, or gastrointestinal transport. For example, oral cancers frequently cause patient demise from direct obstruction of both the esophagus and the pharynx/larynx. A pancreas cancer that obstructs the common bile duct will cause the patient to become jaundiced.

Because malignant tumors contribute to such obstructive consequences and because they often may directly or indirectly interfere with the inflammatory-immune response, they frequently contribute to associated secondary infection of the diseased organ. If the tracheobronchial tree is obstructed, collapsed, or destroyed by malignant growth, the normal clearance of bacteria will be altered and pneumonia will result from entrapped pathogenic organisms. This pneumonia may cause patient death. *Cachexia* is a rather common manifestation of advanced cancer. The cancer patient appears weak and wasted, and rapid weight loss is recorded. This cachexia is probably the result of starvation, tumor obstruction, intestinal impairment, immune impairment and resultant infection, chronic hemorrhage and anemia, and organ malfunction. Perhaps the cachexia is also a sequela of major surgery, irradiation, and chemotherapy, which destroys or injures normal tissues as well as tumor cells.

DIAGNOSIS OF MALIGNANCY

Cancer is diagnosed based on the previously described aberrant social behavior as manifested in distinctive clinical, microscopic, biochemical, immunologic, and radiographic changes. Clinical features (signs and symptoms) are usually the first and most easily detected changes. These may be manifest as apparent tumor growth, color changes, ulcerations, organ dysfunction, hemorrhage, or changes detectable by radiography. Malignant tumors tend to grow rapidly and are usually poorly demarcated from adjacent tissue. Surface cancers tend to ulcerate, are attached (fixed) to adjacent tissue, and feel firm (indurated) to palpation. Intrabony malignancies tend to grow rapidly, perforate rather than expand bony plates, and cause associated changes such as pain, anesthesia (nerve destruction), or marrow destruction. These changes are frequently not specific and can be the result of many other nonneoplastic or benign conditions. Therefore, diagnostic tests are usually necessary. The diagnostic techniques include biopsy. Biopsy, as we previously noted, is the removal of a lesion or portion of a lesion for microscopic interpreta-

tion. We have already noted the histopathologic changes that occur in cancer. Biopsy helps the pathologist determine the tissue of origin of the cancer, and it aids in forming the prognosis based on certain histopathologic criteria. Radiographs are important tests that can help determine location and size, delineate margins, and assess spread of a cancer. Often surgery will also serve to determine size, margins, and spread of the tumor. Surgical staging systems have been devised based on the features we have described, and these help guide prognosis and treatment. For example, an oral cancer of surgical stage I—as determined by histologic, surgical, and radiographic techniques—has a prognosis that is quite good. On the other hand, a stage IV lesion is of tremendous size or has widespread metastasis, or both. The prognosis for such a tumor is usually quite grave. Additional tumor- or tissue-specific techniques such as biochemical, immunologic, cytologic and ultrastructural analysis are quite helpful in diagnosing certain specific cancers.

TREATMENT OF MALIGNANCY

Once a cancer is diagnosed, the treatment is dictated by the combination of its surgical stage, the histopathologic type, the area or areas of involvement, and complicating aspects of health status. The most common treatment for cancer is surgical removal. The primary growth and all metastases must be completely removed to render a cure. Naturally, the smaller and more localized the cancer, the better the chance of achieving a cure. Therefore, early detection is of paramount importance. Surgery can be quite mutilating, and cannot be done in certain vital tissues (such as the brainstem). The surgery itself can cause severe disease; therefore, surgery is not always the appropriate therapy. Radiation therapy is either an alternative or an adjunct to surgery. High-dosage irradiation kills dividing cells (cancer cells, and normal cells that are dividing). Since many cancers are rapidly dividing tissues, serial doses of radiation will destroy the whole tumor or portions of the tumor—as well as some normal cells. This procedure is usually less mutilating and often more acceptable than cancer surgery. However, radiation therapy is less effective in destroying tumor cells, is not effective at all with some specific tumors, and has a total dosage limitation. In addition, many local and systemic side effects such as hair loss, nausea, mucositis, bone marrow depression, and bone destruction can occur. It is not unusual for radiation and surgery to be used in combination. Large tumors may be shrunken with radiation to a size that is manageable for surgery. Alternatively, the bulk of the tumor can be surgically removed, and then radiation therapy may be used to eliminate any remaining viable tumor cells.

Cancer chemotherapy is based on a principle similar to that of radiation—that is, that cancer cells are actively dividing and growing. Most chemotherapeutic drugs like nitrogen mustard or cisplatin either arrest and inhibit cell division or poison cell biochemical mechanisms necessary for cell growth and activity (act as antimetabolites). They therefore inhibit cancer cell growth and spread, and kill many of the existing cells. In the process, these drugs also inhibit growth and division of normal cells and tissues, especially labile tissues. Side effects include loss of hair, nausea and vomiting, kidney damage, and decreased number of blood cells (leukopenia, anemia, thrombocytopenia). Some chemotherapeutic drugs destroy specific tissues (for example, adriamycin destroys cardiac muscle) and can be life threatening. Often these drugs are used in combination so that combined modes of tumor destruction can be exploited. With specific exceptions, chemotherapeutic drugs do not provide a cure for malignancy, since most cancers seem to have mutant cells

that are resistant to the effects of the drugs and that are, in effect, selected by use of these drugs. Chemotherapy, then, is seldom used as a primary cancer treatment, but is better considered a palliative treatment for large or inoperable cancers and widespread tumors. Most recently, chemotherapy has become more promising as a prophylactic agent used to destroy hidden primary or metastatic cancer cells in patients with early-stage, operable cancer.

Many other types of cancer therapy are currently being researched. These modalities include immune stimulation with immune rejection of cancers, specific cytotoxic chemicals or radioactive substances that can attack and destroy tumor cells, antiviral drugs, and new surgical techniques. More importantly, new techniques in identification of high-risk populations, in prevention, and in early detection of cancers give hope that the disease might someday be minimized. Recent research in genome mapping has identified specific oncogenes that lead to cancer susceptibility or directly cause some cancers. These findings may allow identification of individuals who are susceptible for certain types of cancer. Either prophylactic avoidance of carcinogenic and promoting factors, or genetic engineering might help prevent cancer growth in such individuals.

Case Studies

Case 1

K. P. is a 53-year-old woman who developed a lump in the upper outer quadrant of her left breast. The lump was present for at least 3 months, and the skin on the surface was puckered. The lump was fixed to the breast tissues and slightly painful. She gave her physician a history of breast cancer in her mother, maternal aunt, and one of her younger sisters. Her mammogram was highly indicative of malignancy. Biopsy and mastectomy revealed a moderately differentiated adenocarcinoma, and surgery of the axillary nodes revealed cancer in two nodes at level 1. She developed mouth ulcers secondary to her chemotherapy but otherwise did well. Four years later she developed metastatic adenocarcinoma of the lungs and spine. Despite further chemotherapy, K. P. died 8 months later of pneumonia and associated metastatic disease of the lungs.

Case 2

R. S. is a 71-year-old man who worked in the textile industry for 30 years. He developed blood in his urine. Biopsy revealed transitional cell carcinoma of the urinary bladder in surgical stage II. The tumor and a smaller second carcinoma were excised. On follow-up examination 1 year later, four more small malignancies of the bladder were revealed. R. S. received a course of chemotherapy into his bladder. Four years after surgery, he has been told he is free of cancer.

Case 3

A. C. is a 53-year-old man who noticed an ulcer of his lower lip that did not heal. He went to his dentist with a history of pipe smoking for 30 years and exposure to the sun as a roofer. He was of fair complexion and had red hair. Biopsy revealed squamous cell carcinoma, stage I. There was no clinical evidence of lymph node swelling in the submental, submandibular, or cervical area. A wedge-shaped excision of the tumor was made, followed by plastic surgery. He was advised to discontinue his smoking and to protect his lips and face with sunscreen. He is tumor free 5 years after diagnosis.

Case 4

M. A. is a 29-year-old black woman who began to lose weight without dieting. She complained of insomnia and that she kept dropping objects. Physical examination revealed a discrete 2 cm movable lump of her right thyroid gland. Her T_4 levels were elevated. An excisional biopsy resulted in diagnosis of follicular adenoma of the thyroid. Symptoms persisted following surgery, and T_4 levels remained high. A diagnosis of thyroid hyperplasia was followed by surgical removal of the thyroid. M. A. is symptom free 2 years later and is taking thyroid-replacement medication.

Case 1

1. Do you think a family history is important in prevention of breast cancer?
2. What is significant about the lump being "fixed" to the adjacent tissue?
3. Why was surgery performed on the axillary lymph nodes?
4. Does the presence of cancer in the lymph nodes mean the tumor has spread to other sites as well?
5. Why did K. P. develop pneumonia?

Case 2

1. Do certain environmental conditions cause predisposition to some cancers? Name several examples.
2. Explain the term transitional cell carcinoma.
3. Explain the significance of a stage II lesion compared to a stage I lesion. How is this related to size, invasion, and prognosis? Is it important to know the stage of a cancer?
4. Is chemotherapy usually curative for cancer?

Case 3

1. Why is A. C. susceptible to development of lip cancer?
2. Does stage I cancer usually have a good or bad prognosis?
3. What carcinogens and promoters are important in this case?

Case 4

1. Explain the symptoms of an adenoma.
2. Is this tumor malignant?
3. How could a hyperplasia be confused with a benign neoplasm? Could they exist together?
4. Why is she taking thyroid medication?

SUMMARY

- Neoplastic growth is new uncontrolled growth where there is either derepression of normal cellular growth constraints or stimulus of genetic growth factors.

- The stimulus of neoplasia may be environmental or from endogenous defects in cell division.
- Benign neoplasms are characterized by a localized uncontrolled increase in tissue growth. The tumor remains localized and may be injurious but seldom fatal in behavior.
- Malignant neoplasms are characterized by uncontrolled growth and the acquisition of other behavioral characteristics of tumor cells that facilitate invasion and metastasis of cells. This often has fatal consequences.
- A standard nomenclature system can be used to communicate the origin and behavior of a neoplastic growth. Exceptions exist.
- Malignant neoplastic growth can be caused by chemicals, viruses, radiation, inherent genetic factors, and genetic mutations.
- Factors such as hormones, chronic trauma, immune deficiency, nutritional deficiency, and genetic susceptibility can promote cancer formation by carcinogens.
- In many instances, cancer etiology is dependent on multiple hits by carcinogens and the interaction of multiple carcinogens and promoters.
- The pathogenesis of malignancy is based on direct cellular mutation into oncogenes, activation or stimulation of oncogenes, depression of repressor genes, or a combination of these events.
- Individual malignant tumors tend to behave and grow in a somewhat predictable manner. Therefore, knowledge of tumor type, size, and location is important in predicting malignant behavior and forming a prognosis.
- Malignant tumors can be fatal because of direct destruction of tissues, or because of associated hemorrhage, obstruction, infection, immune deficiency, or cachexia.
- The diagnosis of malignancy is often based on an association of clinical and histopathologic data and criteria. Additional information from imaging, chemistry, histochemistry, and immune chemistry can be important.
- Treatment for cancer is usually dependent on removing all malignant cells. Treatment includes surgery, irradiation, chemotherapy, immune therapy, and other modes of killing rapidly dividing and highly metabolic cells. Combinations are frequently used, and prophylactic therapy may help prevent recurrence.

Suggested readings

1. Creech JL Jr and Johnson MN: Angiosarcoma of liver in the manufacture of polyvinyl chloride, J Occup Med 16:150, 1974.
2. Doll R and Peto R: The causes of cancer: quantitative estimates of avoidable risks of cancer in the United States today, J Natl Cancer Inst 66:1191, 1981.
3. Fidler IJ, Gersten DM, and Hart IR: The biology of cancer invasion and metastasis, Adv Cancer Res 28:149, 1978.
4. Kumar V, Cotran RS, and Robbins SL: Basic pathology, ed 5, Philadelphia, 1992, WB Saunders, pp 193-203.
5. Liotta LA: Tumor invasion and metastasis: role of the basement membrane, Am J Pathol 117:339, 1984.
6. Marshall CJ: Tumor suppressor genes, Cell 64:313, 1991.
7. Marx JL: What do oncogenes do? Science 223:673, 1984.
8. Miller JA: Carcinogenesis by chemicals: an overview, Cancer Res 30:559, 1970.
9. Roitt IM: Essential immunology, ed 7, Oxford, 1991, Blackwell Scientific Publications, pp 298-303.
10. Weinberg RA: The integration of molecular genetics into cancer management, Cancer 70:1653, 1992.
11. Wyke J: Strategies of viral oncogenesis, Nature 23:629, 1981.

8 Benign Oral Neoplasms and Premalignant Lesions

IN THIS CHAPTER

1. Oral epithelial tumors
   - Squamous papilloma
   - Verruca vulgaris
   - Keratoacanthoma
2. Oral nevi
3. Oral connective tissue tumors
   - Fibroma
   - Neurofibroma
   - Neurilemoma
   - Granular cell tumor
   - Traumatic neuroma
   - Lipoma
4. Oral premalignant conditions
   - Clinical white patch
   - Epithelial dysplasia
   - Erythroplasia
   - Carcinoma in situ
5. Case studies

After studying this chapter, you should be able to meet the following objectives and define the key terms:

- Identify the oral papilloma and verruca vulgaris clinically.
- Discuss the similarities between keratoacanthoma and lip cancer.
- List common nevi of the skin and describe their typical clinical features.
- Analyze and comment on the relationship between nevi and malignant melanomas.
- Explain the causes of oral fibromas.
- Explain the association between neurofibroma and neurofibromatosis.
- Explain the etiology and pathogenesis of the amputation neuroma.

- Develop a differential diagnosis for a clinical white patch.
- Discuss the significance of the location of a clinical white patch.
- Define epithelial dysplasia and discuss the premalignant potential of dysplasia.
- Define leukoplakia and erythroplasia.
- List the usual lesions that represent clinical erythroplasia.
- Identify the potential risk of malignancy associated with erythroplasia.

Benign oral neoplasms and premalignant lesions represent a relatively large number of oral diseases that, as a group, occur with significant frequency. Within this category are conditions that are quite common, as well as others that are very rare. The focus of this chapter is on those conditions likely to be encountered in clinical practice. The major emphasis in studying these diseases is twofold—namely, we will concentrate on (1) the relationship of the benign neoplasm or lesion to environmental etiologic factors and systemic disease and (2) the potential for transformation of some of these benign lesions into cancer.

ORAL EPITHELIAL TUMORS

Squamous Papilloma

The squamous *papilloma* is a benign neoplasm derived from the surface epithelium of the oral mucosa. It is widely considered to be the most common benign epithelial neoplasm to occur in the mouth. Recent studies of this neoplasm and similar lesions occurring in other areas of the body (such as the skin, larynx, uterine cervix) are providing increasing evidence that the papilloma is often the result of an infection with human papilloma virus (HPV). As such, the papilloma can be considered closely related to the verruca vulgaris or common wart.

The papilloma represents a slow-growing proliferation of stratified squamous epithelium arranged in fingerlike projections, usually growing from a single, narrow, stalklike structure connecting to the underlying oral mucosa. This narrow stalk form of attachment is typical of pedunculated lesions (Fig. 8-1). The fingerlike projections can be readily seen on most specimens. Often, a similarity to the appearance of a cauliflower or fern may be appreciated.

Papillomas show a wide distribution intraorally, most frequently occurring on the palate, tongue, buccal and labial mucosa, and gingiva. For reasons that are not entirely clear, papillomas are most commonly seen on the soft palate. Papillomas may be white or pink, are soft and flexible on palpation, are usually less than 2 cm in diameter, and are generally asymptomatic. Although generally solitary, papillomas on occasion may be multiple.

Treatment of a papilloma consists of local excision including the base or the connecting stalk. Attempted excision leaving a portion of the stalk in all likelihood will permit recurrence of the lesion. Confirmation of the clinical diagnosis depends on microscopic examination of the excised tissue. Oral papilloma has no potential for undergoing malignant transformation (that is, becoming a cancer).

Verruca Vulgaris

The *verruca vulgaris,* also known as the common wart, is a benign epithelial neoplasm produced by infection with certain types of HPV. The verruca vulgaris is far more common on skin than in the mouth, and it shows a predilection for occurring in children and young adults. Verruca vulgaris of the skin typically appears as a nodular or craterlike tumor, generally less than 1 cm in diameter. Common locations include the fingers, and it is not unusual for the patient to complain of local mild to moderate irritation.

Verruca vulgaris of the mouth bears a strong similarity to oral papilloma. It may be pedunculated or show a broad base of attachment to the underlying mucosa (sessile), and it is typically white with either a rough surface or obvious, well-formed fingerlike projections (Fig. 8-2). Oral verruca vulgaris

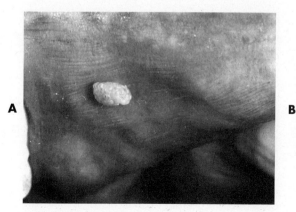
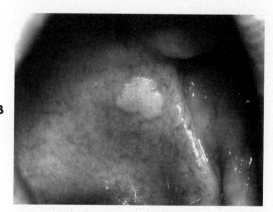

Fig. 8-1   Papilloma. **A,** Papilloma of the upper labial mucosa. **B,** Papilloma of the soft palate.

should be suspected in pediatric patients when (1) multiple white papillary oral lesions are present, and (2) evidence of cutaneous verruca vulgaris is found. This is particularly true if the patient admits to chewing warts, typically situated on the fingers. It is likely that this habit contributes to spread of the virus to the oral mucosa through self-inoculation.

Keratoacanthoma

The keratoacanthoma is a distinctive and unusual benign neoplasm of stratified squamous epithelium. Although relatively rare, its importance to our study of oral disease is based on (1) its clinical resemblance to skin cancer; (2) its predilection for occurrence on sun-exposed skin, most notably the face and lip; and (3) its microscopic resemblance to epidermoid carcinoma.

The specific etiology of keratoacanthoma is unknown; however, the predilection for occurring on sun-exposed skin strongly suggests a relationship to actinic (ultraviolet radiation) tissue damage. Predictably, the keratoacanthoma is more common in people who are constantly exposed to sunlight. The lesion is usually solitary; it generally occurs on the skin of the midface including the cheek and nose, although it sometimes also involves the forehead and ear. It is noteworthy that 8% of keratoacanthomas occur on sun-exposed portions of the lips. These cutaneous lesions are often described as somewhat painful.

Keratoacanthoma has a distinctive pattern of clinical presentation. It is typically umbilicated—meaning that is has a depressed center and a raised border (Fig. 8-3). This border is sharply circumscribed. The central portion of the lesion, rather than being cupped out, may be filled with a hard, rough-surfaced, white to discolored keratin plug. In many respects, these features are similar to those of the most common skin cancers. However, keratoacanthoma is distinctive in that it usually grows to its full size (between 1 and 2 cm in diameter) within 6 months. As will be seen in a subsequent chapter, skin cancers typically grow at a slower rate.

Keratoacanthoma is firm on palpation. Although the lesion often has a central keratin plug, the keratoacanthoma is usually free of ulceration. As a result, clinical "weeping" and formation of crusts and scabs in the absence of a history of direct physical trauma are unusual, and are more likely indicative that the lesion is in fact a skin cancer.

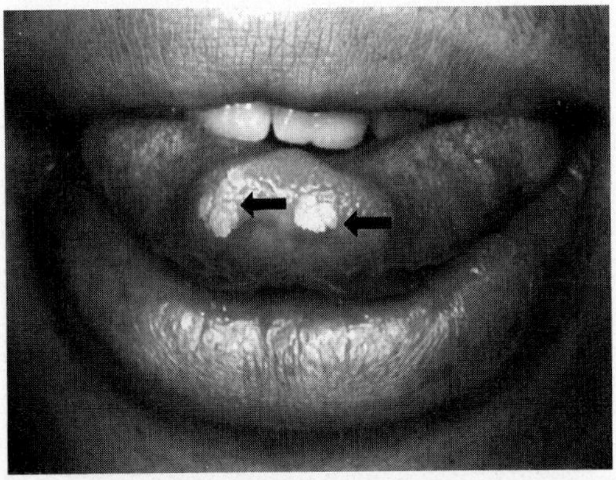

Fig. 8-2 Verruca vulgaris. This young man had warts on his fingers and admitted nibbling the cutaneous lesions.

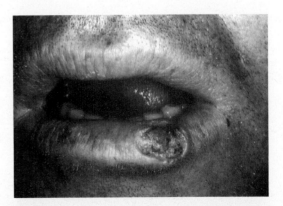

Fig. 8-3 Keratoacanthoma. This cup-shaped lesion of the lower lip developed within months.

It can be appreciated at this point that the keratoacanthoma bears a number of clinical similarities to skin cancer. For this reason, it is recommended that all lesions suspected of being keratoacanthoma be excised and examined microscopically. However, the dilemma may not end there, for—interestingly—the keratoacanthoma closely mimics the histologic appearance of epidermoid carcinoma. Happily, this challenge is one with which the pathologist, rather than the dentist or dental hygienist, must deal. History of rapid growth becomes an important diagnostic factor.

There is some disagreement among investigators as to the overall significance of keratoacanthoma. Many consider the condition entirely benign with no predisposition for malignant transformation. Others adopt a more cautious stance, judging the lesion to be precancerous with a significant potential for malignant transformation. It should be recognized that the keratoacanthoma and skin cancer share common etiologic factors (such as sun exposure) and that both types of lesions occur in similar populations. Certainly close patient follow-up is indicated. Keratoacanthomas are not likely to recur if fully excised, and examples of spontaneous disappearance of keratoacanthomas following partial excision are well documented.

ORAL NEVI

The *pigmented nevus* or *mole* is a very common lesion of the skin. It consists of a benign proliferation of melanin-producing cells situated in the layers of the skin. Such nevi are considered by some authorities to be benign neoplasms characterized, if only theoretically, by uncontrolled and potentially unlimited growth potential. Other investigators take a somewhat less dramatic view and consider pigmented nevi to represent limited, controlled proliferations of essentially normal cells in normal or abnormal locations. Such lesions would satisfy the definition of hamartoma and choristoma, respectively (see Chapter 6). These distinctions carry little practical significance, however, since all of these conditions are benign.

Most of our knowledge of pigmented nevi comes from studies of these lesions occurring on the skin. A variety of specific types of pigmented nevi are known to occur, and these types are distinguished on the basis of clinical and microscopic features. Two of the more common nevi to occur on both skin and oral mucosa are the intradermal nevus (specifically referred to as *intramucosal nevus* when in the mouth) and the *junctional nevus*.

The intradermal nevus is the most common pigmented nevus to affect either skin or oral mucosa. It is far more common on skin than in the mouth, but in either location it typically is manifest as an asymptomatic, soft, sessile, pink to light brown to very dark brown, uniformly colored, dome-shaped, smooth-surfaced nodule (Fig. 8-4). Although generally less than 1 cm in diameter, on occasion they may be somewhat larger, as well as pedunculated and rough surfaced. Cutaneous examples frequently demonstrate outgrowth of hair. The junctional nevus offers a somewhat

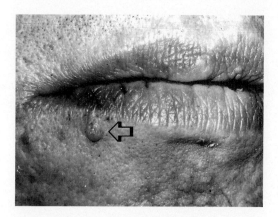

Fig. 8-4 Intradermal nevus. This soft, raised mole has been present without growth for many years.

different clinical appearance, being entirely flat (macular), smooth surfaced, and usually demonstrating brown, uniform pigmentation.

Intraoral pigmented nevi closely resemble their counterparts on the skin, and interestingly show a marked predilection for occurring on the hard palate and gingiva. Most (55%) intraoral pigmented nevi are intramucosal, while only 3% are junctional. Approximately 36% of intraoral nevi are *blue nevi*. The blue nevus bears many clinical similarities to the intradermal/intramucosal nevus and, again, is most commonly found on skin. Oral lesions are usually small, blue to black, uniformly colored, flat, and most frequently located on the palate (Fig. 8-5). Although the histopathology of the blue nevus is peculiar, for our purposes we will consider the blue nevus to be essentially similar to the intradermal and intramucosal nevus.

In evaluating the nature of an unidentified oral pigmented lesion, specific attention should be directed toward the detection of clinical features that are not characteristic of benign nevi (Fig. 8-6). The finding of one or more of these features constitutes evidence that the pigmented lesion may in fact represent either a melanoma or a premalignant melanocytic lesion. These clinical features will be fully discussed in Chapter 9.

Appropriate management of oral pigmented lesions suspected of representing benign nevi consists of local conservative excision. This contrasts markedly with accepted management of cutaneous pigmented lesions suspected of being nevi. As is commonly known, the majority of skin moles are not excised, but merely followed clinically. The justifications for routine excision of suspected oral nevi are as follows. First, oral nevi are far less common than those of the skin. Therefore it becomes more difficult to speak of oral nevi as a "normal" finding, and diagnostic confirmation through microscopic examination is indicated. The second justification is related to the relative numbers of pigmented

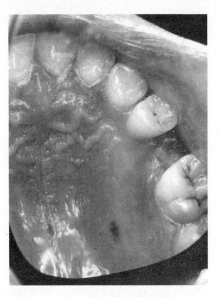

Fig. 8-5 Blue nevus of palate. This is a common location for a nevus.

skin and oral lesions that in fact represent malignant melanoma. Clinical investigators have found that the ratio of benign to malignant pigmented lesions greatly favors the probability of benign nevi on the skin. Intraoral benign pigmented lesions are also far more common than oral melanoma, but the ratio of benign to malignant lesions in the oral cavity is not nearly as favorable. Therefore it has been recommended that a greater degree of caution be used in dealing with oral pigmented lesions, usually leading to a decision to excise the lesion.

A final issue to consider is the question of whether benign pigmented nevi undergo malignant transformation. Authorities on the subject disagree on the answer to this question. Rarely, there have been reported cases of junctional nevi transforming into melanomas. It should be pointed out that malignant melanomas may often begin as small, pigmented lesions whose clinical features do not suggest their more ominous biologic character but rather are quite similar to the features of nevi. At this stage of development, only micro-

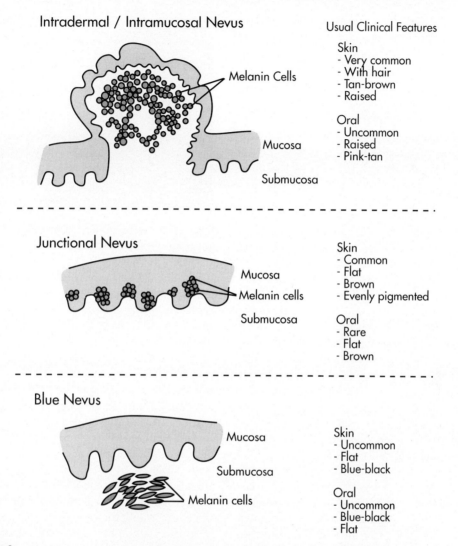

Fig. 8-6 Common nevi can be distinguished both by clinical features and by microscopic examination of the location and features of the melanin cells.

scopic examination can reliably distinguish benign nevi from malignant melanoma and its precursor lesions. The histologic features of pigmented nevi and melanoma are distinctly different. In addition, it must be understood that the true potential for transformation of any excised intradermal or junctional nevus can never be known—for after all, following excision the patient is cured! Perhaps it is best to adopt the view that the pigmented nevus

may, on rare occasions, undergo malignant transformation. However, it should be recognized that this probably accounts for a very small percentage of all oral melanomas.

ORAL CONNECTIVE TISSUE TUMORS
Fibroma

It would certainly be reasonable to interpret the term fibroma to be the proper name for a benign neoplasm of fibrous connective tissue origin. However, a fibroma—as the term is commonly used in connection with an often-encountered soft tissue lesion of the oral mucosa—is generally not considered a neoplasm, but rather hyperplastic fibrous tissue. A somewhat more accurate name for this disorder is fibrous hyperplasia. The fibromas and essentially identical fibrous hyperplasias are discussed in Chapter 13.

Neurofibroma

The neurofibroma is a relatively uncommon benign neoplasm, consisting histologically of a mixture of neoplastic Schwann cells and scattered axons. This neoplasm develops from nerve bundles and larger nerve trunks, producing tumorous expansion. The neurofibroma is much softer on palpation than the surrounding normal oral mucosa and is often described as having a cystic consistency or resembling the texture of adipose tissue. The borders with surrounding normal tissue are somewhat ill defined. The neurofibroma may exhibit a variety of colors, ranging from pale to somewhat yellow, as well as varying shades of brown. The overlying skin or mucosa appears normal (Fig. 8-7).

Cutaneous and mucosal neurofibroma can be said to occur in two separate conditions. The least common of these is as an *isolated lesion,* without any family history of similar or related disease. The more common occurrence of neurofibroma is as a component of the autosomal dominant disorder *neurofibromatosis.* This disease, also known as von Recklinghausen's disease of the skin, is generally characterized by the concurrent presence of skin pigmentations known as café au lait spots (resembling coffee with milk) and multiple neurofibromas (Fig. 8-8). The neurofibromas may take a variety of forms, including localized nodular sessile tumors; segmented, linear, lobular nerve trunk expansions (like "peas in a pod" and classically referred to as plexiform neurofibroma); large, deforming,

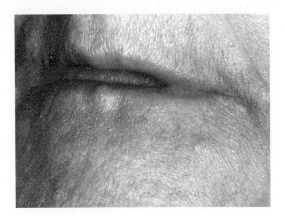

Fig. 8-7 Neurofibroma. This tumor of the lower lip is solitary.

tumorous masses; and small, pedunculated, nodular skin lesions. All of these presentations represent forms of neurofibroma, and on occasion the oral cavity will demonstrate such tumors.

As an autosomal dominant condition, neurofibromatosis often demonstrates a familial history, with a 50% chance of the offspring of an affected parent showing clinical evidence of the disease. Alternatively, the disease may be encountered in patients without any history of a similar disorder in the family. There is wide variation of the clinical expression of this disease, with some individuals only showing café au lait pigmentations; others showing large, deforming tumor masses; and still others with various combinations of these and other associated lesions (such as hirsutism and ocular disturbances).

Isolated neurofibromas pose few dilemmas for patients under most circumstances. Excision establishes the diagnosis, and typically results in a cure. The overall prognosis for the patient with neurofibromatosis is more problematic. Patients with this disorder may have continued growth and development of tumors throughout life. In some cases the functional and cosmetic impact can be devastating. Also of concern is the significant potential for the development of neurogenic sarcoma. This

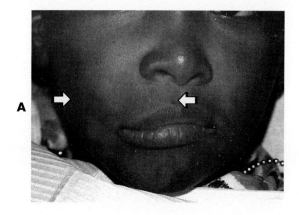 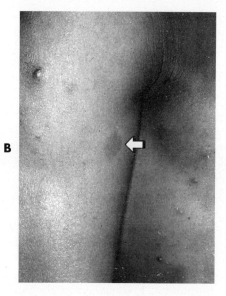

Fig. 8-8 Neurofibromatosis. **A,** A large neurofibroma of the maxilla and right lip. **B,** Multiple neurofibromas of the skin and a café au lait spot on the arm *(arrow).*

neoplasm may develop in preexisting neurofibroma and usually affects large and bulky tumors, particularly if deeply situated. Such malignant neoplasms are aggressive, with significant metastatic potential and leading to poor prognosis.

Neurilemoma

The neurilemoma (schwannoma) is a relatively uncommon benign neoplasm of peripheral nerve tissue that, in contrast to neurofibroma, is composed of a proliferation of Schwann cells without axons. It is typically encapsulated, is firm on palpation, and ranges in color from yellowish to white. These tumors are often somewhat deeply situated, and thus associated color changes may not be apparent (Fig. 8-9). Although usually discovered when less than 2 cm in diameter, longstanding lesions may achieve considerable size. Again, the overlying skin or mucosa appears normal.

While the neurofibroma is usually associated with neurofibromatosis, most neurilemo-

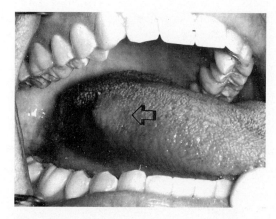

Fig. 8-9 Neurilemoma. This firm, demarcated, submucosal swelling had been increasing in size for years.

mas occur sporadically as solitary tumors. Although neurilemoma may occur in a wide variety of locations, the most common oral location is the tongue. Neurilemoma shows little tendency toward malignant degeneration, and local excision is curative.

Granular Cell Tumor

The granular cell tumor is a relatively common benign oral growth that has a distinctive pattern of clinical presentation. Although it is on occasion seen in a wide range of organs and locations, the majority occur in the tongue. It is typically slow growing, rarely exceeds 1 to 2 cm in diameter, and is usually solitary. When superficially situated, the tumor typically exhibits a distinctly yellowish hue (Fig. 8-10), whereas deeper lesions are without visible color change. When the tumor is situated in the tongue, the overlying lingual mucosa may be normal, but there are often subtle changes of lingual papillae, including reduced number and flattening. Characteristically these tumors are very firm on palpation and are asymptomatic. Currently it is thought that the granular cell tumor represents a proliferation of Schwann cells exhibiting microscopically a peculiar granular cytoplasm. There was a previous theory that it originated in striated muscle tissue. For this reason the name granu-

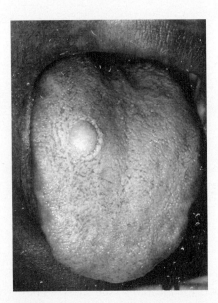

Fig. 8-10 Granular cell tumor. The tongue is the usual location of this tumor.

lar cell myoblastoma has been applied to this condition, a name that continues in wide usage. In addition to granular cells, this tumor is often associated with a hyperplastic proliferation of the overlying mucosal epithelium. This epithelial proliferation microscopically bears some resemblance to epidermoid carcinoma; but it is benign and is referred to as pseudoepitheliomatous hyperplasia (PEH). It must be emphasized that this epithelial change is clinically insignificant and unrelated to oral cancer.

Treatment for granular cell tumor consists of conservative excision. Examples of incomplete excision followed by spontaneous regression have been reported. Recurrence is most unlikely.

Traumatic Neuroma

The traumatic (amputation) neuroma represents a nonneoplastic overgrowth of axons and fibrous scar tissue. It arises following amputation of a peripheral nerve, with the subsequent reparative axon growth impeded by scar tissue formation. The amputated axon bundles attempt to regenerate but cannot find the neurilemmal tracts necessary to guide them back to the receptor sites. The resultant mass of fibrous tissue and axons produces a clinical nodule that is usually well circumscribed, firm, and often painful when palpated.

Traumatic neuroma typically occurs at sites vulnerable to physical trauma, including the lips, tongue, and buccal mucosa. Traumatic neuroma is also reported to occur in the area of the mental nerve in edentulous patients, as well as sporadically at sites of tooth extraction. Treatment consists of conservative excision, and recurrence is uncommon.

Lipoma

The lipoma is a benign neoplasm of adipose tissue that is common in the subcutaneous tissues of the skin but is uncommon in the oral cavity. Lipoma is most commonly found in adults and usually occurs as a solitary tumor of the back, shoulder, or neck. Occasionally, multiple lipomas are observed. Intraoral lipoma is usually solitary, well circumscribed, and soft on palpation. Although usually less than 2 cm when discovered, examples of lipoma have been known to reach considerable size. The lipoma often exhibits a yellowish hue when situated beneath oral mucosa (Fig. 8-11). Another, more common, lesion of the oral cavity, also consisting of mature adipose tissue, is the so-called herniated buccal fat-pad. This represents displaced, anatomically normal adipose tissue, clinically producing a nodular mass of the buccal mucosa. These masses are typically excised for purposes of diagnosis and are not considered to be true neoplasms. Treatment for lipoma consists of conservative excision, and recurrence is uncommon.

ORAL PREMALIGNANT CONDITIONS

Clinical White Patch

The oral cavity, like other mucosal sites of the body, is frequently affected by diseases and conditions that produce flat, white lesions. At the outset it should be emphasized that many contrasting disorders, characterized by widely different etiologies and prognoses, may pro-

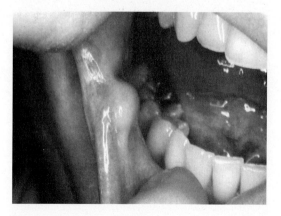

Fig. 8-11   Lipoma. This tumor is soft and yellow.

duce very similar white changes in the oral mucosa. Thus the detection of a white lesion does not in itself indicate a specific diagnosis, but rather suggests one disorder out of a fairly large list of disorders that share this clinical characteristic.

Although the list of disorders that may produce white changes in the oral mucosa is relatively long, fortunately, many of these disorders can be specifically identified clinically through correlation with other forms of clinical and historical data. In this manner the macerated white lesion of the buccal mucosa can be identified as a cheek-chewing lesion in the patient who admits to chronic sucking and chewing on the cheeks (see Chapter 13), and the white lacy lesions observed on the buccal mucosa bilaterally may be recognized as conforming to the clinical pattern of presentation characteristic of the common dermatologic disorder lichen planus (see Chapter 16). However, despite the most rigorous attempts at clinical analysis, there will remain a number of white mucosal lesions that cannot be attributed to specific etiologic factors or placed within recognized clinical patterns of disease. Such white patches are often termed *leukoplakia*—namely, a white patch of the mucosa that cannot otherwise be clinically identified as a specific disease (Fig. 8-12).

Several points regarding clinical white patches should be emphasized. First, leukoplakia is a clinical diagnosis by exclusion, representing white patches that cannot be attributed to specific diseases on a clinical basis. Second, leukoplakia is a clinical lesion that may be produced by a variety of microscopic alterations in the oral mucosa, ranging in origin from entirely innocuous hyperkeratoses to precancerous alterations (dysplasia) and frank cancers (epidermoid carcinoma; see Chapter 9). Unfortunately, the term leukoplakia is used in some medical literature to imply premalignant change (dysplasia). Therefore, we discourage use of this term in favor of

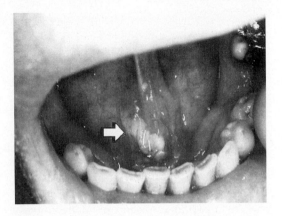

Fig. 8-12 Clinical white patch. This demarcated patch of the lateral and ventral surfaces of the tongue occurred in a pipe smoker. Biopsy of the lesion revealed hyperkeratosis.

the phrase clinical white patch. Even the astute, experienced clinician cannot reliably distinguish between white patches representing these different microscopic features. This limitation in the utility of clinical examination leads us to a third important point regarding white patches. The clinical inability to determine which white patches are or will become cancer requires us to suspect all white patches of representing premalignant lesions. This perspective demands careful and meticulous clinical management of all unexplained oral white lesions. The white color is produced by reduced visibility of the underlying normal microvasculature (such as capillaries and venules). These structures are hidden by the increased thickness of the epithelium, including thickened keratin layer (as in hyperkeratosis) and thickened spinous cell layer (as in acanthosis).

Epithelial Dysplasia

It has been indicated previously that some lesions clinically identified as white patches will be found, upon biopsy and microscopic examination, to be premalignant lesions. *Epithelial dysplasia* is defined as a microscopic disruption in the normal pattern of epithelial maturation. By experience, it has come to be recognized that this disruption in maturation is indicative of a significant risk for malignant transformation. Epithelial dysplasia is not cancer, and in the strictest sense is not a neoplasm. It is a tissue (surface epithelium) change that exhibits morphologic criteria suggesting early inappropriate genetic expression, and it is considered an intermediate stage between normal epithelium and cancer. If epithelial dysplasia is diagnosed, it can be anticipated that a certain percentage (25%) will transform into cancer—even if the stimulus is removed. Not all dysplasias transform, and some even disappear after removal of the stimulus. We are unable to predict either clinically or microscopically exactly which dysplasias will behave in what manner (Fig. 8-13).

It is fortunate that most epithelial dysplasias do exhibit clinical features. This permits early detection and elimination prior to the development of cancer. Because it is common for dysplastic mucosa to produce excess surface keratin, epithelial dysplasia usually produces a white patch (Fig. 8-14). Hyperkeratosis alone is not considered to represent epithelial dysplasia. Although epithelial dysplasia may be detected as a white patch, this disorder is not associated with symptoms, such as pain or swelling. The absence of symptoms is extremely significant, for it means that the patient will virtually never have a chief complaint about the lesion. Detection of these premalignant lesions is entirely the responsibility of the oral health care worker. Epithelial dysplasia tends to occur in specific areas of the mouth, correlating closely with sites most susceptible to oral cancer. These include the floor of the mouth, the ventral and lateral surfaces of the tongue, the soft palate, and tonsillar pillars. Not only do dysplasias occur most frequently in these locations, but white patches in these locations are far more likely to represent epithelial dysplasia

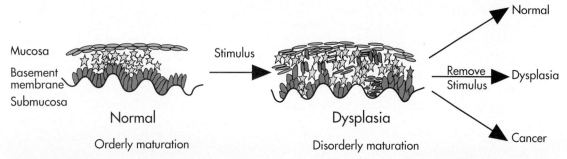

Fig. 8-13 Microscopically normal tissue may be induced by a stimulus to begin disorderly maturation (dysplasia). In time, after removal of the stimulus, dysplasia may progress back to normal, may remain as dysplasia, or may progress to cancer.

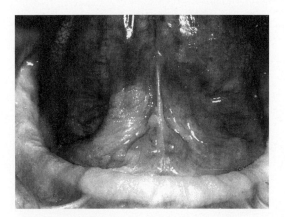

Fig. 8-14 Epithelial dysplasia. This white lesion of the floor of the mouth is present in a cigarette smoker.

(or cancer) than similar lesions situated in areas such as the buccal mucosa, gingiva, or hard palate. However, an unexplained, persistent white patch must be rigorously evaluated, regardless of location.

While location of a white patch correlates with the likelihood that it represents premalignancy or malignancy, other features such as degree of whiteness and size of the lesion are of little predictive value. However, three clinical features that are important are presence of associated redness, nodularity or induration, and ulceration. The presence of a nonpainful, velvety red component (erythroplasia) in a

white lesion greatly increases the likelihood that dysplasia or cancer is present (Fig. 8-15). The finding of nodularity or induration (firmness on palpation) suggests that more is present beneath the surface than merely a hyperkeratosis. The possibility that underlying invasive cancer is present should be carefully considered. In a similar fashion, ulceration in a white lesion may provide an indication that a local destructive disease process such as cancer, infection, or other necrosis may be present. Such lesions require close scrutiny and rigorous follow-up.

It is widely accepted that the etiology of epithelial dysplasia is essentially similar to that of oral epidermoid carcinoma. Thus, factors such as heavy exposure to smoked and smokeless tobacco, heavy alcohol consumption, and, in the case of the vermilion border, sun damage are usually contributory.

The histopathologic features of epithelial dysplasia include a variety of changes that represent a disruption in the normal pattern of epithelium maturation. These features constitute changes from the normal appearance of the oral mucosa and are the following: (1) loss of the usual orderly stratification of the epithelium, (2) keratinization in the deeper layers (dyskeratosis), (3) increased and abnormal mitotic activity, (4) mitoses in the superficial layers, (5) hyperchromasia, (6) nuclear and cellular pleomorphism, and (7) other subtle changes. These microscopic characteristics are similar to those noted in carcinomas; however, epithelial dysplasias do not show evidence of cellular invasion or metastasis.

It is apparent that a diagnosis of epithelial dysplasia is made on a microscopic basis. The diagnosis is based upon an assessment of the number and severity of alterations present. Frequently, the pathologist will qualify the diagnosis of dysplasia by attaching such descriptive terms as mild, moderate, or severe. In essence, this represents a subjective assessment of the likelihood that the dysplasia will become cancer if untreated. As explained in Chapter 7, one can envision the microscopic aberrations seen in epithelial dysplasia as markers of abnormal cell behavior. Changes in cell and tissue morphology mirror altered biologic behavior. Even greater loss of control resulting in malignant neoplastic disease is thus foreshadowed.

Treatment of epithelial dysplasia usually requires thorough removal of the affected tissue. The most commonly employed technique is surgical excision. Alternatively, the use of lasers is increasing with advances in that technology. Probably as important as removal of the dysplastic tissue is the elimination of any environmental agents representing etiologic factors in the disease. Regrettably, most of the etiologic factors are tied to chemical dependencies (alcohol dependism, nicotine addiction), and the difficulties in modifying such dependent behaviors are well known. Education of the patient concerning the connection between carcinogenic agents, epithelial dysplasia, and cancer is required. However, a holistic approach to patient care mandates that competent professional aid be sought for dealing with related nicotine- and alcohol-dependent behavior. In the case of actinic etiology, use of hats and sunscreens can be most effective.

Finally, close periodic follow-up is required. It must be recognized that in most cases wide areas of the oral cavity have been subject to the same etiologic factors as the area of dysplastic tissue. Risks of incomplete excision with recurrence, as well as development of new lesions, are considerable. These risks are especially increased in patients who fail to achieve a change in their habits in relation to carcinogenic agents such as tobacco, alcohol, or sunlight.

Erythroplasia

Erythroplasia is represented by a red patch that cannot be diagnosed as a specific disease

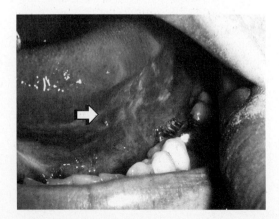

Fig. 8-15 Epithelial dysplasia. This red and white area occurred in a nonsmoker. It was proven to be dysplasia by biopsy.

on the basis of clinical analysis. As in the case of its white counterpart, the diagnosis of erythroplasia is clinical rather than histologic and is made by exclusion. There are a number of conditions that can produce a red mucosal change. As in the case of mucosal white lesions, many of the possible conditions may be diagnosed or strongly suspected on the basis of identification of concurrent, related findings. Nonetheless, following rigorous clinical analysis, there will remain a small number of asymptomatic, red, velvety patches that cannot be specifically attributed to an identifiable clinical disorder. Should such a lesion be found to be persistent (generally, lasting for 2 weeks or more), then it may be termed an erythroplasia (Fig. 8-16).

As indicated previously, erythroplasia is typically asymptomatic, although the presence of symptoms such as pain do not always rule out the diagnosis. Erythroplasias occur with greatest frequency in locations considered typical of oral cancer. Thus they are encountered most commonly in the floor of the mouth, tonsillar pillars, the soft palate, and the lateral and ventral surfaces of the tongue. Any persistent unexplained red patch of the oral mucosa, regardless of location, must be considered to represent an erythro-

plasia and be managed appropriately. The combination of a persistent red patch with a white patch, nodularity and/or induration, or an ulcer should be cause for great concern. More than 90% of erythroplasias are actually premalignant or malignant epithelial lesions. Erythroplasia is most commonly found in patients who are heavy users of tobacco and alcohol. However, a negative history in this regard should not reduce one's suspicions concerning an unexplained, chronic red patch.

Considerable study has been devoted to erythroplasia. A very significant number of these lesions have been found, on histologic examination, to represent severe dysplasia, carcinoma in situ, or frank epidermoid carcinoma. As carcinoma in situ most characteristically manifests itself clinically as an erythroplasia, we will consider this lesion in greater detail.

Carcinoma in Situ

Despite what the name might suggest, carcinoma in situ is not a cancer. It represents the most severe form of epithelial premalignancy, with complete disruption of epithelium maturation throughout its entire thickness. All of the histopathologic features of epithelial dysplasia enumerated previously may be found in carcinoma in situ. However, the degree of maturation disruption is so severe that no surface keratin is produced. The complete absence of keratin renders the epithelium transparent to light, thus enhancing the visibility of underlying small blood vessels. This is the basis of the clinical redness so characteristic of erythroplasia. Although carcinoma in situ is defined by a complete disruption of the maturation sequence, no cellular invasion of the submucosa is present. Therefore, it is the property of invasion that separates carcinoma in situ from epidermoid carcinoma (see Chapter 9).

Patients with carcinoma in situ must be regarded as being at great risk for the development

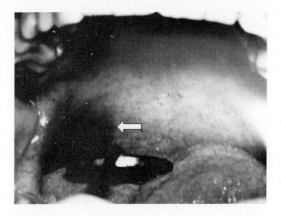

Fig. 8-16 Erythroplasia. This red velvety lesion proved to be a carcinoma in situ.

of oral cancer, because carcinoma in situ will most likely develop into squamous cell carcinoma. Treatment of carcinoma in situ is therefore much like that of any other form of epithelial dysplasia. Complete eradication of the lesion is required, with conventional or laser surgical procedures indicated. Close periodic follow-up for recurrence, thorough oral soft tissue examinations for new lesions, and awareness of development of any unusual symptoms involving the upper aerodigestive tract (such as hoarseness, chest pain, bloody sputum, dysphagia) are indicated. Alterations in substance-dependent behaviors are also exceedingly important.

Case Studies

Case 1

R.G. is an 8-year-old boy who was receiving routine dental care. On oral examination, the dental team noted a 1.5-cm, poorly demarcated submucosal growth on the left dorsal-lateral surface of the tongue. The child thought the lesion had been present for 1 year. Biopsy revealed that the tumor was a plexiform neurofibroma. A physical examination by the physician revealed a second, similar but smaller, tumor of the right shoulder area and café au lait pigmentations of the trunk (three), the left upper arm, and the back. A thorough family history revealed that one sibling of three had two café au lait spots. The proband's father and paternal grandmother also exhibited several café au lait spots, and the paternal uncle had died at age 47 from "nerve cancer." A diagnosis of neurofibromatosis was made, and the patient was referred to a developmental disease clinic.

Case 2

M.C. is a 59-year-old woman who admitted to 40 pack years of cigarette smoking (years of smoking x packs per day=pack years). She came for routine dental care with an asymptomatic, white, rough lesion of the midline floor of the mouth measuring 1 cm in diameter. The patient was unaware of the presence of the lesion, which

was detected on oral examination. No other mucosal lesions were noted. The patient was advised to discontinue smoking; however, she did not comply with directions. Incisional biopsy revealed moderate dysplasia. Excision of the lesion was done with laser surgery, and healing was noneventful. The area healed with no scarring. Follow-up revealed a new, white, 1-cm plaque of the right lateral surface of the tongue 2 years later. Excisional biopsy revealed hyperkeratosis. M.C. began smoking cessation using a transdermal nicotine patch. One-year follow-up revealed no new or recurrent lesions.

Case 3

B.D. is a 64-year-old man who went to a veteran's hospital dental clinic for dental and denture care. He had 50 pack years of smoking history but had discontinued smoking 3 years previously. Oral examination revealed a red, velvety, asymptomatic, 3-cm patch of the left surface of the soft palate and anterior pillar area. The lesion had not been noticed on thorough inspection 1 year previously. Biopsy revealed carcinoma in situ. Excisional surgery and grafting had good result, with no recurrent lesion of the area 1 year later. A second, 0.8-cm, red and white lesion of the left lateral surface of the tongue developed 18 months after discovery of the first lesion. Excisional biopsy resulted in a diagnosis of severe dysplasia. Healing has been normal, and B.D. is examined every 3 months by the dental team.

Case 1

1. Why was a physical exam necessary following the diagnosis of plexiform neurofibroma?
2. Is the combination of neurofibromas and café au lait spots significant? Why?
3. Is the family history predictable? Is this pattern consistent with autosomal dominant transmission?
4. Is there any association between neurofibromatosis and cancer?
5. How can this disease be prevented in future generations?

Case 2

1. Do you think smoking had an etiologic relationship with the white lesion (dysplasia)?
2. Does this patient have cancer?
3. Does this patient have a predisposition to develop cancer if the dysplasia is untreated? Does the patient have predisposition if the dysplasia is removed?
4. What type of cancer develops from dysplasia?
5. Do you think the hyperkeratosis of the tongue is related to smoking?

Case 3

1. Does a history of heavy smoking (50 pack years) increase the risk of B. D. developing oral cancer?
2. Is carcinoma in situ a form of cancer?
3. What is the expected outcome of carcinoma in situ?
4. Is the second lesion (severe dysplasia) unexpected?
5. Why is B.D. placed on a 3-month recall schedule?

SUMMARY

- Papillomas and warts of the mouth are quite similar in appearance and are considered viral in origin.
- The keratoacanthoma clinically and microscopically resembles a well-differentiated skin cancer.
- Nevi or moles of the oral cavity are uncommon pigmented tumors that seldom become malignant.
- Oral neurofibromas are commonly a component of neurofibromatosis, an autosomal dominant condition in which multiple and disfiguring tumors may develop.
- Neurilemomas and lipomas are slow growing and well demarcated.
- Granular cell tumors are usually slow growing and usually found on the tongue. The surface

is often covered with pseudoepitheliomatous hyperplasia.
- Traumatic neuromas result from amputation and attempted tumorous regrowth of a severed nerve bundle.
- Oral clinical white patches may represent a spectrum of diseases ranging from hyperplastic to premalignant and malignant. White lesions in high-risk oral areas and high-risk patients are more likely to represent malignancy.
- Leukoplakia is a term that means different things to different people; therefore, its use is discouraged.
- Epithelial dysplasia is a sometimes premalignant change in tissue that is characterized by increased division and abnormal maturation of cells. Dysplasia is not invasive and should not be considered malignant. Some dysplasia will progress into cancer, even if the stimulus is removed.
- Erythroplasia is represented by a red clinical patch that cannot otherwise be classified as a specific disease. Erythroplasia is usually premalignant or malignant.
- Carcinoma in situ usually presents itself as a clinical erythroplasia. This premalignant lesion can be expected to become malignant if left untreated.

Suggested readings

1. Buchner A, Hansen L: Pigmented nevi of the oral mucosa: a clinicopathologic study of 36 new cases and review of 155 cases from the literature. Part II: analysis of 191 cases, Oral Surg Oral Med Oral Pathol 64:676, 1987.
2. Eversole LR, Laipis P: Oral squamous papillomas: detection of HPV DNA by in situ hybridization, Oral Surg Oral Med Oral Pathol 65:545, 1988.
3. Lever WF, Schaumburg-Lever G: Histopathology of the skin, Philadelphia, 1983, Lippincott, pp 681-687.
4. Pindborg JJ, Jolst O, Renstrup G, and Roed-Petersen B: Studies in oral leukoplakia: a report on the period prevalence of malignant transformation in leukoplakia

based on a follow-up study of 248 patients, JADA 76:767, 1968.

5. Rubenstein A: Neurofibromatosis: a review of the clinical problem, Ann NY Acad Sci 486:1, 1986.

6. Shafer WG and Waldron CA: Erthroplakia of the oral cavity, Cancer 36:1021, 1975.

7. Sist TC Jr and Greene GW: Traumatic neuroma of the oral cavity. Report of thirty-one new cases and review of the literature, Oral Surg Oral Med Oral Pathol 51:394, 1981.

8. Waldron CA and Shafer WG: Leukoplakia revisited, a clinicopathologic study of 3256 oral leukoplakias, Cancer 36:1386, 1975.

9 Oral Cancer

After studying this chapter, you should be able to meet the following objectives and define the key terms:

- Recognize the most common sites for formation of intraoral squamous cell carcinoma.
- Identify the high-risk patient for oral squamous cell carcinoma.
- Differentiate oral squamous cell carcinoma from verrucous carcinoma by appearance, location, and etiology.
- List other diseases and lesions that may lead to oral cancer.
- Describe common clinical features of early intraoral squamous cell carcinoma.
- Describe common clinical features of late intraoral squamous cell carcinoma.
- Identify predisposing factors for lip cancer.
- Predict routes of metastasis of oral cancer.
- Predict modes of management and rehabilitation based on clinical data (size, location, stage) of oral cancer.
- Recognize and anticipate complications of treatment for oral cancer.
- Predict the behavior of verrucous carcinoma.
- Recognize common basal cell carcinomas by location, clinical appearance, and patient profile.
- Alert the patient to suspicious skin lesions.
- Identify the clinical signs and symptoms of antral carcinoma.
- Differentiate types of melanoma by location, cause, and clinical features.
- Recognize the clinical features that distinguish melanomas from benign pigmented lesions.
- List the primary bone malignancies that most commonly occur in the jaws.
- Distinguish clinical and radiographic features of osteosarcomas of the jaws from those of benign growths.

- Identify the oral signs and symptoms of leukemia.
- Anticipate oral problems associated with leukemia and leukemia therapy.

Oral cancer is one of the most significant diseases that dental health care workers may encounter in their patients. You will bear a major responsibility in this regard. By virtue of your training and professional role, you, as a dental hygienist, are well positioned within the U.S. health care delivery system to contribute to the early diagnosis and appropriate management of oral cancer. Increasingly, the dental hygienist is called upon to provide pre- and post-cancer oral health care appropriate to the special needs of oral cancer patients. A clear understanding of oral cancer and its therapy is requisite to the effective provision of this care.

In the United States, oral cancer occurs much less frequently than do cancers originating at sites such as the breast, lung, and colon. Oral cancer accounts for approximately 4% of all cancer (excluding common skin cancer). Yet if one considers the entire head and neck as an anatomic region, the number of primary malignancies arising in the oral cavity is far greater than that originating in any other head-and-neck location. Oral cancer is more than twice as common as cancer arising in the central nervous system, and nearly 3 times more common than cancer of either the larynx, thyroid, or esophagus. The vast majority of oral cancers arise from the oral mucosa, producing distinctive clinical changes that may be detected by direct visual examination. These clinical signs permit early detection by the oral health care worker, thus facilitating early diagnosis, prompt therapy, and an improved prognosis.

SQUAMOUS CELL CARCINOMA

Squamous cell carcinoma (SCC) of the oral cavity is a specific form of oral cancer composed of squamous cells that often produce keratin. Also known as epidermoid carcinoma, this tumor is defined by its microscopic appearance and is the most common form of cancer to arise in the mouth. SCC is not unique to the oral cavity, also occurring as a primary cancer in a variety of organs and tissues including the lung, esophagus, larynx, uterine cervix, and skin. It is very important to understand that while squamous cell carcinomas arising in these various locations closely resemble one another histologically, the clinical behaviors may be highly dissimilar. Thus SCC of the skin is generally considered a moderately aggressive but usually curable neoplasm, whereas SCC of the esophagus carries a very poor prognosis. Oral SCC demonstrates specific characteristics of clinical behavior and prognosis that distinguish it from histologically similar tumors arising in other locations. We will also see that the specific oral site of origin has an impact on SCC clinical and prognostic features.

Etiology

The major etiologic factors prevalent in the United States that significantly contribute to the development of oral SCC are tobacco, alcoholic beverages, and, in the specific case of lip cancer, sunlight. Numerous epidemiologic investigations provide strong evidence for the etiologic role of tobacco in SCC. These studies indicate that pipe and cigar smoking carry the greatest risk, followed by cigarette smoking and then smokeless tobacco (snuff, chewing tobacco). Pipe smoking is specifically linked to development of SCC of the lower lip, and to a lesser but still significant degree, intraoral SCC. Long-term cigarette smoking not only greatly increases the risk of oral SCC, but increases the risk of cancer throughout the upper aerodigestive tract and lung. Habitual use of snuff and chewing tobacco also increases the risk of oral SCC, although it is clear that their carcinogenic effects are expressed after a longer exposure than in the cases of cigarettes and pipes. Habitual heavy alcoholic beverage consumption is strongly correlated with an elevated risk of oral SCC, a risk that increases with increased beverage consumption and that is greatly potentiated through concurrent use of tobacco.

Geographic and social factors correlate with the use of tobacco and alcohol, and exposure to sunlight. In specific regions of the southeastern United States, use of snuff among women is endemic, and oral cancer rates in this population are significantly elevated. In recent years a major increase in habitual cigarette smoking among women has been observed. This social change has been associated with a substantial increase in the incidence of oral SCC in the female population. Higher rates of lip and skin SCC are seen in populations with greater annual sun exposure. Exposure to solar radiation is influenced by geography and prevailing weather patterns, but also by social customs involving sunbathing and personal esthetics values. Use of *pan,* a combination of tobacco leaf, spices, betel nut, and slaked lime, is endemic in large populations living in India and Southeast Asia. Within some of these groups oral SCC has been reported to be the most common form of cancer, contrasting with the prevalance of lung, colon, and breast cancer observed in the United States. Significant etiologic cofactors in intraoral SCC include Plummer-Vinson syndrome, chronic atrophic mucosal disorders, and genetic predisposition. Plummer-Vinson syndrome is discussed in Chapter 18 and represents a symptom complex in which iron deficiency anemia appears to produce a greatly increased risk of oral SCC. As this syndrome is significantly more common among Scandinavian women, it is not surprising to see an elevated rate of occurrence of oral SCC in this geographically defined population. The relationship between chronic atrophic mucosal diseases and SCC is in some cases clearly defined, and in other cases hotly debated. Discoid lupus erythematosus commonly produces permanent atrophic damage

to the lower lip, rendering the lip vulnerable to the damaging effects of sunlight. Patients so affected experience an increased incidence of lip cancer. The relationship between oral SCC and atrophic lichen planus (see Chapter 16) is far less clear-cut. Authorities are divided as to whether lichen planus significantly contributes to the development of SCC. A recent estimate in the literature suggests that oral SCC arises in 1.5% of cases of lichen planus. The overall contribution of lichen planus to the larger problem of oral SCC would seem minimal.

Genetic predisposition is difficult to evaluate in relation to oral SCC, but its role should not be overlooked. There are a number of rare but well-defined genetic disorders that are associated with a significantly increased rate of oral SCC (for example, Fanconi's anemia and dyskeratosis congenita). The genetic basis of neoplasia was discussed in Chapter 7 and it was pointed out that a large measure of the observed variation in susceptibility to neoplastic disease has a genetic basis.

A short discussion should be offered concerning a number of etiologic agents that are frequently mentioned in connection with oral SCC, but whose actual contribution is either of debatable significance or unknown. Chronic oral candidal infection (Chapter 5) has been repeatedly implicated in the development of oral cancer, though numerous epidemiologic investigations have failed to provide rigorous support. Tertiary syphilis has long been cited as a major etiologic factor in oral SCC, and specifically that of the dorsal surface of the tongue. While a significant number of patients with tertiary syphilis did indeed develop oral SCC, claims of the etiologic contribution of Treponema pallidum infection to oral SCC development is compromised by the recognition that many of these patients also received arsenical drug therapy. This therapy carries a significant risk for producing oral SCC in its own right. Viral infection has also long been investigated as a possible etiologic

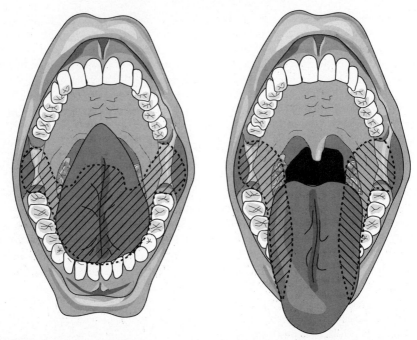

Fig. 9-1   The shaded areas of the mouth represent the most frequent location of intraoral squamous cell carcinoma.

factor in oral SCC. While most investigators no longer consider the herpes simplex virus a significant etiologic factor, there is mounting evidence that human papillomavirus contributes to the development of at least some forms of oral cancer. Finally, mention should be made of etiologic roles of chronic trauma and poor oral hygiene (which may lead to sepsis) in oral SCC. Chronic trauma and sepsis have long been cited as contributory to oral SCC. We have previously noted that chronic trauma may be a cancer promoter in other organ systems. Patients with oral cancer frequently exhibit poor oral hygiene and are likely to complain of local trauma from the expanding tumor. These findings in oral cancer patients are probably best considered associated clinical findings. The association with oral SCC appears circumstantial and cannot be taken as evidence of an etiologic link. Indeed, the areas of most frequent chronic trauma

(that is, buccal and labial mucosa) have a relatively lower cancer incidence.

Clinical Features

Oral SCC occurs in both male and female populations, but is twice as common in the former. Although SCC is chiefly a disease of middle-aged and older adults, no age group is completely spared. This disease usually occurs in individuals with a history of heavy tobacco usage and alcohol consumption, or in the case of lower lip cancer, sun exposure. However, cases are encountered in individuals without clinical or historical evidence of exposure to known oral cancer etiologic factors.

Approximately one third of the cases of oral SCC arise at the vermilion border of the lip. The other intraoral mucosal sites include, in order of frequency, the floor of the mouth, lateral surface of the tongue, and retromolar area including associated gingiva and soft palate. This horseshoe-shaped zone (Fig. 9-1) seems more susceptible to carcinogens from derivatives of smoke pooling in saliva that accumulates in these areas. Therefore, these areas may be exposed to carcinogens for longer periods of time. In addition, these tissues are void of a protective layer of keratin, making them more susceptible to carcinogenesis. Squamous carcinomas of the gingiva and buccal mucosa are less common and more frequently specifically associated with smokeless tobacco—resulting from long-term direct contact with these products. Carcinoma of the highly keratinized (protected) hard palate and dorsal tongue are very rare.

Oral SCC exhibits a wide range of clinical features; however, a number of important common characteristics may be described that are seen early in this disease. These characteristics include the following: (1) color, texture, and surface changes (such as raised or corrugated areas); (2) a general absence of symptoms (such as pain and burning); (3) a tendency to produce a fixed, indurated texture in the surrounding soft tissues as the tumor invades; and (4) presentation as a chronic ulcer that fails to heal. It is likely that the most common clinical pattern of presentation of early oral SCC is an asymptomatic, flat, red patch (that is, erythroplasia). Advanced oral SCC often shares many of the clinical features of the early disease, but in addition demonstrates clinical features such as development of a firm, obvious, tumorous mass. The tumor is typically ulcerated, and its growth pattern may be primarily outward and superficial (exophytic), or invasive and indurated (endophytic). Other clinical features of advanced oral SCC include invasion into adjacent bone with loosening of teeth; poorly delineated radiolucent bone destruction; severe pain; development of palpable, discrete swellings in the submandibular, submental, and cervical regions (representing lymph node metastatic disease); and tumor growth bridging the

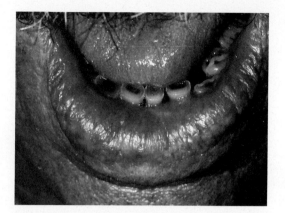

Fig. 9-2 Sun-damaged lip. The lower lip appears chronically swollen and blotchy in coloration.

tongue and floor of the mouth, resulting in loss of mobility of the tongue and slurred speech. While the clinical features of advanced oral SCC appear dramatic and obvious, it must be emphasized that all too often, early *and* even moderately advanced oral SCC may be difficult to detect clinically. Since early detection and diagnosis is the key to improved prognosis, thorough examination is mandatory—especially in high-risk patients.

SCC of the Lip

Oral SCC of the vermilion border typically occurs in the context of a sun-damaged lower lip. The upper lip is less commonly involved, because it is not in as direct a path of exposure to ultraviolet light. The sun-damaged lip is typically encountered in middle- to older-aged individuals of generally fair complexion. Their history typically includes extended occupational (as in farming, construction) or recreational (as in boating, golf) sun exposure. Clinical examination of the sun-damaged lip reveals a blotchy white change in the vermilion border that is free of significant crusting scabs, ulcers, or nodularity (Fig. 9-2). The junction between hair-bearing skin and the vermilion border appears smudged or obscured, and the lip often appears swollen and slightly everted. Biopsy at this stage might show hyperkeratosis, atrophy, or dysplasia. Early SCC arising on the lower lip may appear as a small, asymptomatic area of crusting, oras a callus-like thickening (Fig. 9-3). Patients will often be aware of the condition, but may consider it merely a shaving cut or chapped lip. With continued growth, an obvious crusted ulcer develops (Fig. 9-4) and palpation will reveal an indurated tumor mass. Lip

SCC can become large, very destructive, and disfiguring.

Intraoral SCC

Oral SCC of the lateral and ventral surfaces of the tongue, floor of the mouth, gingiva, buccal and labial mucosa, and palate often appears to arise in white plaques, erythroplasia, and combined red and white lesions. As discussed in Chapter 8, white patches and erythroplasia may represent premalignant lesions, and at the time of discovery may histologically represent epithelial dysplasia, carcinoma in situ, or SCC. Thus in its earliest clinical presentation, oral SCC may appear as an asymptomatic red or white flat patch (Fig. 9-5). Alternatively, oral SCC may appear as a fibrin-coated, yellow to white ulcer that fails to heal (Fig. 9-6). With continued growth, clinical presentations such as further ulceration, red and white surface fissuring (Fig. 9-7), limitation of tongue mobility, invasion of the adjacent jaw bone, and lymph node metastases (Fig. 9-8) may be seen.

On occasion, oral SCC may be quite advanced and invasive, yet its appearance so deceptive as to obscure its true nature. This is particularly true of SCC arising in the gingiva.

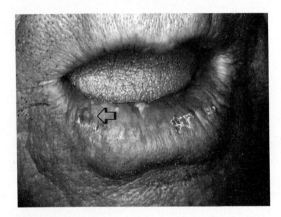

Fig. 9-3 Early lip cancer. Several crusted, ulcerated, and white thickened areas are apparent. The ulcer (*arrow*) is early squamous cell carcinoma. The crusted areas are dysplastic.

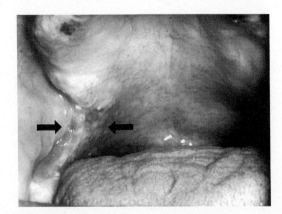

Fig. 9-5 Squamous cell carcinoma of retromolar area. This red and white patch (*arrows*) was determined by biopsy to be malignant.

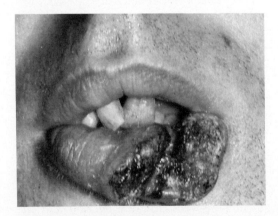

Fig. 9-4 Squamous cell carcinoma of the lip.

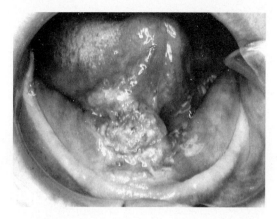

Fig. 9-6 Squamous cell carcinoma, floor of the mouth. This chronic ulcer failed to heal, and there is limited tongue mobility.

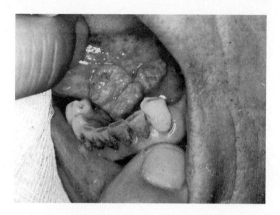

Fig. 9-7 Squamous cell carcinoma, floor of the mouth. This cancer is raised and fissured. Note the tobacco stains on the teeth.

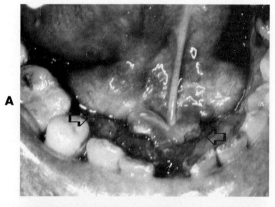

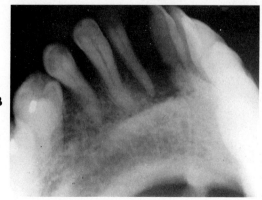

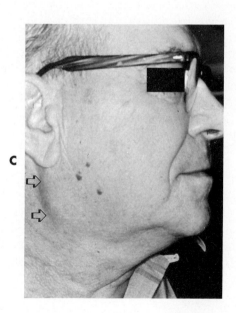

Fig. 9-8 **A,** Squamous cell carcinoma of gingiva. **B,** Radiograph shows tumor invasion about socket No. 25. **C,** Lymph node metastasis is apparent.

It is characteristic for these tumors to produce a granular, red surface change, but in other respects to mimic the general architecture of the gingiva. The clinical features in many respects are similar to those of a chronic gingival inflammatory disorder, and thus may be initially misdiagnosed and treated as such. Gingival SCC often exhibits minimal exophytic growth, but rather is highly endophytic, invading the underlying jaw. Gingival SCC may invade the jaw via the periodontal ligament, producing a loose tooth and radiographic changes that in combination may also closely mimic advanced periodontal disease (Fig 9-8). Failure of the extraction site to heal following removal of the tooth may represent the first clinical evidence that cancer is present.

Behavior

Oral SCC is a neoplasm that is characterized by relentless growth and invasion into all surrounding tissues. The growth rate is highly unpredictable and may change during the course of the disease. The tumor has a significant potential initially for lymphatic metastasis to regional lymph nodes, followed ultimately by a systemic, hematogenous dissemination and metastasis to organs such as the lungs and liver. The risk of regional and distant metastasis appears to increase in proportion to the size of the primary tumor at the time of diagnosis.

In addition to these general behavioral characteristics, oral SCCs exhibit a variation in clinical behavior that correlates to the specific site of origin. These features will be covered later, in the discussion of prognosis.

Treatment

Treatment of oral SCC is directed toward two major goals: (1) cure (control of primary disease) and (2) management of metastatic disease. Control of primary disease is critical in all forms of cancer, as it prevents continued tumor invasion with its resultant destruction of normal organ and tissue function, airway obstruction, uncontrollable hemorrhage, and infection. In cases where primary disease is not advanced and is still confined to a small area, attempted removal of the tumor is more likely to be fully successful, and may entirely prevent metastatic disease. It is for these two reasons that early detection and diagnosis of oral SCC is critical to patient welfare. Treatment choices for control of primary disease include surgical resection and radiation. In most cases these therapeutic choices are equally effective. Decisions on whether to use surgery, radiation, or various combinations of these therapeutic modes in controlling primary disease are based on such factors as tumor size and location, surgical accessibility of the tumor, and general health status of the patient. Successful surgical therapy is dependent on achieving a complete excision of the entire tumor. Often this requires resection of large portions of tissue, with microscopic examination of the surgical margins to confirm that no tumor cells are present. Radiation therapy typically entails exposing an area of the patient's mouth and jaws to a dose of radiation that is likely to kill all of the tumor cells in the primary location. The size of the area exposed to radiation is controlled by the dimension of the beam or port, and the radiation is often delivered in partial (fractionated) doses over several weeks in order to maximize tumor killing while preventing as much damage as possible to normal adjacent tissues.

Treatment of the primary site includes not only elimination of tumor, but restoration of structure and function. In many cases the elimination of an oral SCC requires removal of the tongue, a jaw, a portion of a cheek including buccal mucosa and skin, or a palate. Some of these defects may be corrected by use of maxillofacial prosthodontic appliances. In other situations in which significant portions of soft and/or hard tissues have been removed, plastic surgical and microsurgical procedures (referred to as free tissue transfers) are used for restoration of function and, to some degree, acceptable appearance. One example might involve an individual with a cancer of the anterior area of the floor of the mouth, with tumor invasion of both the mandible and the adjacent skin. Following surgical excision the defect is eliminated by transferring a portion of the patient's scapula (or toe!) with attached skin and blood vessels (vascular pedicle) to the tumor surgical site. The vascular pedicle is attached to available local blood vessels, the bone is sectioned and reassembled to approximate the shape of the segment of missing mandible, and the skin is sectioned into segments whose shapes and dimensions match both the facial skin and oral mucosa defects. The tissue is fixed in place with sutures and wire ligatures, and healing is allowed to occur. The patient's dentition can then be further reconstructed by fabrication of a special dental prosthetic device. Reconstructive techniques such as these have made it possible to attempt surgical removal of tumors that in the past would have been considered inoperable because of the resultant severe postoperative deformity and loss of function.

Treatment of regional lymph node metastasis is also accomplished via surgical and radiation therapy. When metastasis to regional lymph nodes is considered probable or is clinically apparent, the patient may undergo a surgical lymph node dissection (such as "radical neck procedure"). This may be followed by postoperative radiation to the area to kill any remaining tumor cells. Once a tumor has metastasized to regional lymph nodes, the likelihood of achieving a complete cure is relatively remote. Again, early detection of oral SCC, prior to metastasis, offers the best hope of a satisfactory outcome.

Disseminated metastatic disease is usually managed with chemotherapy. The goal of chemotherapy is enhancement of the quality of life, as well as prolongation of life. Cure is not possible with currently available chemo-

therapeutic regimens. Chemotherapy treatment may extend over long periods of time and may be intermittent, dependent upon response of the tumor to the drugs and the ability of the patient to tolerate the therapy.

Treatment of oral SCC includes management of oral complications of surgery, irradiation, and chemotherapy. The role of maxillofacial prosthodontics and reconstructive surgery in eliminating surgical defects and restoring function has been briefly described. Therapeutic irradiation and chemotherapy can lead to a number of disorders and functional problems including oral mucositis and ulceration, secondary bacterial and fungal infection, and—particularly in reference to head and neck radiation therapy—xerostomia, dental caries, and osteoradionecrosis. Specific pre- and posttreatment oral interventions and patient education are recommended as part of a coordinated team (physician-dentist-dental hygienist) approach to the treatment of oral SCC. The dental team may become directly involved in administration of special dental prophylaxis, fluoride therapy, and oral hygiene instruction.

With successful cancer therapy the dental team should anticipate ongoing involvement in the care of these patients. Perhaps the most important contribution the dental hygienist can make to the care of a patient with a history of treated oral cancer is continued vigilance for clinical signs of either tumor recurrence or development of new cancers within the upper aerodigestive tract and lung. As the majority of these cancers result from a regional generalized exposure to tobacco constituents (such as smoke, polycyclic hydrocarbons) or alcohol, it is probable that large areas of mucosa have been damaged and predisposed to malignant transformation. The likelihood of development of second cancers is greatly increased in these patients, this observation representing the basis of the *field theory of cancerization*. Patients treated for oral SCC should not be looked on as cured, but rather as controlled. Every return appointment for oral care should include a thorough oral examination with neck palpation and review of general signs and symptoms.

Prognosis

The prognosis of oral SCC is dependent on a number of factors. Probably most important is the determination of the surgical stage as described in Chapter 7. A second important prognostic factor is location of the primary tumor. SCC of the vermilion border of the lower lip has the best prognosis of all oral SCC, and its prognosis is significantly better than that of SCC of the labial mucosa. SCC of the anterior lateral surface of the tongue has a better prognosis than that of the posterior surface of the tongue. Cancers in anterior, easily examined areas of the oral cavity are more likely to be detected when the lesion is small—a factor that improves prognosis.

It is often suggested that the histologic grade of SCC has an impact on prognosis. Histologic grade refers to tumor cell differentiation—that is, the extent to which these cells resemble mature normal squamous cells and produce keratin. Well-differentiated tumors closely resemble normal keratinizing squamous cells and are considered low-grade, whereas poorly differentiated tumors lack these histologic features and are high-grade lesions. Clinical experience indicates that histologic grade does not always accurately predict tumor behavior. With the exception of the case of the very poorly differentiated, anaplastic high-grade tumor, histologic grading is not nearly as important a predictor of tumor behavior as surgical stage and location.

VERRUCOUS CARCINOMA

Verrucous carcinoma is considered a specific form of SCC that exhibits a very high level of differentiation and a low potential for metastatic spread. This latter characteristic is responsible for both the relatively conservative therapy indicated for the tumor and its generally favorable prognosis.

Etiology

Smokeless tobacco products are strongly implicated in the etiology of oral verrucous carcinoma, with by far the leading culprit being chewing tobacco. Because of its common use, the most common cause of verrucous carcinoma is combustible tobacco. However, the greatest risk of developing this cancer is associated with habitual use of smokeless tobacco. The recent increase in use of smokeless tobacco as a "macho" social habit makes it likely that there will be a long-term increase in incidence of verrucous carcinoma. Recently the use of smokeless tobacco was banned by minor league baseball teams to help reduce the incidence of oral diseases, including verrucous carcinoma, associated with this subcultural habit. Verrucous carcinoma is not limited in its occurrence to the oral cavity, as it also may arise from nasal and paranasal sinus mucosa, genital mucosa, and skin. It is probable that a variety of etiologic factors are involved. Recently, evidence of human papillomavirus infection has been observed in verrucous carcinoma of the genital mucosa. The contribution of this virus to oral verrucous carcinoma is not as yet defined.

Clinical Features

The buccal vestibule and adjacent maxillary and mandibular gingiva are sites for the vast majority of oral verrucous carcinomas. Occasional cases are seen at other oral mucosal sites. The majority of cases are encountered in men over the age of 50, reflecting both the long duration of smokeless tobacco exposure required for tumor development, and the cultural restriction of tobacco chewing to adult men. The location of the lesions also directly corresponds to the usual locations where chewing tobacco "quids" or the snuff "dip" is placed—"between the cheek and the gum." Increasing use of smokeless tobacco in pediatric populations may reduce the usual age of appearance of verrucous carcinoma in the future.

Verrucous carcinoma draws its name from its highly characteristic clinical appearance, that of a very rough-surfaced, white, shaggy exophytic tumor (verrucous meaning warty) (Fig. 9-9). It typically has a broad-based attachment without the clinically prominent tendency toward induration associated with typical oral SCC.

Behavior

The growth pattern of verrucous carcinoma is one of invasion without significant potential for metastasis. Its growth can be described as slow but relentless, invading and destroying all tissues at its periphery. In this manner its biologic behavior closely resembles that of at least two other neoplasms discussed in this text—basal cell carcinoma (discussed later in this chapter) and ameloblastoma (discussed in Chapter 14). Rarely, verrucous carcinoma of long-standing duration evolves into squamous cell carcinoma. When this occurs, the behavior becomes more aggressive and metastasis is more likely.

Treatment and Prognosis

Accepted treatment for verrucous carcinoma consists of complete surgical excision. De-

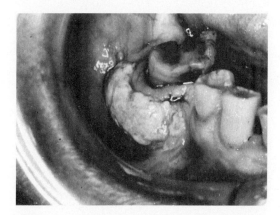

Fig. 9-9 Verrucous carcinoma of the gingiva. Note dental abrasion from associated tobacco-chewing action.

pending on the size of the tumor, surgery may be radical or conservative. Radiation therapy is less effective and in rare instances may actually stimulate tumor growth. Given the very low metastatic rate, lymph node dissection is rarely required for curative therapy, and indications for chemotherapy are extremely uncommon. Following definitive therapy, verrucous carcinoma patients face many of the same problems observed with oral SCC—including loss of function, and radiation therapy side effects when this treatment mode is used. Appropriate application of reconstructive and restorative techniques and continuing preventive dental care are therefore indicated. Field cancerization in the oral cavity applies to these patients, and periodic thorough oral examination is required. Fortunately, the prognosis for patients with fully excised verrucous carcinoma is excellent.

BASAL CELL CARCINOMA

Basal cell carcinoma (BCC) represents one of the most common forms of cancer to occur in humans. It is the most common cancer to occur in the head and neck, and exceeds the incidence of all other primary cancers of this region by nearly a factor of 4. This cancer of the skin is generally slow growing, destructive, and invasive, although metastasis only very rarely occurs. The term rodent ulcer is occasionally applied to this tumor when the lesion is particularly large and destructive; however, the neoplasm is unrelated to animal bites.

Etiology

Sun exposure is strongly correlated to development of basal cell carcinoma. Greater duration and intensity of exposure leads to an increased incidence of these tumors, and the incidence is increased among people with fair complexion and in populations living in areas that favor sun exposure. Since considerable sun exposure is necessary to produce neoplastic transformation, it is not surprising that this is primarily a disease of the elderly.

Therapeutic radiation exposure and severe thermal burns can also increase the risk of subsequent development of basal cell carcinoma. Both sunlight and ionizing radiation cause genetic damage to epithelial cells, contributing to neoplastic transformation (see Chapter 7). Not surprisingly, increased rates of basal cell carcinoma are seen among individuals with inherited disorders in DNA replication or repair (such as xeroderma pigmentosum). The *basal cell nevus syndrome* (see Chapter 14) is an inherited condition in which large numbers of basal cell carcinomas may appear at a relatively early age, on both sun-exposed and sun-shielded skin sites.

Clinical Features

As noted earlier, basal cell carcinoma typically appears on chronically exposed, sun-damaged skin of elderly persons, with a significant male predilection. A large percentage of these tumors occur on the skin of the midface area and are thus readily detectable through careful clinical examination. Basal cell carcinomas typically produce a yellowish or pearl-like, firm nodular elevation of the skin, over which distinct dilated blood vessels may be discerned (Fig. 9-10). Because of the invasive character

of the tumor, the overlying skin usually ulcerates and crusts while the tumor is small, and the skin around the tumor may feel indurated on palpation. With continued growth the tumor will invade bone and other tissues, and produce major disfigurement (Fig. 9-11).

Considerable variation in appearance of basal cell carcinoma may be observed. The condition is frequently multifocal, giving an additional example of field cancerization. Patients with a history of BCC can be expected to develop new primary tumors at a later date unless sunscreens or shields are used regularly. In some cases the tumor exhibits increased pigmentation, and it may at times resemble melanoma.

Treatment and Prognosis

The usual treatment for basal cell carcinoma is surgical elimination. Small lesions are often curetted; whereas in other cases, routine excision, cryotherapy, or electrosurgery may be employed. Therapeutic radiation is also an effective treatment. Topical chemotherapy can be useful for small lesions.

Given the very low metastatic potential, the prognosis of basal cell carcinoma is generally excellent. However it must be emphasized that early diagnosis and prompt treatment are imperative. These tumors are not generally

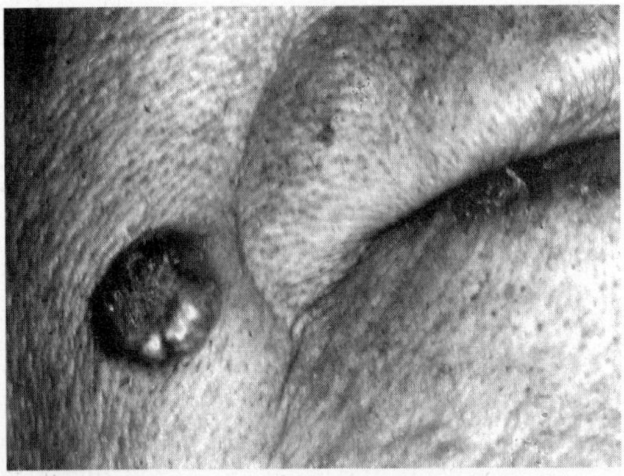

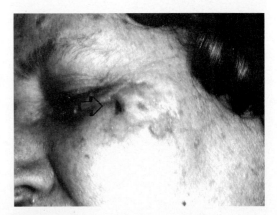

Fig. 9-10 Basal cell carcinoma of the face. This pearly ulcer has been growing for 4 years.

Fig. 9-11 Basal cell carcinoma. One margin is invading the region of the eye (*arrow*).

painful until advanced, and examples of cases where these tumors have been ignored by patients until inoperable are all too common. Some basal cell carcinomas exhibit unusually aggressive growth characteristics, adversely affecting prognosis. One of the more common reasons for a poor prognosis in basal cell carcinoma is related to site of origin. Basal cell carcinomas originating near the bridge of the nose are so positioned as to enable early invasion into the ethmoid sinus. Once this occurs, surgical control is difficult to achieve.

ANTRAL CARCINOMA

Antral carcinoma is a relatively uncommon but significant form of head and neck cancer. Its origin is close to the oral cavity, and this neoplasm frequently produces a variety of oral manifestations. A majority of these tumors are squamous cell carcinomas arising presumably from the antral epithelial lining. The cause of antral carcinoma is largely unknown. This neoplasm is generally asymptomatic in its early stages and is usually discovered only after it has become significantly advanced with extensive local invasion. Direct cancerous spread may produce prominent dental problems, including sore teeth, loosened and shifted teeth, swelling of the palate and gingivobuccal sulcus, failure of dental extraction sites to heal, and trismus. Alternatively, invasion medially toward the nose often results in symptoms of nasal obstruction with unilateral stuffiness, unusual nasal discharges, and hemorrhage. Tumor extension toward the orbit may result in eye displacement and visual disturbances such as double vision. Facial swelling, facial nerve palsy, and headaches are among the other diverse symptoms this tumor may produce. Some lesions produce symptoms such as sinusitis or perceived toothache. Apical and panoramic radiographs may show antral radiopacity and destruction of the antral wall. However, many more common, less severe antral lesions (sinusitis, polyps) may ap-

pear as radiodense areas of the maxillary sinuses. Antral carcinomas usually carry a poor prognosis because they are discovered at relatively late stages of growth.

MALIGNANT MELANOMA

Malignant melanoma represents a cancer of melanin pigment–producing cells (melanocytes). These cancers most commonly occur on the skin, but have been observed in a wide range of locations including the eye, upper respiratory tract, oral cavity, esophagus, and rectum. Chief areas of concern to the dental team include melanoma of the skin and oral cavity; therefore, comments will be largely restricted to melanomas affecting these locations.

Malignant melanoma constitutes 2% of all cancer (excluding basal cell carcinoma of the skin) and represents the third most common cancer of the head and neck following oral cancer and primary tumors of the brain. Cutaneous melanomas are more common in fair-skinned individuals and occur with greatest frequency in geographic regions receiving the largest amounts of sunlight. Similar complexion- and sunlight-related factors have already been described in connection with basal cell carcinoma and SCC of the skin.

It is currently recognized that malignant melanoma is not a single form of cancer, but rather occurs as several distinct malignant neoplastic diseases that differ in pattern of clinical presentation, histologic appearance, and prognosis (Table 9-1). We will discuss four types of melanoma: superficial spreading, malignant lentigo, acral lentiginous, and nodular types. *Superficial spreading melanoma* is a form of melanoma whose development is favored by sun exposure. However, it also rarely occurs intraorally and in this site is unrelated to sun damage. The tumor typically begins as a gradually enlarging premalignant flat pigmentation of the skin or mucosa termed superficial spreading melanoma in situ.

TABLE 9-1

Melanoma

Type	Location	Oral occurrence	Growth	Prognosis
Superficial spreading	Sun-exposed skin	++	++Horizontal ++Vertical	Depends on depth and stage
Malignant lentigo	Sun-exposed skin— especially face	—	++++Horizontal +Vertical	Excellent, usually early stage
Acral lentiginous	Hands, feet, mucous membranes	+	+Horizontal ++Vertical	Depends on depth and stage
Nodular	Sun-exposed skin	+	++++Vertical	Poor, usually late stage

This enlargement occurs as a result of the spread of neoplastic melanocytes along the epithelium–connective tissue junction—a pattern of spread that is termed horizontal or radial growth. Such horizontal growth may continue for a number of years, only to begin connective tissue invasion through vertical growth. Clinical features, common to many cancers, including tumor formation, ulceration, and bleeding, now become apparent. The neoplasm is capable of metastasis.

Malignant lentigo melanoma shares many clinical similarities with superficial spreading melanoma, including origin in a premalignant horizontal growth phase in this case termed *malignant lentigo* or Hutchinson's freckle. Malignant lentigo has a very strong predilection for sun-exposed areas, often occurring on the face of men, and is not believed to occur in the mouth. The horizontal phase may last for up to 30 years, after which the development of vertical growth, invasion, and metastatic potential may occur.

Acral lentiginous melanoma shares with superficial spreading melanoma and malignant lentigo melanoma an origin in a horizontal growth phase, with subsequent development of vertical growth and metastatic potential. This peculiar form of melanoma has a predilection for the acral parts of extremities (hands, feet), often occurring in nail beds. It appears to be unrelated to sun exposure and contrasts with other types of melanoma by

showing a predilection for occurrence in black people. This form of melanoma is also seen in the mouth. *Nodular melanoma* may also occur on the skin or intraorally. Rather than appearing initially as a macular, horizontally spreading lesion, nodular melanoma begins as an invasive cancer displaying only vertical growth.

Clinical Features

As mentioned previously, most melanomas originate in premalignant, flat, slowly enlarging pigmented macules of several years' duration. These lesions show a tendency to change shape with horizontal growth. Margins are often irregular, and variation in intensity of pigmentation is typical (Fig. 9-12). In time, nodularity, ulceration, crusting, and bleeding may develop, indicating invasive malignant vertical growth. In rare cases melanomas first appear as obvious, aggressive tumorous growths. Both patterns of clinical presentation may be seen on skin and oral mucosa. Melanomas often show variation of coloration, with combinations of brown, black, blue, purple, and red. Shape remains irregular, and advanced lesions demonstrate induration as well as metastasis. The aforementioned clinical features and changes help distinguish the melanomas from the much more common nevi and other fairly common pigmented skin lesions that we have not discussed. A change in size, irregularity of margins, irregular coloration, ulceration, or ac-

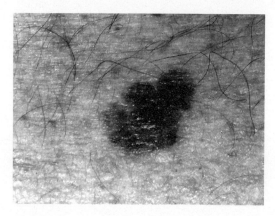

Fig 9-12 Superficial spreading melanoma of the arm. Note the central nodule (verticle growth) and blotchy coloration.

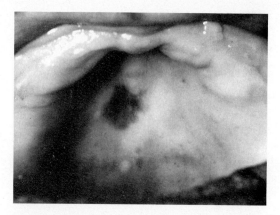

Fig. 9-13 Superficial spreading melanoma of palate. The margins are irregular and the lesion color is variable.

quired nodularity in a pigmented lesion should always be considered ominous, and the patient should be referred appropriately. Oral melanoma shows a striking predilection for beginning on the hard palate and gingiva, although occurrence in other areas—including lip and buccal mucosa—may be encountered. Growing pigmented areas of the skin and mucosa and all pigmented areas of the gingiva and palate should therefore be closely evaluated (Fig. 9-13).

Treatment and Prognosis

The primary treatment for melanoma is surgical excision, although adjunctive chemotherapy is also often used. Prognosis for oral melanoma is not favorable and is significantly worse than that of skin melanoma. Prognosis of cutaneous melanoma is closely tied to the depth of neoplastic invasion, as well as to specific type of melanoma (such as acral lentiginous, superficial spreading). (See Table 9-1.) Melanomas in the horizontal growth phase seldom metastasize, and those in vertical growth metastasize more readily. Therefore, malignant lentigo has an excellent prognosis (mostly horizontal growth), whereas nodular melanoma (with only vertical growth) has a poor prognosis. Oral melanomas tend to

be diagnosed later than skin melanomas and thus show advanced invasion, probably accounting for the less favorable outcome. In addition, surgical excision of oral melanoma offers technical difficulties that are significantly greater than those encountered in dealing with melanomas of skin. These considerations underscore the importance of early diagnosis of oral melanoma, and the requirement that all unexplained focal oral pigmentations be excised and evaluated microscopically.

Differential Diagnosis of Pigmented Lesions

Oral pigmented lesions are relatively common findings, and they represent a variety of generally benign vascular and melanotic lesions, as well as foreign body implantations. A summary list of oral pigmented lesions is given in Table 9-2.

SARCOMAS

Cancers of connective tissue origin are exceedingly rare in the oral cavity. This notwithstanding, the variety of sarcomas encountered in the mouth and jaws is considerable, showing origin from such tissues as fibrous

TABLE 9-2

Oral pigmented lesions

Lesion	Common location	Color	Growth	Other characteristics	Occurrence
Amalgam tattoo	Gingiva, ridge	Black, gray	None	50% radiopacity	Common
Varix	Ventral surface of tongue, floor of mouth	Blue, black	None	Often multiple	Common
Hemangioma Capillary Cavernous	Lip, buccal mucosa	Red, purple	Slow	Blanch with pressure	Uncommon
Freckle	Lip	Brown	None	Uniform color	Uncommon
Nevus Intramucosal Blue	Palate, gingiva	Brown-tan, blue-black	Slow	Uniform color	Rare
Melanoma Superficial spreading Acral lentiginous Nodular	Palate, gingiva	Brown-black	Radial, radial-vertical, vertical	Mottled color, raised appearance, ulceration	Very rare

connective tissue, fat, smooth and striated muscle, nerve, bone, cartilage, and bone marrow. Three examples of sarcoma exhibiting a significant rate of occurrence in the oral cavity will be discussed.

Osteosarcoma

Osteosarcoma is defined as a malignant neoplasm of bone-producing cells. It is the second most common primary malignancy of the skeleton, representing approximately 20% of all primary cancers occurring in bone. The most common location is in the long bones, particularly near the knee joint. Average age of occurrence is approximately 17 years. Roughly 5% of osteosarcomas originate in the jaws, with essentially equal rates of involvement of the maxilla and mandible. Average age of occurrence of osteosarcoma of the jaw is at least a decade older than that of long-bone osteosarcoma. Common clinical features of jaw os-

teosarcoma include swelling, pain, and loosened teeth. A classic radiographic finding in osteosarcoma of the jaw is symmetrical widening of periodontal ligament spaces around individual teeth located in the area of the tumor. This widening in all likelihood represents neoplastic invasion of the tumor into the periodontal ligament, with destruction of the periodontal ligament and lamina dura. Other radiographic features include ill-defined, destructive change with areas of radiolucency attributable to cellular proliferation and radiopacity attributable to calcification of bone produced by the tumor.

Osteosarcoma of the jaw has a 5-year survival rate that ranges from 25% to 40%. Treatment consists of radical excision such as mandibulectomy or maxillectomy. Chemotherapy has been noted to be of limited value. It has been reported that the most common cause of failure in treatment of this tumor is failure to fully excise the primary tumor. In time, these oral osteosarcomas metastasize, usually to the lung and brain. Many of these features differ from those of osteosarcoma of long bones, where a poorer overall prognosis is observed and treatment failure is more commonly due to early metastatic disease.

Multiple Myeloma

Multiple myeloma is a malignant neoplasm of plasma cells. As a malignant tumor of bone marrow origin, it is considered a sarcoma, representing the most common primary malignancy to occur in bone. As the name implies, multiple myeloma typically appears as a disseminated disease of the skeleton. Interestingly, the vast majority of cases show involvement of the maxilla and mandible. This disease appears at a mean age of 63, and there is a slight male predilection.

The malignant plasma cells of multiple myeloma generally produce abnormal amounts of a single antibody or portion of an antibody. The production of an identical antibody product by the neoplastic cells lends support to the concept that this neoplasm is derived from the cloning of a single neoplastically transformed cell. The abnormal immunoglobulin product can be detected in the serum and is termed the monoclonal immunoglobulin protein or M spike. This protein may also appear in the urine, where it is called the *Bence Jones* protein. Thus both serum and urine analysis can provide diagnostic evidence of this disease.

The radiographic features of multiple myeloma, particularly as they affect the skull, are considered highly characteristic. The sharply delineated, cleanly "punched-out" radiolucencies of the skull are very distinctive. In the jaw, the lesions of multiple myeloma are typically radiolucent, ill defined, and destructive (Fig. 9-14). Associated clinical features may include pain, jaw expansion, pathologic fracture, numbness, loose teeth, and soft tissue swelling. Such radiographic and clinical features are not specific to multiple myeloma, but

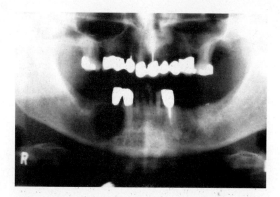

Fig. 9-14 Multiple myeloma. This lesion was rapid growing and caused paresthesia in a patient with a history of myeloma.

indicative of an aggressive, destructive disease process in the jaws. A wide variety of cancers, as well as severe localized jaw infection (See Chapter 12), can produce many of the same disease manifestations.

Treatment for multiple myeloma involves use of chemotherapeutic agents, as well as radiation. The prognosis is generally poor, with less than 20% of patients living 5 years following diagnosis.

Leukemia

Leukemia represents a group of malignant neoplastic disorders involving circulating cancerous white cells that originate in the bone marrow. These diseases differ according to affected cell (such as lymphocyte, neutrophil) and severity of disease onset (acute versus chronic). A wide range of clinical signs, symptoms, and responsiveness to treatment are observed.

The major impact of leukemia occurs at the level of the bone marrow. Leukemic cells gradually crowd out normal bone marrow, thus preventing the formation of other infection-fighting white blood cells, oxygen-carrying red blood cells, and platelets. Thus the major clinical manifestations of leukemia include uncontrollable bacterial infections, anemia, and severe hemorrhage. Leukemic cells often appear in large numbers in the circulating blood; but because they are malignant, they lack function. These cells, however, may retain a degree of normal responsiveness, moving to organs where their normal counterpart cells might ordinarily be found. Thus, a lymphocytic leukemia often shows lymph node and liver enlargement resulting from accumulation of neoplastic lymphoid cells, and the spleen often becomes enlarged in myelogenous (granulocytic) leukemia. The gingiva often becomes inflamed, swollen, hemorrhagic, and ulcerated as a result of secondary infections, platelet deficiency, and accumulation of leukemic cells. Gingival lesions are readily confused with other forms of gingivitis including ANUG (trench mouth), hormonal gingivitis, and HIV gingivitis. (See Chapter 17).

The oral health management of leukemic patients is not dissimilar to that of patients with immunologic deficiencies and bleeding disorders. Both the disease and the treatment often lead to impairment in inflammation, deficiency in defense against infection and poor hemostasis. Remember that the chemotherapeutic agents used to treat leukemia often may also damage the bone marrow. Many of the principles listed in treatment of oral cancer patients also apply in this situation. Coordinated health care, with close communication with the oncologist, is essential to patient well-being.

Case Studies

Case 1
A.B. is a 49-year-old man with 40 pack years' smoking experience and a moderate to heavy alcohol intake. He went for routine dental treatment. Oral examination revealed a painless, slightly ulcerated white plaque of the left ventral surface of the tongue that was 1 cm in size. Adjacent areas showed red and white patches. The ulcer margins were white and firm. No enlarged lymph nodes were palpable in his neck.

Biopsy revealed well-differentiated squamous cell carcinoma of the tongue with dysplasia of adjacent tissues. Further excision and dissection of the left-side neck nodes revealed only the primary site of carcinoma with no lymph node involvement (stage I). Skin grafting was used to correct the intraoral defect. A.B. has discontinued smoking and alcohol intake, and his condition is watched closely by his dentist and oncologist for development of oral lesions. Five years after surgery, he is tumor free and complains only of intermittent edema of the left side of the face.

Case 2
K.B. is a 60-year-old male dentist who noted a brown-black mole on his arm that slowly enlarged and formed a nodule over a 1-year period of time. The mole had been present for at least 4 years. Excision revealed a superficial spreading melanoma in vertical (nodular) growth phase. A swelling of the axillary area was surgically and diagnosed as metastatic melanoma. K.B. is now 1 year beyond surgery and has completed a course of chemotherapy and immune therapy. He is closely examined by his oncologist and has retired from dental practice—largely because of side effects from his therapies.

Case 3
C.S. is a 50-year-old male farmer who has used smokeless tobacco as a dip between his cheek and gum since he was 14 years old. He complained to his dentist of a rough irritation of this area. Oral examination revealed a white, warty, raised growth measuring 3.5 cm and involving his right buccal vestibule, buccal mucosa, and mandibular buccal gingiva. Radiographs showed bone loss around teeth No. 29, 30, and 31 corresponding to the clinical areas of the white lesion. Biopsy revealed verrucous carcinoma invading the deep submucosa and bone. Excisional surgery and a block mandibular resection followed to excise the cancer. Skin grafts, bone grafts, and reconstructive surgery have followed. Physical examination revealed no evidence of metastasis. He is tumor free 4 years after definitive surgery.

Case 4

M.G. is a 45-year-old blond-haired white woman who went for annual dental care. The dental personnel noted a raised, firm, white nodule of the skin of the right cheek that had not been present 1 year previously. M.G. gave a history of frequent, intense suntanning for cosmetic purposes. Her complexion was fair. She was referred to her physician, who removed the lesion. A diagnosis of basal cell carcinoma was rendered. The lesion site healed adequately. M.G. has had two new BCCs removed from her nose and right cheek within the past 3 years, and she monitors her skin closely.

Case 1

1. What cancer risk factors are present for A.B.?
2. Are the symptoms, color, and location typical for oral cancer?
3. Why the interest in the lymph nodes of the neck?
4. What is meant by stage I cancer? How does stage affect the prognosis and treatment?
5. Explain the presence of edema of the face.

Case 2

1. What signs and symptoms indicate that a mole (nevus) may be malignant (melanoma)?
2. What is meant by vertical growth phase? Is this a good prognostic sign?
3. Explain the rationale for chemotherapy and immune therapy.
4. Based on what we know about K.B., what is the prognosis?
5. What do you think caused the melanoma to form?

Case 3

1. Does smokeless tobacco have a relationship to oral cancer? If so, what types of cancer would you expect?

2. Are the size, color, texture, and location consistent with that expected for verrucous carcinoma?
3. Do verrucous carcinomas invade bone?
4. Do verrucous carcinomas metastasize?
5. Do verrucous carcinomas ever transform into other forms of cancer?

Case 4

1. Does the fair complexion of M.G. predispose her to skin cancer?
2. What is the likely cause?
3. Do basal cell carcinomas usually metastasize?
4. Are basal cell carcinomas frequently multiple?
5. What are the common locations for basal cell carcinomas?
6. What was the dentist's responsibility? Should the dentist remove the lesion? Should the dentist be concerned with the lesion?

SUMMARY

- Most intraoral cancers are squamous cell carcinomas and occur in adults who use tobacco and drink heavily. Squamous cell carcinomas of the lip are associated with chronic sun exposure in fair-skinned individuals.
- Intraoral squamous cell carcinomas most commonly originate in the floor of the mouth, the ventral surface of the tongue, and retromolar areas. The mucosa in these areas is not protected by keratin, and carcinogen-saturated saliva from smoking tends to accumulate in these areas.
- Early squamous cell carcinomas usually appear as white patches, erythroplasias, or speckled red and white lesions. Less commonly, lesions appear as chronic ulcers.
- Late squamous cell carcinomas may be raised or flat and are frequently ulcerated. These cancers tend to be indurated and fixed to adjacent tissues.
- Surgical excision is the usual primary treatment for oral squamous cell carcinoma.

Large defects are corrected with grafts and prosthetic appliances. Radiation therapy is useful in reducing tumor mass and as an adjunct for surgery. Chemotherapy is reserved for cases with widespread metastasis.

- Oral cancer usually first metastasizes to the regional cervical lymph nodes.
- Numerous oral side effects can result from surgical, radiation, and chemical treatment of cancers.
- Patients with oral squamous cell carcinoma have an increased risk of developing a second primary cancer—especially of the oral region.
- Oral verrucous carcinoma is usually slow growing and does not metastasize. The tumor is frequently wartlike.
- Oral verrucous carcinoma is associated with smoking and use of smokeless tobacco. The prevalence is greatest in smokeless tobacco users. Verrucous carcinomas are most commonly located on the gingiva, vestibular mucosa, and buccal mucosa, the zones of smokeless tobacco contact.
- Basal cell carcinomas occur on sun-exposed skin and do not occur within the oral cavity. They tend to be invasive but not metastatic.
- Antral carcinomas are usually of squamous cell type. They may manifest themselves clinically as tooth pain or tooth mobility and thereby mimic common oral diseases and infections. Panoramic radiographs are useful in identifying these tumors.
- Most forms of malignant melanoma are related to sun exposure. The behavior of melanomas depends on type, depth of invasion, and amount of spread of the tumor.
- Oral melanomas are rare and usually carry a poor prognosis because they tend to be of the more aggressive types and because they are frequently diagnosed at a late stage.
- Osteosarcomas of bone cause painful swellings that can mimic periodontal and periapical infections.
- Multiple myeloma occurs as punched-out lesions of the jaws and other bones in older individuals. Abnormal blood and urine proteins serve as a diagnostic marker of myeloma.
- Some leukemias cause hypertrophic gingivitis, acute ulcerative gingivitis, and oral bleeding tendencies. Leukemia therefore must be considered when these conditions persist.

Suggested readings

1. Ackerman LV: Verrucous carcinoma of the oral cavity, Surgery 23:670, 1948.
2. Boring CC, Squires TS, and Tong T: Cancer statistics 1993, CA Cancer J Clin 43:7, 1993.
3. Lever WF and Schaumburg-Lever G: Histopathology of the skin, ed 6, Philadelphia, 1983, JB Lippincott, pp 708-714.
4. McDonald JS and others: Acral-lentiginous melanoma of the oral cavity, Head and Neck Surg 6:257, 1983.
5. Moore C: Smoking and cancer of the mouth, pharynx, and larynx, JAMA 191:283, 1965.
6. Osserman EF, Merlini G, and Butler VP Jr: Multiple myeloma and related plasma cell dyscrasias, JAMA 258:2930, 1987.
7. Silverman S Jr, editor: Oral cancer, New York, 1985, American Cancer Society.
8. US Department of Health and Human Services: The health consequences of smoking: a report of the surgeon general, Public Health Service, Centers for Disease Control, 1986.
9. US Department of Health and Human Services: Smokeless tobacco or health: an international perspective, Monograph No 2, Public Health Service, National Cancer Institute, 1992.
10. Zarbo RJ: Malignant non-odontogenic neoplasms of the jaws. In Regezi JA and Sciubba J, editors: Oral pathology: clinical-pathologic correlations, ed 2, Philadelphia, 1993, WB Saunders, pp 438-442, 451-456.

10 Hemodynamics and Circulatory Disturbances

IN THIS CHAPTER

1. Edema
2. Congestion
   - Passive congestion
   - Heart failure
3. Hemorrhage
4. Blood pressure regulation
   - Hypertension
   - Shock
   - Syncope
5. Vascular disease
   - Atherosclerosis
   - Other types of arteriosclerosis
6. Thrombosis
   - Arterial thrombosis
   - Phlebothrombosis
7. Ischemia and infarction
8. Embolism
   - Venous embolism
   - Arterial embolism
9. Heart disease
   - Ischemic heart disease
   - Valvular heart disease
10. Case Studies

After studying this chapter, you should be able to meet the following objectives and define the key terms:

- Discuss the common causes of edema of tissues and spaces.
- Explain the etiology and pathogenesis of left-sided heart failure.
- Explain the etiology and pathogenesis of right-sided heart failure.
- List common causes of hemorrhage based on interference with the mechanisms of clotting.

- Define hypertension.
- Define the subtypes of hypertension.
- Discuss the theories of pathogenesis of hypertension.
- List the types of antihypertensive drugs and match them to their actions.
- List the common pathologic sequelae of hypertension.
- Identify the causes of shock.
- Describe the causes and pathogenesis of syncope.
- List the major and minor risk factors for atherosclerosis.
- Explain the pathogenic mechanisms of atherosclerosis and correlate them to risk factors.
- Differentiate atherosclerosis from arteriosclerosis by cause and by sequelae.
- Define thrombosis and embolism.
- List common factors that lead to thrombosis.
- List the usual and pathologic sequelae of thrombosis and embolism.
- Explain passive congestion.
- Predict the routes of travel of emboli of venous and arterial origin.
- Define ischemic heart disease and distinguish the subtypes.
- Recognize valvular heart conditions that lead to bacterial endocarditis.
- Select conditions of heart valves that call for premedication of a patient before dental treatment.
- Define ischemia and infarction of tissues and list the common sequelae.

The circulatory system is a closed system that supplies nutritious oxygenated blood to the tissues, exchanges these vital substances with the tissue, and returns waste products and gases to be detoxified or eliminated. Although somewhat leaky (semipermeable) at some levels, the circulatory system must remain intact, and the blood should be within certain pressure limits in order for it to infiltrate (perfuse) the organs and tissues that require nutrients and oxygen. Under normal conditions, fluid and molecules are exchanged with the tissues. This exchange depends on several biophysical functions that regulate fluid flow through small vessel walls.

EDEMA

To review briefly, fluids are forced from the circulatory system when the concentration of molecules within blood decreases, causing water to escape into the tissues (decreased osmotic pressure), when the concentration of molecules in tissues increases, or when the hydrostatic pressure of the blood in the venules and capillaries increases (as with obstruction of a vein). The fluids escape through pores of the capillaries and venules and accumulate within the tissues and body cavities (Fig. 10-1). Such derangement of watery fluid within the tissues and cavities is termed *edema*. We addressed the concept of edema

Causes of Edema

Inflammation

↑ Hydrostatic pressure

  - Venous obstruction (1)

  - Heart failure

↓ Osmotic pressure

  - ↓ Protein in blood (2)

Lymphatic obstruction

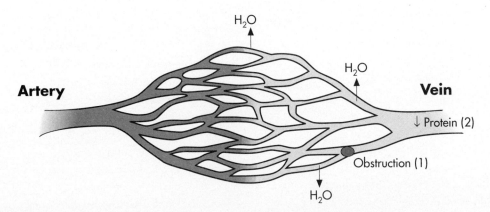

Fig. 10-1 Causes of edema of tissues *(1)* include increased hydrostatic pressure secondary to venous obstruction and *(2)* reduced vascular osmotic pressure secondary to decreased blood protein. Inflammation and lymphatic obstruction can also result in local edema.

previously when we discussed the cardinal signs of inflammation. Edema results in swelling of the tissues, fluid accumulation in spaces and organs, occasional pain of the tissues and some associated dysfunction of the organ secondary to the physical presence of increased water within the tissues. Congestion of the blood vessels is a frequent parallel to edema.

Primary causes of edema in dentistry include inflammation and lymphatic obstruction. Inflammation is usually secondary to infection, trauma, or a surgical procedure. The pathogenesis includes vasodilation, congestion, permeability, and exudation, as discussed previously. Edema associated with lymphatic obstruction occurs when there is blockage or interference within the lymph nodes or lymph channels that drain an anatomic site, as the neck nodes and lymphatics drain the face and mouth. Surgical removal of the neck nodes secondary to mouth or throat cancer (see Chapter 9) or occlusion of these nodes secondary to chronic infection or cancer spread might result in *lymphedema* (edema from lymphatic obstruction) of the face. Both inflammatory exudative edema and lymphedema result in local swelling confined to the areas of inflammation or drainage, respectively.

As mentioned earlier, edema can also result from increased pressure within venules or capillaries. This increased hydrostatic (water) pressure is commonly the result of interference with the venous return of blood. Venous return may be impeded by such events as partial venous occlusion, compression of veins, increased venous pressure, or failure of the heart to drain the veins (Fig. 10-1). For example, individuals who work in an upright position for hours at a time without significant muscular movement will frequently suffer from edema of the lower legs, ankles, and feet. The oft-heard "I can't wait to get home and get my feet up" suggests that relief is accomplished by postural change. Indeed, long-term

gravitational pressures on blood resulting from the upright posture, compounded with poor venous valvular function caused by lack of muscular activity, increase the hydrostatic pressure within the ankles and legs and results in edema—with relief gained by exercise, support hose, and postural change.

It is apparent that if a mass were to obstruct a major vein, the hydrostatic pressure in the distal system would increase and edema would result. For example, in pregnancy, the fetus frequently creates a partial external obstruction of the inferior vena cava, resulting in congested veins and edema of the legs. Likewise, a tumor of the lungs might block the pulmonary venous return, resulting in pulmonary edema and fluid accumulation within the thorax (hydrothorax). As we will discuss more fully in this chapter, heart failure is a consequence of several common pathologic conditions (Fig. 10-2). When the heart is weakened by these diseases, the heart fails to pump the blood forward, the heart chambers become congested, and the blood backs up into the venous system. This phenomenon is termed backward heart failure. If the left side of the heart is diseased, oxygenated blood flow to the tissues will be decreased, and the hydrostatic pressure will increase in the pulmonary veins (Fig. 10-3). Pulmonary edema and hydrothorax will result—as in the case of the obstructed pulmonary vein described earlier. Likewise, if the right side of the heart is diseased and weakened, less blood will be pumped to the lungs and blood will back up into the vena cava. The increased hydrostatic pressure will cause edema of the internal organs and extremities drained by the vena cava—especially the ankles and feet, where gravity increases the hydrostatic pressure further (Fig. 10-4). A patient with left ventricular failure frequently develops severe acute pulmonary edema and may even drown from this consequence. When consulting with physicians, we often are told that a patient has

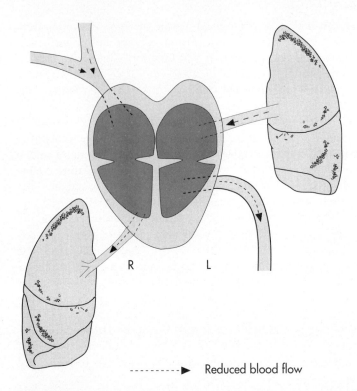

Left Ventricular Disease
Ischemic heart disease
Chronic ishemic
heart disease
Myocardial infarct
Hypertensive heart disease
Valvular disease
Rheumatic disease
Congenital
Cardiomyopathy

Right Ventricular Disease
Primary (rare)
Right ventricular failure
Emphysema
Left ventricular failure
Chronic obstructive
pulmonary disease

- - - - - - - - - ▶ Reduced blood flow

Fig. 10-2 When the heart fails to pump, forward blood flow is decreased in the aorta and pulmonary arteries. Likewise, the vena cava and pulmonary veins are not drained at optimum levels with resultant congestion and edema of the draining organs. The common causes of heart failure are listed.

one-pillow to four-pillow orthopnea. Four-pillow orthopnea indicates that a patient can sleep comfortably only when supported by four pillows to prevent edema of the lungs from choking the patient. By using four pillows, the patient elevates the upper body so that the edema drains to the base of the lungs and difficulty in breathing is reduced. The diagnosis of four-pillow orthopnea then, indicates that the patient has severe *left-sided* heart failure resulting in severe chronic pulmonary edema. Such a patient might best receive dental treatment in a hospital setting where the heart can be monitored. Special positioning in the dental chair may also be necessary. Likewise, a patient with *right-sided* heart failure may demonstrate grade 1 to 4+ pitting edema of the ankles, depending on the severity of the heart disease. Again, a patient with

severe right-sided heart disease may present a diagnosis from his or her physician of grade 4+ edema of the ankles as a measure of the severity of the heart problem (Fig. 10-3). The dental treatment plan might be altered because of knowledge of this condition.

Decreased plasma osmotic pressure or increased fluid retention by tissues may result in a systemic edema—termed *anasarca*. Anasarca results as a consequence of such conditions as retained water secondary to kidney failure or decreased plasma proteins (hypoalbuminemia) secondary to albumin loss or reduced albumin synthesis. In acute kidney disease, normal glomerular water excretion may be reduced; and water is thereby retained in the blood. Albumin decrease is a common sequela of types of kidney failure when albumin is lost in the urine (albuminuria) and in

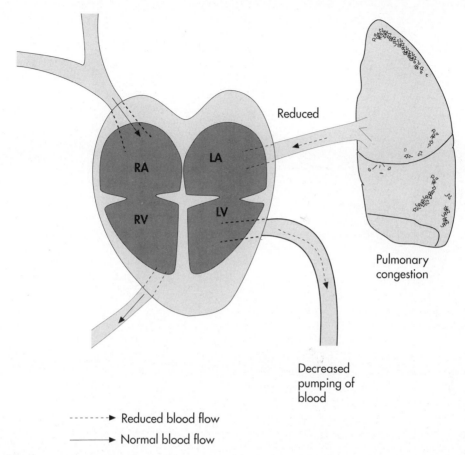

Reduced

RA   LA

RV   LV

Pulmonary
congestion

Decreased
pumping of
blood

- - - - - ▶ Reduced blood flow

———▶ Normal blood flow

Fig. 10-3   In the left-sided heart failure, the pulmonary venous return is reduced and the lungs become congested.

types of liver disease such as cirrhosis (scarring) when the liver fails to manufacture sufficient protein for the blood. Protein starvation (kwashiorkor) also results in hypoalbuminemia. The diluted blood from water retention of hypoalbuminemia has a decreased plasma osmotic pressure; therefore, water (edema fluid) easily leaks from the blood into the tissue. Loose tissues such as the periorbital skin and eyelids are especially affected but all tissues will become edematous to some extent. Patients with liver cirrhosis, frequently caused by alcoholism or chronic hepatitis, develop generalized edema and edema of the

peritoneal cavity. The peritoneal edema results from a combination of increased hydrostatic pressure in the portal system secondary to obstructive liver scarring, and to decreased plasma osmotic pressure. Individuals with kidney disease can develop severe anasarca due to albuminuria and water retention.

A nomenclature is frequently used for tissues or cavities that are edematous. Sometimes terms designate the cause of the edema, as with lymphedema or inflammatory edema; sometimes terms suggest location, such as ankle edema, renal edema, or pulmonary edema; and occasionally, terms suggest

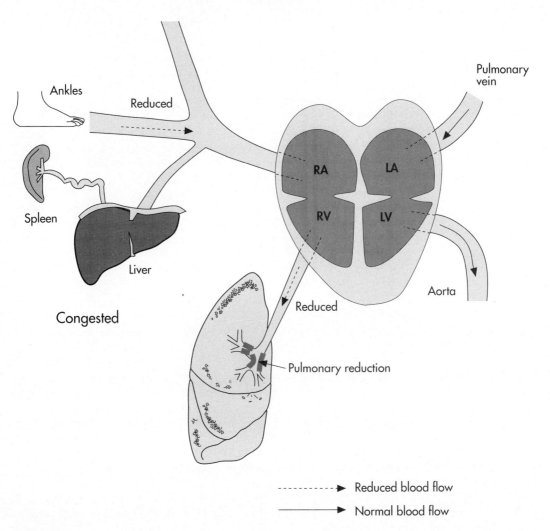

Fig. 10-4 In right-sided heart failure, the return of blood in the vena cava is reduced and congestion and edema of the peripheral organs occurs. Pulmonary vascular reduction frequently causes right-sided heart failure.

appearance, as with pitting edema. When fluid appears within body cavities, the prefix hydro- is used in conjunction with the designation for the area—for example, hydrothorax, hydro-pericardium, hydroperitoneum (also known as ascites), and hydrocele of the testicle. Edema of tissues is seldom harmful by itself. However, if edema is significant in some tissues such as the lungs or brain, it can inhibit function or increase the risk of infection. The major signifi-cance of edema, however, is that it is an indication of severe associated disease—such as infection, heart failure, obstruction, kidney fail-ure, or cirrhosis—and therefore the patient with edema may be at risk from the attendant disease.

CONGESTION

Congestion of tissues and organs frequently is associated with edema and usually is caused by some of the same circumstances. Congestion is defined as an increased volume of blood within the vascular system of a tissue. Congestion usually imparts a red discoloration to tissue, and swelling is a common component. We tend to classify tissue congestion as active or passive based on cause. We have discussed *active congestion* as an important component in acute inflammation. In active congestion, vasoactive substances such as histamine and PGE cause vasodilation and sludging of blood resulting in hyperemia within vessels. This congestion is usually acute and short-lived. When the vasoactive substances are no longer released or are detoxified, the congestion subsides. Occasionally, certain vasoactive secretions from tumors cause vasodilation and congestion. Psychoneurogenic influences (as with blushing, flushing) can also cause acute active congestion of blood vessels.

Passive Congestion

Passive congestion is an important and common sequela of *venous* obstruction. In this long-term condition, tissues become congested, small hemorrhages are common, and edema is usually apparent. At first the tissues appear swollen and red-purple. Causes include the occlusion of a vein with a clot (thrombus), constriction of veins by tumor or mass, and failure of the left or right side of the heart to empty the venous system (heart failure). When congestion is chronic and significant, the sludging of blood may interfere further with perfusion of the tissue. As a result, tissues may atrophy from loss of cells, and resultant scarring may occur. Hemosiderin—a blood breakdown product—accumulates within the atrophic scarred tissue and within tissue macrophages. At this point, the shrunken, firm tissue often appears brown-red because of the congestion and hemosiderin pigments. The function of the chronically congested tissue is diminished because of the atrophy and scarring.

Heart Failure

To better understand passive congestion and edema of tissue, we need to further consider the concept of heart failure. Diseases such as arteriosclerosis, viral myocarditis, mitral and aortic valvular disease, and hypertension can considerably weaken the left side of the heart. As previously described, the weakened left ventricle of the heart cannot empty the pulmonary veins, and passive congestion and edema of the lungs occurs. The patient compensates for the edema and orthopnea with pillows. However, the congestion becomes chronic. Over a period of years, scarring and pigmentation increases within the fine alveolar structures, and the tissue becomes thickened, dense and discolored with hemosiderin (a condition known as brown induration). Numerous hemosiderin-laden macrophages, termed heart failure cells, accumulate within the alveoli. Respiration is impaired, and arterioles degenerate and become less elastic, resulting in increased pulmonary arterial pressure. Chronic left-sided heart failure therefore can result in pulmonary dysfunction.

Chronic right-sided heart failure usually does not result from primary disease of the right side of the heart, but rather most commonly results from diseases of the lungs that increase the pulmonary vascular resistance and thereby increase the pulmonary arterial pressure. Such common chronic diseases as emphysema, brown induration (caused by left ventricular failure), asthma, and chronic bronchitis increase the blood pressure of the pulmonary artery. The right ventricle of the heart has difficulty pumping against the increased pressure; therefore, there is backup and passive congestion of the right ventricle, atrium, and vena cava. The result is chronic passive congestion of the systemic organs, especially the legs and ankles. When the condition persists for years, atrophy and scarring of the spleen and liver (cardiac cirrhosis) may result, with associated dysfunction. Pitting ankle edema, intestinal congestion, and swollen jugular veins may also be common signs and symptoms. Can you trace left-sided heart failure through the lung and right side of the heart to the liver and ankles? Use Figs. 10-3 and 10-4 to help. In most instances, the dental team is not responsible for diagnosis of such conditions as hemodynamic problems and heart failure. We are, however, responsible for reacting to information gathered with the health history and patient examination, and for providing correct treatment based on this information.

HEMORRHAGE

The vascular system is a closed system that allows for fluid exchange but not gross volumetric blood loss. When gross blood loss occurs, a state of disease often results. When blood loss is acute, the blood pressure may drop. The result of a major blood pressure decrease may be poor tissue perfusion—hence anoxia, degeneration, and necrosis of tissue (see Chapter 2). When blood loss is chronic, anemia can result. Anemic patients are weak, tired, and pale because of the insufficient oxygen-carrying capacity of the blood. Mechanisms exist to help prevent blood loss from the vascular system, to stop extravasation of blood when vascular integrity is lost, and to repair the damaged vessels. In dentistry, bleeding (hemorrhage) is a common condition presented for dental treatment and a common complication of dental treatment. Therefore, we must all be familiar with the mechanisms of hemorrhage prevention and control and the common causes that lead to hemorrhage.

There are three primary mechanisms by which the body controls bleeding and maintains vascular integrity. These mechanisms are vasoconstriction, clot formation, and clot and blood vessel interactions. All three mechanisms must be working adequately to control hemorrhage.

We have discussed vasoconstriction of arterioles previously (Chapter 3) in relationship to the early stages of acute inflammation. Remember, when injury and necrosis occur within tissues, an axon reflex results. This reflex causes the arterioles supplying the injured tissues to constrict. In many instances, the necrosis involves blood vessels and therefore bleeding is a component of the injury. Vasoconstriction immediately limits the blood circulated through the injured vessels and forces collateral noninjured vessels to open, thereby preventing the loss of blood. Although this mechanism is both of minor significance and short-lived, it provides an immediate "small bandage" until the more slowly activated, more important major mechanisms of hemorrhage control can take effect.

A clot is a plug that forms about a vascular break and is composed of activated proteins and cells of the circulatory system. This fibrin plug not only acts to stop flow from a blood vessel but also serves as a framework for healing and repair of the blood vessels and surrounding tissues (see Chapter 3). Clots are formed primarily from the protein fibrin and entrapped sticky blood cells (platelets). Products of tissue necrosis and changes in the vascular lining caused by tissue damage initiate a series of events that activate soluble blood proteins. These events ultimately result in formation of the insoluble gelatinous protein *fibrin* that forms the matrix of the clot. You have previously studied fibrin formation and realize that the activation of blood factors XII, XI, X, IX, etc., is a cascade of events that ultimately results in fibrin formation (Fig. 10-5). Efficiently, factor XII also initiates the formation of kinins for the inflammatory process and the formation of plasmin, a substance that will slowly dissolve the clot when it is no longer necessary. If any of the numbered clotting factors are absent or resistant to activa-

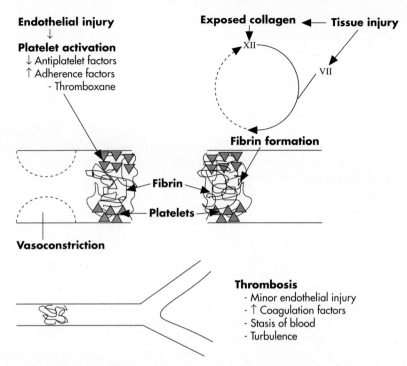

Fig. 10-5 Adequate hemorrhage control is mediated by clot formation. The formation of an occlusive clot depends upon vasoconstriction, platelet activation and adherence, and fibrin formation. Failure of any of these mechanisms allows for hemorrhage. A thrombosis occurs when these mechanisms are activated within an intact vessel.

tion, clot formation will be absent, impaired, or delayed, and the patient will bleed after vascular damage or even spontaneously. Later we will discuss several common situations in which this occurs. Blood platelets are also entrapped and give additional structure and strength to the clot. Since platelets do not normally adhere to each other, or to vascular walls, they must be activated to do so. Products released from the damaged vascular lining such as prostaglandins (see the discussion of inflammation in Chapter 3) provide for such platelet aggregation and hence clot formation. If this activation is blocked, a fibrinous clot will form more slowly and might soon fragment. Bleeding will most likely result.

Blood vessel wall and clot interaction is the third important mechanism to control hemor-

rhage. This series of events is directed by a very complicated series of physical and chemical interactions. Normally the cells that internally line the blood vessels (endothelial cells) exert antiplatelet factors. We certainly do not want to initiate clotting when there is no vascular damage (see section on thrombosis later in this chapter), or the vessel will be plugged. However, when vessel walls are damaged, these endothelial anticlotting factors are diminished, and new platelet adherence factors are activated as products of the endothelial damage. This reaction allows for platelet adherence to the endothelial wall at the site of damage. These platelets help activate and elaborate factor XII and other factors of the fibrin cascade and are responsible for adherence of the fibrin clot to the damaged vessel wall (Fig. 10-5). Again, if there is inhibition of this process, the clot might break loose or be poorly formed and bleeding will result.

Once again, there is a system of nomenclature that helps to describe the clinical presentation of hemorrhage. The suffix *hema-* is frequently used to denote bleeding; thus hematuria designates blood in the urine, hematemesis denotes bloody vomit, hemoptysis denotes bloody nose, and hemopericardium describes blood within the pericardial space. A hematoma is a focal swelling caused by hemorrhage within a tissue (bruise). When hemorrhage occurs within the skin or mucous membranes, it is named by the size of the area involved. Thus, petechiae denotes pinpoint hemorrhage, purpura denotes larger patches, and ecchymoses describes hemorrhagic patches in excess of 2 cm in diameter.

We are well equipped in the dental office to anticipate, prevent, and control hemorrhage. Limited surgical procedures, pressure, suturing, application of coagulants, and other therapies exist and are commonly used. Serious bleeding consequences of dental treatment are therefore rare. Hemorrhage becomes a severe problem, however, when the patient has coexisting conditions that interfere with the normal hemostatic mechanisms that control hemorrhage. Rare genetic conditions such as hemophilia (factor VIII deficiency) are well known and can lead to both postsurgical hemorrhage and spontaneous bleeding. Two drugs, warfarin and heparin, are commonly used for stroke patients and dialysis patients. These drugs render the patient thrombin deficient and therefore can promote posttreatment hemmorhage. Patients with platelet deficiencies likewise will have hemorrhage problems. Since platelets participate in clot formation (platelets activate clotting factors), clot stability, and clot adherence to vessel walls, any quantitative or qualitative deficiency can be expected to cause such problems. *Thrombocytopenia* (thrombocyte: platelet, penia: deficiency) is a rather common bleeding disorder caused by leukemia and

certain drugs and medications, and as an early consequence of HIV infection. Finally, we have covered the role of prostaglandin formation in platelet adherence and clot-endothelium interactions. Medications that contain aspirin inhibit formation of these prostaglandins, with hemorrhage a possible side effect. Dental patients frequently take high-dose or long-term aspirin products for dental pain, arthritis therapy, or prevention of certain vascular diseases such as heart attack and stroke. All these patients are at increased risk for posttreatment hemorrhage—even after a very minor treatment.

BLOOD PRESSURE REGULATION

The vascular system is a relatively closed system, and circulation is dependent on a functional pump (heart). The heart imparts an internal pressure to the system. The pressure is dependent on the volume of blood, the constriction or relaxation of the vessels, and the volume being pumped by the heart (Fig. 10-6). A reduction in cardiac output, a relaxation of the peripheral blood vessels, or a reduction in blood volume will result in low blood pressure (hypotension) or no blood pressure (shock) unless the condition is corrected or there is compensation through one of the other mechanisms. Likewise, if there is increased cardiac output, increased vasoconstriction, or increased blood volume, high blood pressure (hypertension) will result. Both hypotension and hypertension can lead to disease and even death.

We need to review regulation of these mechanisms to better understand the pathogenesis, sequelae, and treatment of hypertension and shock. Cardiac output is dependent on the strength and number of heartbeats per minute. Heart rate is initiated by an internal rate within the heart (atrium) itself and governed by external innervation. Both the internal and external controls can be adjusted by endogenous hormones, exogenous drugs, and electrophysical stimuli. The strength of the

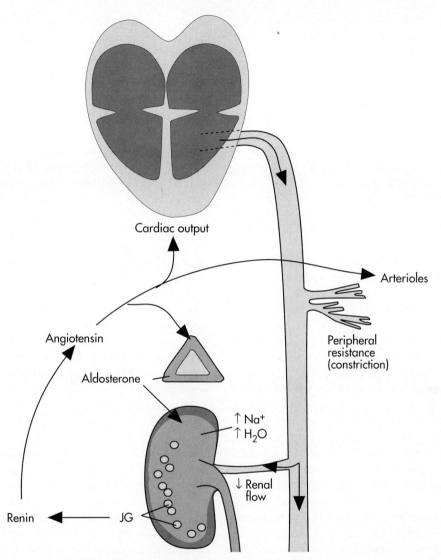

Cardiac output

Arterioles

Angiotensin

Peripheral
resistance
(constriction)

Aldosterone

↑ Na$^+$
↑ H$_2$O

↓ Renal
flow

Renin ◄——— JG

Fig. **10-6** Blood pressure regulation depends on interactions of total blood volume, peripheral resistance, and cardiac output. The renin-angiotensin system helps regulate volume through sodium and water retention, peripheral resistance through vasoconstriction of arterioles, and cardiac output through frequency and force of heartbeat.

heartbeat is also dependent on similar internal and external regulation. Any defect or modification of this system might result in increased or decreased blood pressure—depending on the type of modification.

Blood volume depends on the amount of blood and the amount of fluid in the blood. We have already noted that hemorrhage can acutely reduce blood volume and lead to hypotension or shock. Occasionally, fluid volume will be lost due to osmotic disturbances. Quite commonly, fluid volume is reduced by lack of resorption of water in the kidney. Such diseases as Addison's disease (hypoaldosteronism) and diabetes insipidus (caused by decreased antidiuretic hormone), and many common diuretic medications (promoting water loss) contribute to increased water loss and resultant hypotension. The opposite also might occur. Patients with chronic kidney disease, hyperaldosteronism, or salt retention may exhibit hypertension.

The volume of the vascular compartment is regulated chiefly at the level of the arterioles (peripheral resistance). Although small, arterioles are very numerous and have dense muscular walls with by far the greatest capacity for constriction or dilation of any of the vessels. Therefore, the large volume of blood within arterioles can be readily altered. The kidneys seem to play a vital role in arteriole contraction-dilation and blood pressure regulation. Tissues within the kidneys called juxtaglomerular (JG) apparati monitor the blood flow and blood pressure. When the renal blood flow decreases, the JG responds by secreting renin. Renin begins a series of interactions that results in activation of angiotensin and secretion of aldosterone. Angiotensin in turn causes constriction of arterioles, and aldosterone causes retention of sodium and water at the level of the kidneys (Fig. 10-6). Either way, blood pressure is increased. Naturally, opposite feedback reactions help reduce blood pressure (Fig. 10-6). Patients with chronic or acute renovascular disease may develop hypertension as a result of increased renin-angiotensin activity. Individuals given vasoconstrictor type of medications may also develop hypertension. Normal blood pressure is considered to be approximately 120/80 when measured at the arm. The biologic regulation necessary to maintain a normal pressure is a complex interaction of these three systems.

Hypertension

Hypertension is an extremely common pathologic condition that affects millions of people and leads to disease and death. The majority (90%) of individuals with hypertension have *essential* or idiopathic *type*. Essential hypertension tends to occur in families, is more common among blacks, and is confined almost exclusively to adults. As the name implies, the cause is unknown; although certainly the renin, angiotensin, and aldosterone systems play a role in the etiology. The condition itself is silent; therefore, it must be detected by the physician, dental personnel, or patient without attendant signs and symptoms.

About 10% of patients with hypertension have *secondary* or nonessential *type*. This hypertension results from chronic kidney disease, hormone-secreting tumors, Cushing's disease, or other known conditions that stimulate the mechanisms of blood pressure regulation.

Patients whose sustained hypertension exceeds 140 mm Hg systolic or 90 mm Hg diastolic (some adjustment is allowed for age) have benign hypertension. Although this level seldom causes acute disease, the sequelae of long-term benign hypertension are considerable. Benign hypertension can lead to hypertensive kidney disease and hypertensive heart disease and is a major risk factor in formation of several types of arteriosclerosis and their sequelae. It is a pathologic condition that must be detected, diagnosed, and treated—or serious disease and death will follow. When patients exhibit long-term hypertension, the arterioles of the kidneys are damaged, and this leads to a thickened condition termed arteriolosclerosis. The thickened, damaged arterioles are responsible for reduced renal blood flow—which, in turn, may increase renin secretion and vasoconstriction, thereby further increasing the blood pressure. Long-term hypertension applies pressure to the walls of large- and medium-sized arteries and coronary arteries. This tension contributes to formation of atherosclerosis. We will discuss the outcomes of this most serious disease later in this chapter. Remember that hypertension causes atherosclerosis; however, atherosclerosis seldom causes hypertension. What are the causes of hypertension?

Finally, long-term hypertension puts a chronic increased load on the left side of the heart. The heart muscle must work harder to pump blood to the periphery against the pressure. Like most muscles, the cardiac muscles hypertrophy in response to the increased work load, and the heart enlarges (cardiomegaly). Although larger, this heart is not necessarily stronger and needs more nutrients and oxygen from its own coronary circulation. In addition, associated atherosclerosis of the coronary arteries might further reduce cardiac output and contribute to passive congestion. The condition is termed hypertensive heart disease and is the second most common cause of heart failure today.

Blood pressure that exceeds 120 mm Hg diastolic (the second of the two numbers) on a sustained basis is termed malignant hypertension. Such a high blood pressure will invariably be fatal within 1 to 2 years unless intervention occurs. Death is usually the result of stroke or kidney failure. Malignant hypertension frequently is of secondary type.

Hypertension affects up to 30% of the adult population. It can be treated medically using drugs that reduce cardiac output (beta-blockers), promote renal discharge of water (diuretics), or inhibit activation of angiotensin (ace inhibitors). These are some of the most commonly prescribed medications today. These medications may elicit side effects such as dizziness or lethargy. For example, a patient taking antihypertensive agents may faint or become dizzy when moved from the horizontal position of a dental chair to the upright position (orthostatic hypotension). Care should be taken to allow for accommodation to this change before the patient is dismissed.

Shock

Mild forms of hypotension usually do not exhibit clinical signs and symptoms and have no major pathologic sequelae. In fact, blood pressures below 100/70 are not uncommon in normal young women. Mildly hypotensive individuals tend to have a lower rate of arteriosclerosis and stroke. Severe hypotension (*shock*), however, can be a serious or even fatal pathophysiologic condition. Shock tends to be classified by cause. *Hypovolemic* shock usually results from acute hemorrhage associated with trauma. *Cardiogenic* shock results from decreased cardiac output secondary to heart disease or a constrictive pericardium. *Anaphylactic* shock occurs as a result of massive histamine and leukotriene release in an allergic reaction, resulting in systemic vasodilation and bronchoconstriction (see Chapter 4). *Septic* shock occurs as a result of toxin release by the microorganisms of massive infection causing vasodilation and hemorrhage. Finally, *neurogenic* shock occurs in response to pain, crushing injury, and hemorrhage (as in a severe automobile accident), yielding both blood volume decrease and vasodilation (See Table 10-1).

When a patient exhibits shock, the tissues are not perfused with oxygenated blood. The body attempts to compensate with such

TABLE 10-1

Shock

Type	Cause
Anaphylactic	Type 1 hypersensitivity (allergy)
	Drugs
	Insect bites
	Foods
Hypovolemic	Loss of blood volume
	Hemorrhage
	Exudation
Cardiogenic	Reduced cardiac output
	Heart failure
	Restrictive
Septic	Septicemia
	(from massive infection)
Neurogenic	Traumatic injury
	Fear, pain, crushing injury

hormonal secretions as corticosteroids and epinephrine, but this reaction is often inadequate unless the cause of the shock is immediately corrected. The poorly perfused tissues become weakened and begin to degenerate. The brain and kidneys seem especially susceptible, with damage occurring in less than 10 minutes in severe cases. The blood became acidic from lack of oxygen to the tissues, and the acidosis can contribute further to the seriousness of the condition. The state of shock itself must be corrected by such means as removal of the cause (through hemorrhage control, antihistamine injection, cardiopulmonary resuscitation), rapid infusion of intravenous fluids to increase blood volume (5% sugar water, blood transfusion), and use of basic solutions (sodium bicarbonate) to neutralize the acidosis. In most cases, shock can be controlled with these measures.

Syncope

Syncope is considered by some to be a mild form of shock and is very common in the dental office. Fright and pain predispose certain individuals to syncope. During syncope, the neurogenic influences of fear elicit a physiologic pooling of blood in the visceral vessels with associated decrease in circulation or pressure to the brain. As a result, the patient will become dizzy, appear ashen about the face, begin to sweat profusely, and ultimately lose consciousness. Recovery is usually spontaneous, although lowering the head and raising the extremities facilitates increased circulation to the brain. Syncope is sometimes confused with other forms of shock (such as that caused by allergy to an injection). Special care may be necessary to prevent falling and injury in affected dental patients.

VASCULAR DISEASE

Vascular diseases are extremely common in the adult population. These diseases and their sequelae constitute the most common causes of death in the United States. In addition, vascular diseases are a major cause of patient disease; they cause or contribute to such common diseases as chronic heart failure, stroke, brain atrophy, and senility and are an important component of aging. Almost every dental patient will have some degree of vascular disease. Evidence of such disease is often documented in early childhood. Vascular disease should be considered in planning the treatment and carrying out the therapy of the dental patient. The patient's health history, physical appearance, and oral status will give clues to the patient's vascular status.

Arteriosclerosis is the most common of the vascular diseases and affects most adults. The term arteriosclerosis literally means hardening of the arteries. Three common conditions cause such hardening of the arteries. These are atherosclerosis, medial calcific sclerosis, and arteriolosclerosis.

Atherosclerosis

Atherosclerosis is the type of arteriosclerosis that hardens arteries by causing cholesterol and lipids to accumulate within walls. This leads to thickening and scarring of the inside walls of large elastic arteries (aorta) and medium-sized muscular arteries. The disease begins at an early age and is progressive. This progression can result in arteries that become almost entirely occluded as a result of the internal vascular wall thickening (Fig. 10-7). Naturally, tissue supplied by the affected artery will thus become atrophic, degenerated, or even necrotic (infarcted) from the loss of blood supply—unless alternative or collateral circulation is available. In addition, the thickened vessel wall may become ulcerated (leading to thrombosis) or weakened (leading to ballooning or aneurysm). We will discuss these complications later.

The mechanism of atherosclerosis has been studied intensely. We understand that there are a combination of risk factors that predispose one to the disease. Major risk factors

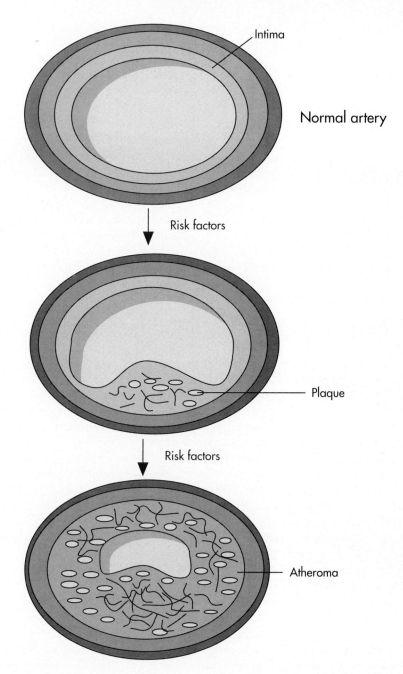

Intima

Normal artery

Risk factors

Plaque

Risk factors

Atheroma

Fig. 10-7 The atherosclerotic artery develops a tumor like plaque composed of proliferative smooth muscle cells, inflammatory cells, and cholesterol products. The atheroma may grow to considerable size and will reduce blood flow to the tissues.

include diabetes mellitus, hypertension, hyperlipidemia (high blood cholesterol and lipids), and cigarette smoking. In this author's opinion, a family history of atherosclerosis also constitutes a major risk factor. Lesser but still important risk factors include increasing age, poor diet, anxious personality, sedentary lifestyle, and chronic stressful situations. The degree of atherosclerosis depends on the type, intensity, and number of risk factors. Since most of these factors are environmental and can be managed to some extent, the progression of atherosclerosis may be prevented or reduced through risk factor controls.

The pathogenesis of the disease is complicated. We know that the artery lining (endothelial cells) and smooth muscle of the intimal artery walls become very proliferative and accumulate excessive amounts of cholesterol and other lipids. The lipids may initiate a low-grade chronic inflammatory reaction with proliferation of lipid-laden macrophages, fibrosis, and scarring. The tumorous lesion resulting is termed an atheroma (lipid growth) or plaque (Fig. 10-7). This plaque slowly progresses, enlarges, continues to scar, and frequently calcifies. The atheroma bulges into the lumen of the artery and thereby restricts blood flow (Fig. 10-7). The endothelial surface may ulcerate and even bleed into the vessel lumen.

The exact cause of plaque formation is unclear and is probably multifactorial. Humans and laboratory animals who have sustained high blood levels of either cholesterol or cholesterol-containing low-density lipoproteins (LDLs) tend to develop severe atherosclerosis at an early age. It could be speculated that the endothelial cells and muscle cells of the vessels are unable to transport and catabolize high levels of these lipids, resulting in accumulation of lipids in the vessel wall. This accumulation initiates cell damage, macrophage activity, proliferation of muscle cells, and scarring of the vessel wall. Many of the risk factors—such as heredity, diabetes, and smoking—raise blood cholesterol levels, thereby leading to atherosclerosis. It is further known that when the endothelium of the walls of the arteries is slightly injured, the vessel walls react with endothelial and smooth muscle cell proliferation and accumulation of lipids with resultant inflammation and scarring. Thus a plaque is formed. Again, factors such as hypertension, smoking, diabetes, and hyperlipidemia can cause such endothelial injury. Finally, platelet activity and clot formation also seem to play an important role in plaque formation. When the endothelium is injured by risk factors, the degenerating endothelium will lose some of its platelet-inhibiting and anticoagulant factors—thereby allowing for intravascular clot (thrombus) formation on the injured vessel wall (review clot formation). The now-attached platelets and monocytes release growth factors like those utilized in repair of tissues. These growth factors stimulate the endothelial and muscle cells to proliferate and the macrophages to accumulate lipids. A consequential chronic inflammatory response leads to plaque formation, scarring, and calcification. The thrombus itself might organize into scar tissue and contribute to the bulk of the atheroma. Once again, most risk factors (smoking, hypertension, diabetes) increase the chance of injury and thrombosis and therefore may contribute to atherosclerosis through this mechanism. Which of these three mechanisms (lipids, injury, thrombosis) is actually pathogenic? Probably all work together in contributing to plaque formation.

Other Types of Arteriosclerosis

The other types of arteriosclerosis play a much lesser role in contributing to disease and death. *Medial sclerosis* is very common but seldom causes disease. We have previously discussed arteriolosclerosis and its relationship to hypertension. This form of arteriosclerosis is important—especially as it involves kidney arterioles—as a result of hypertensive disease.

THROMBOSIS

Arterial Thrombosis

Arterial thrombosis is a major sequela of atherosclerosis. Thrombosis is defined as the formation of an intravascular blood clot. The clot may block the artery (occlusive thrombus) or merely attach to the wall of a vessel or heart chamber (mural thrombus) without causing occlusion. Either way, it can be expected to limit or stop the blood flow to the organ being supplied by the artery. The organ will either become weakened from lack of oxygen and nutrients (ischemia) or become necrotic (infarction) from anoxia. A thrombus forms in an atherosclerotic vessel either because of damage to or ulceration of the artery wall that allows for activation of factor XII and platelet adherence, or because of increased turbulence or sludging of blood as a result of restriction of blood flow by the narrowed artery (Fig. 10-5).

Although atherosclerosis is one of the most common causes of thrombosis, other causes exist. Common causes include other sources of endothelial injury such as trauma, slowing and stasis of blood flow in a vessel or heart chamber, turbulence of blood flow, and hypercoagulability of the clotting constituents (Fig. 10-5). We have already noted that atherosclerosis of arteries causes stasis, turbulence, and endothelial injury that readily leads to thrombosis. We have previously described the activation of platelet aggregation and fibrin formation by endothelial injury, and we have noted that blood that is turbulent or sludging is predisposed to clotting.

Certain conditions exist in which blood constituents become hypercoaguable. Women who take estrogen-based birth control pills and smoke cigarettes are vulnerable to thrombus formation in the arteries and veins. Certain malignant tumors excrete clotting factors that cause multiple thrombi to form. A pathophysiologic state termed *disseminated intravascular coagulopathy* commonly occurs in patients who suffer from widespread necrosis (as from septicemia, metastatic tumor necrosis, acute heart failure). The released necrosis factors activate clotting precursors so that thousands of clots will form in the patient's arterioles. The result is usually devastating and terminal.

Phlebothrombosis

A number of additional common conditions can lead to thrombosis. The term *phlebothrombosis* designates thrombosis of veins. Veins are rarely affected by arteriosclerosis. However, when veins become congested or inflamed, the resultant stasis and endothelial injury will readily lead to thrombosis. Phlebothrombosis can become a major problem in the deep leg veins of inactive or hospitalized individuals because of congestion and stasis of blood. Phlebothrombosis also may occur following intravenous venipuncture or surgical procedures involving large veins, or in the pelvic veins of the mother subsequent to delivery of the placenta. Several major sequelae of phlebothrombosis can occur, including passive congestion and embolism.

The majority of all thrombi—be they arterial or venous in position—will dissolve. Remember, when clotting mechanisms are activated, clot-dissolving mechanisms (such as fibrinolysin) are also initiated. The majority of all thrombi do not cause disease and simply dissolve, leaving a patent vessel. Some thrombi organize—that is, granulation tissue forms within the clot. The granulation tissue matures to form new blood vessels (recanalization) and minimal scar tissue. The formerly obstructed vessel reopens and the circulation is restored. We have already described the sequelae of ischemia and infarction that can accompany thrombosis of arteries if alternative or collateral circulation is not present. In phlebothrombosis, when alternative circulation is not adequate, passive congestion and edema of the distal tissue is a common sequela. (Review the signs, symptoms, and sequelae of passive congestion described previously.) Finally, thrombi of veins, heart chambers, and large arteries can be dislodged from their attachments to the blood vessels. These thrombi can fragment and move through the circulatory system. They will lodge in small-diameter vessels, thereby obstructing these vessels. This phenomenon is termed *embolism,* and a thrombus that travels and lodges is termed a *thromboembolism.*

ISCHEMIA AND INFARCTION

Ischemia of tissue occurs when that the tissue has become deficient in blood from its local arterial supply or when the demand of the tissue for oxygenated blood exceeds the capacity of the vascular supply. The resulting nutrient and oxygen deficit may cause cell degeneration or long-term tissue atrophy. If the degree or ischemia is great, cell necrosis from anoxia is likely. Ischemic necrosis of tissue is termed *infarction.* Atherosclerosis is a common cause of ischemia and atrophy. Both severe atherosclerosis and thrombosis frequently result in infarction of the tissue (Fig. 10-8). The degree of ischemia and the occurrence of infarction are dependent on a number of variable factors. These factors include (1) the amount and degree of vascular damage, (2) the presence of a collateral or dual circulation, (3) the requirement of the tissue for oxygen, and (4) the association of coexisting systemic or local disease. For example, total occlusion of a coronary artery by thrombosis or atheroma might not yield infarction or even ischemic degeneration of heart muscle if another collateral vessel supplies and meets the demand of the tissue (Fig. 10-8). If however, the patient exercises strenuously—thereby increasing heart rate and demand—the tissue will become ischemic and perhaps infarct. Likewise, if the collateral circulation is also compromised by atherosclerosis or if the oxygen-carrying capacity of the blood is diminished (anemia), the cardiac muscle supplied by the occluded vessel will most likely become ischemic or infarcted (Fig. 10-8).

We previously noted that coagulation necrosis is the usual outcome of infarction of most tissues. Ischemic tissue becomes shrunken and hypopfunctional and is susceptible to further infarction. Infarcted tissues lose function and are structurally weakened. For example, if a small area of infarcted cardiac muscle is in a conduction bundle, a fatal arrhythmia might result. If a large area of cardiac muscle of the interventricular septum is infarcted, a perforation and hemorrhage between chambers might occur. If most of the left ventricular heart muscle is infarcted, acute heart failure will occur or chronic heart failure might result after the infarction has scarred. Similar morbid changes can occur in the brain (as with stroke) and most other organ systems.

EMBOLISM

Embolism exists when a solid, liquid, or gaseous mass travels within the circulatory system from the point of origin to a remote location and impacts at that location. The majority (95% to 99%) of emboli are thromboembolic that originate from either venous, cardiac, or arterial thromboses. Less common types of embolism include fat from atheromas, bone marrow from bone fracture, nitrogen gas from deep sea diving, and amniotic fluid droplets at childbirth.

Venous Embolism

Emboli that arise in the venous system will travel until they reach a narrow vascular bed. Since venous blood circulates through the right-side chambers of the heart to the lungs, most venous emboli lodge in the pulmonary arteries, arterioles, and capillaries (Fig. 10-9). Previously we have noted that phlebothrombosis of deep leg veins is common in debilitated individuals. These thrombi can be easily dislodged by physical activity. The fragments of thromboemboli will travel through the iliac veins, inferior vena cava, right atrium, right

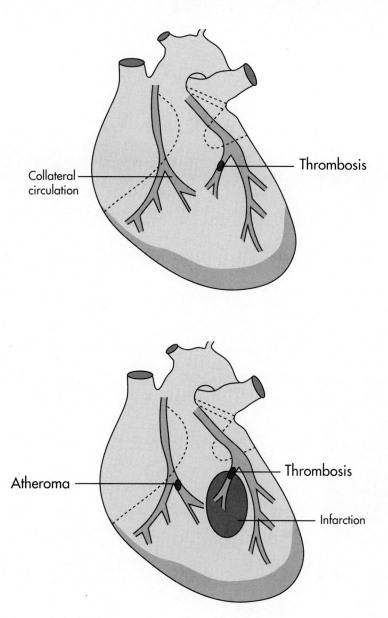

Collateral circulation

Thrombosis

Atheroma

Thrombosis

Infarction

Fig. 10-8 When collateral circulation is adequate, a coronary thrombosis will not infarct the heart muscle. However, if there is inadequate or reduced collateral circulation, the same thrombosis will cause an infarction.

ventricle, and pulmonary arteries and lodge in the pulmonary arterioles. Because the leg veins are large and flaccid, these emboli may be large and, following fragmentation, numer-ous. As a result, the sequelae of the pulmonary thromboembolization may include acute pas-sive congestion of the right side of the heart and infarction of the lungs. If the patient—

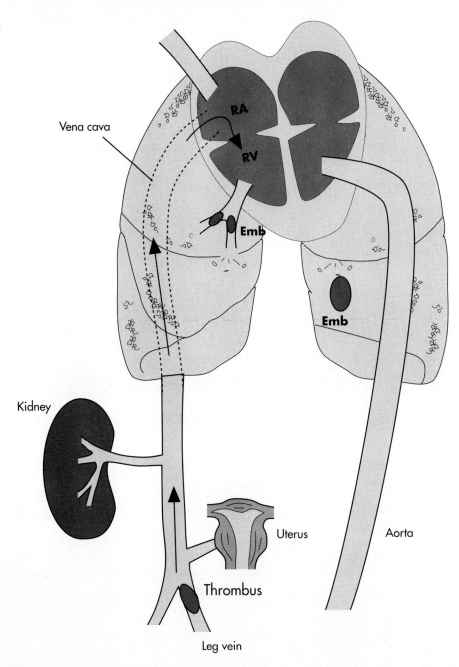

Fig. 10-9 Emboli that originate in the veins of the leg, uterus, or kidney will most likely travel through the right side of the heart and lodge in the pulmonary circulation.

who was already incapacitated—has preexisting lung disease or heart failure, death might follow. Most hospitals and nursing homes attempt to prevent such phlebothrombosis from occurring by keeping the patients active, using support hose to enhance venous circulation, and using anticoagulants when possible.

Arterial embolism

Thrombi that originate in heart chambers, valves, and large arteries can also fragment, dislodge, and embolize. The arterial circulation will carry those emboli to smaller-diameter arteries, arterioles, and capillaries, where they will impact. Sequelae include dissolution and recanalization, or more pathologically significant ischemia and infarction of tissues.

HEART DISEASE

Ischemic Heart Disease

Heart disease is the most common cause of death in the United States. There are numerous causes of heart disease. We will discuss several of the more important types. The most common pathologic heart condition is *ischemic heart disease* (IHD). As the name indicates, the pathogenesis is based on reduction of blood flow (ischemia) to cardiac muscle from the coronary arteries. The most common cause of ischemic heart disease is plaque formation in the coronary arteries—vessels that are especially susceptible to atherosclerosis. Four clinical conditions have been classified as types of ischemic heart disease (Fig. 10-10). *Angina pectoris* is the condition that is characterized by recurrent chest pains and discomfort resulting from ischemia of coronary muscles. There is no apparent infarction (necrosis) of heart muscle. The severity of pain varies but is usually greater in association with exercise. Patients who have angina pectoris are uncomfortable and anxious about their condition. The pain

can be confused with the symptoms of more severe myocardial infarction. Symptoms of angina can be controlled with coronary artery–dilating medications such as nitroglycerin tablets or patches. The dental patient with angina pectoris should be evaluated to make sure that he or she is medicated. Since these patients have ischemic heart disease, we must be cognizant that more serious subtypes can develop or coexist.

Sudden cardiac death (SCD) is a subtype of ischemic heart disease in which acute coronary artery obstruction and ischemia causes an altered heartbeat (arrhythmia). This typically leads to complete heart failure (cardiac arrest). Unless corrected immediately by cardiopulmonary resuscitation (CPR), death within an hour is likely. At time of autopsy, it is discovered that most SCD victims had severe—but previously silent—coronary artherosclerosis.

Myocardial infarction (MI) is the form of ischemic heart disease that occurs when a focal section of the heart becomes necrotic and coagulated because of either severe atherosclerosis or coronary thrombosis. Myocardial infarction can result in acute cardiac failure or chronic arrhythmia. Patients who survive (75%) are at risk for additional MI or SCD. When the patient survives, the infarcted muscle heals by scarring—leading in some cases to congestive heart failure. Myocardial infarction is the most important cause of death from ischemic heart disease.

Chronic ischemic heart disease (CIHD) is a slowly developing chronic condition causing long-term diffuse cardiac muscle degeneration and necrosis with subsequent fibrosis. The heart becomes atrophic and cardiac output is reduced. Patients seldom experience chest pain characteristic of angina pectoris, and rarely have arrhythmia. The condition results in weakness and congestive heart failure, and death may result from severe congestive heart failure or the development of MI or SCD.

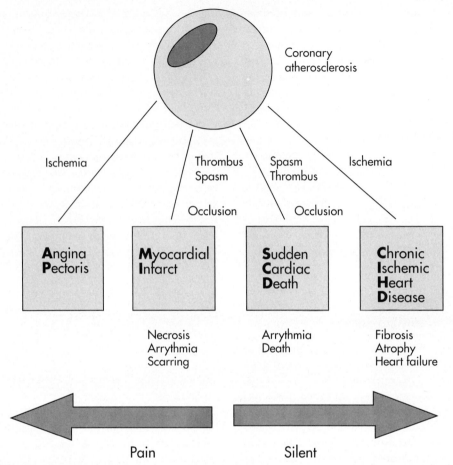

Fig. 10-10 Ischemic heart disease can lead to morbidity in four ways, which can be distinguished by clinical manifestations and tests.

Ischemic heart disease can frequently be prevented by reducing the risk factors for atherosclerosis. When coronary atherosclerosis has already begun, the incidence of IHD and thrombosis can be reduced medically (with coronary vasodilators), surgically (with bypass surgery, coronary artery dilatation) and with anticoagulants (aspirin, warfarin). Abnormalities in cardiac output and arrhythmias are also frequently treated medically. Evaluation of the dental patient's coronary-cardiac status and medications is mandatory for proper dental care.

Valvular Heart Disease

The knowledge of valvular heart disease is necessary for correct dental treatment. Certain valvular conditions such as mitral stenosis, rheumatic heart disease, mitral valve prolapse (click, murmur, Barlow syndrome), and prosthetic valvular replacement can predispose the patient to *bacterial endocarditis* (Fig. 10-11). Routine dental procedures such as scaling, surgery, extractions, and probing will cause a transient bacteremia of nonvirulent oral organisms in most patients. If the individual has a

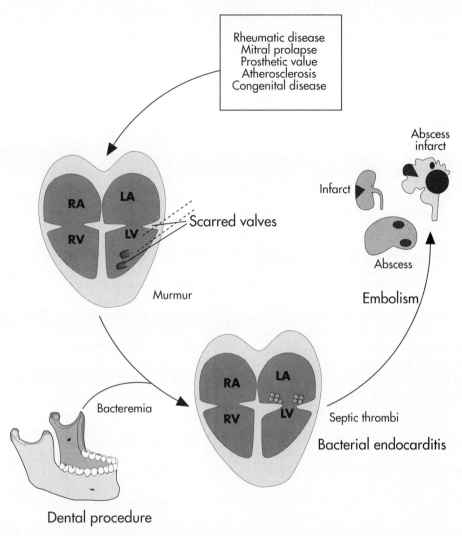

Fig. 10-11 Scarred mitral or aortic valves are susceptible to infected thrombosis following a dental procedure. These septic thrombi can cause valvular damage or embolize to organs of the body where they cause infarctions and infections.

murmur, it may represent one of the previously listed diseases. The damaged heart valve is susceptible to bacterial colonization and septic thrombosis from the bacteremia. The infected valve and endocardium can become weakened, and the infected thrombi may embolize to the systemic organs, where they will infect or infarct the tissues. Historical knowledge of a murmur or of the aforementioned diseases allows the dental practitioner to premedicate with antibiotics and prevent the complications of bacterial endocarditis.

Case Studies

Case 1

H.G. is a 78-year-old female dental patient who lives in a nursing home. Her health history includes heart attacks at 64, 65, and 68 years of age. She has resided in the nursing home for the past 10 years and has been hospitalized twice for congestive heart failure. She is taking medications to stimulate a stronger heartbeat [Lanoxin]), to reduce edema (furosemide [Lasix]), and to replace potassium. She has been confined to a wheelchair for 8 years because of fatigue, weakness, and instability. She has three-pillow nocturnal orthopnea and grade 3+ pitting edema of both ankles. She is quite forgetful and has recently misplaced her partial denture. Her dental treatment plan is conservative, and her partial denture will not be replaced according to this plan.

Case 2

B.A. is a 59-year-old male diabetic patient whose condition is controlled with insulin injection. He has 78 pack years of smoking experience. His father and brother both died of myocardial infarction by age 50. He has suffered with angina pectoris for the past 5 years, controlled somewhat with a nitroglycerin skinpatch. His wife canceled his dental appointment because he is hospitalized with a recent heart attack. After 14 days his arrhythmia persists, and he remains hospitalized. He has recently developed three-pillow orthopnea and bronchopneumonia.

Case 3

C.B. is a 38-year-old man who on his health history gives a diagnosis of end-stage autoimmune kidney disease. He is presently awaiting a kidney transplant. His medicated blood pressure at his dental visit is 220/160. The dentist has previously postponed elective dental surgery because of hypertension. After measurement of blood pressure, C.B. is immediately referred to his physician and his surgery is again deferred.

Case 4

R.Z. is a 49-year-old man who has been taking beta-blockers and diuretics for the past 6 years to control hypertension. His blood pressure at his dental appointment is 110/75. After extensive scaling and polishing lasting for 1 hour, R.Z. is moved to the upright position and dismissed. When leaving the chair, he feels unsteady and quite dizzy. He is placed in a horizontal position for 10 minutes and feels quite comfortable but embarrassed. After slowly getting up, R.Z. leaves the office without incident.

Case 5

A.M. is a 68-year-old woman who is being treated for chronic ischemic heart disease, hypertensive heart disease, and diabetes and is now bedridden. On the fourth day of confinement, A.M. develops swelling of the right calf and ankle, and pain in the right leg. Suddenly, 2 days later on her way to the bathroom, she develops difficulty in breathing and suffers cardiac arrest. Cardiopulmonary resuscitation and emergency medical services are necessary. In the emergency room, chest radiography reveals large occlusive emboli of the right and left pulmonary arteries. Surgical removal fails, and A.M. dies of cardiogenic shock 3 hours after hospitalization.

Case 1

1. Do you think H.G.'s history of heart attack contributes to the pathogenesis of congestive heart failure?
2. Explain the fatigue and weakness based on the given information.
3. Explain three-pillow orthopnea and its probable origin.
4. Explain bilateral ankle edema and its probable origin.
5. Draw and explain the evolution of her ankle edema.
6. Would you consider certain dental procedures or medications to be risky for H.G.?

Case 2

1. What risk factors for heart disease are present? Why did B.A. develop symptoms at age 54?

2. What, if any, is the association between angina pectoris and myocardial infarction (heart attack)?
3. Is arrhythmia often a consequence of myocardial infarction?
4. Explain the possible pathogenesis of his pulmonary disease.

Case 3

1. Why might C.B.'s blood pressure be so high?
2. Are there any immediate or long-term risks associated with this hypertension?
3. Why does the dentist measure blood pressure?
4. Why was oral surgery deferred?

Case 4

1. How do beta-blockers and diuretics control hypertension?
2. Why might R.Z. become dizzy?
3. Is the hypertension controlled?
4. Should the dentist continue to monitor blood pressure at future appointments?

Case 5

1. What is chronic ischemic heart disease?
2. What is hypertensive heart disease?
3. Do you think A.M. has atherosclerosis? Arteriolosclerosis?
4. What was the most likely site of origin of the emboli?
5. Can emboli cause cardiac arrest? How?

SUMMARY

- Edema of tissues usually is caused by the leakage of watery fluid from intact vessels. Common causes of edema include vessel permeability secondary to inflammation, increased hydrostatic pressure from venous obstruction or heart failure, decreased osmotic pressure in blood serum, and obstruction of the lymphatic drainage of the tissue.
- Vascular congestion usually is accompanied by tissue edema. Chronic congestion can lead to atrophy, fibrosis, and hemosiderin pigmentation of the tissues.
- Heart failure causes congestion and edema of the tissues drained by the affected chamber of the heart. Left heart failure yields congestion and edema of the lungs. Right heart failure causes edema and congestion of the liver, spleen, intestines, and ankles.
- Left ventricular failure usually results from myocardial or valvular disease. Right ventricular failure usually results from pulmonary hypertension.
- Hemorrhage is controlled by vasoconstriction, platelet-endothelium adhesion, and activation of clotting proteins with resultant fibrin clot formation.
- Agents that interfere with the clotting mechanisms will leave the patient susceptible to hemorrhage.
- Blood pressure is regulated by cardiac output, hormonally controlled water retention, and the volume of the vascular system. Reduction in any of these mechanisms can result in low blood pressure and an increase can result in high blood pressure.
- The kidneys play a pivotal role in regulating blood pressure through the renin-angiotensin system and through water retention.
- Hypertension is usually essential, or idiopathic.
- Hypertension leads to atherosclerosis, hypertensive kidney and heart disease, stroke, and other pathologic sequelae.
- Medications that reduce cardiac output, inhibit angiotensin, and increase kidney excretion are useful in controlling hypertension.
- Shock results from acute loss of blood pressure caused by vasodilation and leakage or reduced cardiac output. Allergy, hemorrhage, heart failure, sepsis, and neurogenic factors can cause shock.
- Shock leads to severe metabolic tissue changes and therefore must be reversed by endogenous mechanisms or external intervention.
- Atherosclerosis is primarily a disease of arteries caused by a combination of major and minor risk factors.

- The pathogenesis of atherosclerosis is based on vascular injury and repair, thrombosis, and lipid infiltration of artery walls.
- Atherosclerosis can lead directly to tissue ischemia and infarction or indirectly to thrombosis with resultant ischemia and infarction.
- Thrombosis occurs when there is stasis, turbulence, vascular injury, or hypercoagulability within an intact blood vessel. The majority of thrombi dissolve or organize without causing disease.
- Venous thrombi can cause passive congestion and can embolize—usually to the lungs.
- Arterial thrombi can lead to ischemia and infarction of tissues.
- Ischemia of tissues leads to degeneration, atrophy, and necrosis of tissues. Ischemia can be caused by vascular reduction, thrombosis, or increased tissue demand.
- Infarction of tissues is dependent on the degree of ischemia and the amount of collateral circulation.
- Ischemic heart disease usually results from coronary artery atherosclerosis. Subtypes include sudden cardiac death, myocardial infarction, angina pectoris, and chronic ischemic heart disease.

Suggested readings

1. Bisno AL: Group A streptococcal infections and acute rheumatic fever, N Engl J Med 325:783, 1991.
2. Castelli WP: The triglyceride issue: a view from Framingham, Am Heart J 112:432, 1986.
3. Council on Dental Therapeutics, American Heart Association: Preventing bacterial endocarditis: a statement for the dental professional, JADA 122:87 1991.
4. Hawiger J: Formation and regulation of platelet and fibrin hemostatic plug, Hum Pathol 18:111, 1987.
5. Kannel WB, McGee D, and Gordon T: A general cardiovascular risk profile: the Framingham study, Am J Cardiol 38:46, 1976.
6. Kaplan NM: Systemic hypertension: mechanisms and diagnosis. In Braunwald E, editor: Heart disease, ed 3, Philadelphia, 1988, WB Saunders Co., pp 819-848.
7. Kumar V, Cotran RS, and Robbins SL: Basic pathology, ed 5, Philadelphia, 1992, WB Saunders Co., chapter 4.
8. McMahon SW and others: Mitral valve prolapse and infective endocarditis, Am Heart J 113:1291, 1987.
9. Perloff JK and Child JS: Clinical and epidemiologic issues in mitral valve prolapse: overview and perspective, Am Heart J 113:1324, 1987.
10. Quinn EL: Bacterial endocarditis, Postgrad Med 44:82, 1968.
11. Ross R: The pathogenesis of atheroslcerosis: an update, N Engl J Med 314:488, 1986.
12. Young JB, Pratt CM, and Luchi RJ: Coronary heart disease. In Rose LF and Rose KD, editors: Internal medicine for dentistry, ed 2, St Louis, Mosby, pp 462–477.

11 Developmental Diseases

IN THIS CHAPTER

After studying this chapter, you should be able to meet the following objectives and define the key terms.

- Differentiate autosomal dominant, autosomal recessive, and sex-linked recessive inheritance patterns.
- Define the Philadelphia chromosome and recognize its significance in certain leukemias.
- Name diseases resulting in chromosomal abnormalities of deletion and addition.
- Explain the possible role of genetics in susceptibility to some common diseases and infections.
- Define genotype, phenotype, dominant, recessive, genetic penetration, and expression.
- Relate examples of environmental factors that cause developmental diseases.
- Discuss polygenic diseases and the role of environmental factors in disease expression.
- Recognize common oral developmental diseases by location, appearance, history, and behavior.
- Define developmental cysts and classify them by location or origin.
- Recognize the common developmental conditions of teeth.
- Discuss the clinical findings in amelogenesis imperfecta and dentinogenesis imperfecta.
- Relate dentinogenesis imperfecta to osteogenesis imperfecta.
- Recognize the significance of supernumerary teeth, dens in dente, and dental dilaceration.
- Distinguish forms of tooth discoloration by clinical findings and history.
- Define delayed eruption and explain the significance of its relationship to local and systemic diseases.
- Recognize dental tori and exostoses.

Each individual is unique based on the presence and combination of genetic material available and the activation or repression of that material. Physical appearance, biochemical function, behavioral attributes, personality, and disease susceptibility are all to an extent determined by this combination of genetic material found on the 44 paired autosomes and two sexual chromosomes. These traits are passed down as recombinations and mixtures of the genetic material of the two parents. However, occasional spontaneous changes (mutations) of genetic material occur.

The environment also frequently plays an important role in determination of the physical and behavioral attributes of individuals. Environmental influences can derepress or suppress existing genetic material to allow for expression of various genes. These genes directly influence the biochemical and anatomic development and function of tissues. For example, identical (monozygotic) twins share essentially the same genetic makeup in the same combinations (genotypes). Twin studies show that monozygotic twins raised in the same environment have similar appearance, are usually the same height and weight, have similar intelligence, and frequently contract comparable diseases based on contact with injurious agents. The degree of concordance (similarity) is much less for nonidentical (dizygotic) twins and approximates that for siblings. Dizygotic twins and siblings, however, have a greater degree of concordance of anatomic, behavioral, and pathologic features than do nonrelated (adopted) children who live in a similar environment. Separated monozygotic twins that are raised in dissimilar environments still acquire numerous physical, behavioral, and pathologic similarities—exceeding the degree of concordance of siblings, though showing less similarity than if they had been raised in the same environment. For example, identical twins usually experience caries in the same locations on the teeth and in roughly simultaneous fashion. Separated identical twins have greater variation, based on environmental differences (sugar diet, hygiene). There are also concordant studies showing that separated identical twins tend to develop more similar lifestyles, vocations, habits, and even so-called environmental diseases, when compared to nonsiblings living within the same environment. Of course, some environmental influences (A-bomb) can be so enormous in consequence that they will influence any circumstance—no matter the genotype of the involved individual.

Genetic diseases are disorders resulting in cell injury and dysfunction attributable to abnormal gene arrangements. Genetic diseases may result from *chromosomal abnormalities,* where chromosomes or portions of chromosomes are either duplicated or missing. Genetic diseases can also result from *mendelian* abnormalities, where specific defective genes are present and code for cellular injury and dysfunction. These mendelian disorders are inheritable and therefore are passed down through generations of families. Finally, genetic diseases may result from disorders of *polygenic* (multiple gene) combination. These disorders usually are manifest only when environmental injury affects the genetically susceptible individual.

CHROMOSOMAL ABNORMALITIES

Abnormal numbers of chromosomes almost always lead to serious disease or death. As cells divide mitotically or meiotically, errors in chromosome separation can occur. Such accidents can result in chromosomal deletion or addition. Either way, the result is usually deleterious—too much is often as bad as too little. For example, trisomy 21 (Down's) syndrome is a common chromosomal abnormality which is more likely to occur in children when mothers give birth after age 35. In this condition, the affected child is born with an extra chromosome 21 (three) rather than the normal matched pair. The extra genetic material results in numerous abnormalities including mental retardation, mongoloid facial features, growth and bone development deformities, heart defects, and other problems. Dental problems such as macroglossia and cleft palate frequently co-exist with this condition. Trisomy 21 syndrome is usually the result of chromosomal nondisjunction (failure of paired chromosomes to pull apart) during cell division.

Turner's syndrome is a chromosomal abnormality resulting from deletion of an X chromosome in a female embryo. As a result the child has XO genotype rather than having a normal XX female combination. Short stature, webbing of the neck, abnormal edema of the face, and a lack of secondary female sexual characteristics occurs. Interestingly, in rare cases, girls are born with extra X chromosomes (XXX). These individuals are female, but are also sterile and have numerous developmental disturbances (Fig. 11-1).

In Klinefelter's syndrome, an X chromosomal nondysjunction usually results in an XXY (47) individual who appears as a male (Fig. 1-11). The additional X chromsome causes hypogonadism with sterility and feminization of the secondary sexual appearance.

Disease can also result from deletion, addition, or displacement of fragments of chromosomes. A good example of chromosomal displacement occurs when portions of chromosome 22 are substituted for or become attached to chromosome 9. The newly added fragment combines with chromosome 9, and the so-called Philadelphia chromosome (22-) is formed. About 90% of individuals who develop chronic myelogenous leukemia (white cell cancer) show evidence of the Philadelphia chromosome. The chromosome, however, is extremely rare in the normal non-leukemic population. This example, then, provides evidence that chromosomal translocation can cause disease and that some cancers have a genetic etiology (Fig. 11-2). An increased incidence of leukemia is also associated with Trisomy 21 syndrome.

MENDELIAN DISORDERS

Mendelian diseases are coded by the genetic information available at a specific site on a chromosome. The presence and arrangement of the coded genetic material of an individual is termed the *genotype*. The functional and anatomic expression of the genetic material is termed the *phenotype*. If an individual inherits the genes for brown eye color, that individual will have the genotype for brown eyes—even if born without eyes. If an individual has the genotype for brown eyes and is born with brown eyes, that individual has both the genotype and phenotype of brown eye color. Mendelian genetic characteristics are passed down through generations. An abnormal gene area (locus) may code for an abnormal biochemical reaction resulting in abnormal cellular structure and function. Since all gene loci are paired, the genetic disease can be the result of one major (*dominant*) abnormal gene or two lesser (*recessive*) abnormal genes. The presence of a dominant gene will almost always dictate function. That is, if the dominant gene is abnormal, the function is also abnormal. Using our previous example, the gene for brown eyes is dominant over the gene for blue eyes. If the genotype includes either two dominant brown eye genes or one brown eye gene and one recessive blue eye gene, the phenotype will be for brown eyes. If the genotype of an individual has paired blue recessive genes, the phenotype will be for blue eyes (Fig. 11-3).

Most mendelian genetic diseases are the consequence of gene mutations resulting in biochemical or structural abnormalities. Since some of these mutations are compatible with survival (sublethal), they can be passed down through generations in a mathematically predictable manner. Dominant genetic disorders are typically expressed in every generation.

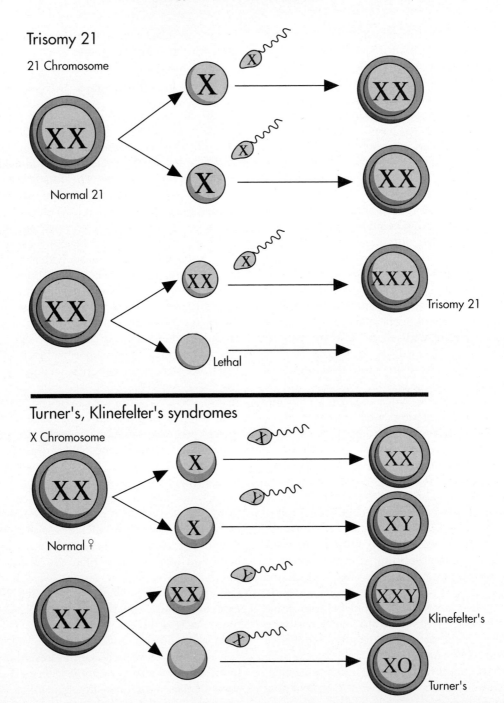

Fig. 11-1 Trisomy 21 results from failure of duplicated chromosomes 21 to separate during cell division. In Klinefelter's syndrome the failure of the x-chromosome to separate during cell division results in an XX genotype. In Turner's syndrome an x-chromosome is deleted during cell division, resulting in an XO genotype.

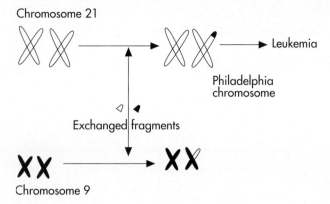

Fig.   11-2   The Philadelphia chromosome is formed when fragments of chromosome 9 are displaced on chromosome 21. This figure shows exchange of chromosomal fragments between these two chromosomes.

Although these disorders may cause serious disease, they are seldom fatal before the age of paternity or maternity. Recessively inherited disorders, on the other hand, usually skip a generation or multiple generations and frequently cause serious illness and even death when present. Recessive genetic diseases and traits are transferred by carriers, that is, individuals who are genotypically heterozygous and therefore not phenotypically affected. For example, one brown-eyed heterozygote may have a blue-eyed child if she marries another brown-eyed heterozygote (25% chance) or if she marries a blue-eyed homozygote (50% chance) (Fig. 11-3). Can she have blue-eyed children with a brown-eyed homozygote? (Answer: No.)

Although we can and frequently do predict the mathematical chance of mendelian genetic disorders and traits developing from genotypically determined parents, other factors play an important role in prediction of genetic transmission. One of these factors is termed *penetrance*. All individuals who carry a dominant gene do not necessarily exhibit the phenotype coded by that gene. Such a gene is said to lack penetrance—that is, the gene is not phenotypically expressed. Theoretically, rare instances occur where genotypic heterozy-

gotes for brown (dominant) eyes have blue eyes because the brown dominant gene lacks penetrance. In some diseases, the lack of penetrance is common—probably because more than one pair of genes codes for the normal structure and function.

Phenotypic features are expressed in mendelian genetic disorders; however, in some patients this *expression* may be very mild and even difficult to detect. A patient who has an autosomal dominant condition for numerous freckles and polyps can be said to have mild expressivity of the phenotype if he or she only has one freckle and a few polyps. This patient has the genotype for disease but does not express the phenotype with the typical severity or quantity.

There are several subtypes of mendelian disorder, which we will discuss in some detail. The box on page 175 provides further illustration of these different types.

Autosomal Dominant Disorders

As previously noted, autosomal dominant types of disorders may occur when one overriding (dominant) gene in a pair is present. These conditions phenotypically occur in every generation and are seldom lethal. Rarely,

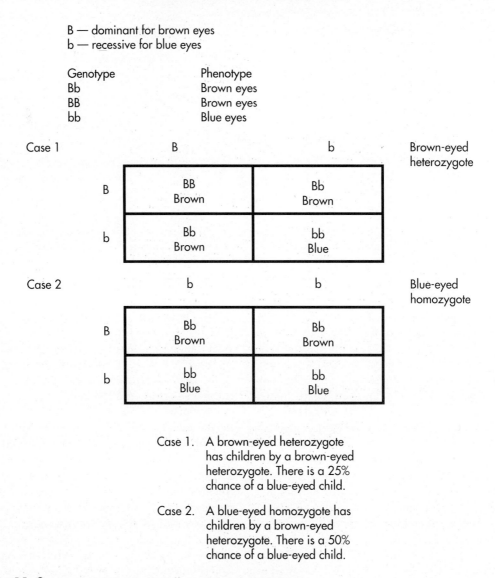

B — dominant for brown eyes
b — recessive for blue eyes

Genotype	Phenotype
Bb	Brown eyes
BB	Brown eyes
bb	Blue eyes

Case 1 — B — b — Brown-eyed heterozygote

	B	b
B	BB Brown	Bb Brown
b	Bb Brown	bb Blue

Case 2 — b — b — Blue-eyed homozygote

	b	b
B	Bb Brown	Bb Brown
b	bb Blue	bb Blue

Case 1. A brown-eyed heterozygote has children by a brown-eyed heterozygote. There is a 25% chance of a blue-eyed child.

Case 2. A blue-eyed homozygote has children by a brown-eyed heterozygote. There is a 50% chance of a blue-eyed child.

Fig. 11-3 Autosomal dominant and recessive transmission.

the conditions may appear to skip generations because of lack of penetrance or mild expressivity. Autosomal dominant osteogenesis imperfecta serves as a good model for this type of disorder. This genetic condition results from an autosomal dominant mutant gene that interferes with the biochemistry of collagen maturation (see the chart on page 175). As a result, affected individuals demonstrate poorly collagenized connective tissues, including those of the bones, teeth, and eyes. The clinical expression is thin, weak bones that easily fracture (brittle bones); malformed, dysfunctional dentin in all teeth (opalescent teeth); and blue-colored sclera of the eyes resulting from thin scleral connective tissues. Bone fractures occur at early ages, are multiple, are usually associated with very low

Chart 1: Mendelian disorders

Autosomal dominant—One gene (dominant) in the pair dictates the abnormal phenotype (osteogenesis imperfecta)

Gene A   brittle bones
Gene a   normal bones

Genotype	Phenotype
AA homozygous	brittle bones
Aa heterozygous	brittle bones
aa homozygous	normal bones

Autosomal recessive—The dominant gene dictates a normal phenotype; the recessive gene dictates an abnormal phenotype (cystic fibrosis)

Gene C   normal secretion
Gene c   abnormal secretion

Genotype	Phenotype
CC homozygous	normal secretion
Cc heterozygous	normal secretion (carrier)
cc homozygous	abnormal secretion

Sex-linked recessive—The recessive gene is located on the X chromosome only; the Y chromosome is void of the gene pair; the recessive gene dictates abnormal phenotype (hemophilia).

X_H normal factor VIII
X_h lack of factor VIII
Y   no code for VIII

Genotype	Phenotype
$X_H X_H$	normal, female
$X_H Y$	normal, male
$X_H X_h$	normal, female (carrier)
$X_h Y$	male, lack of factor VIII (hemophilia)

Codominant—Both genes of the pair are dominant and share equally the phenotype expression (ABO blood)

Gene A   A blood antigen
Gene B   B blood antigen
Gene O   void, no antigen

Genotype	Phenotype
AA	Type A blood
AB	Type AB blood
BB	Type B blood
AO	Type A blood
BO	Type B blood
OO	Type O blood

grade trauma, and may be lethal to the fetus or neonate. Dental problems can also be considerable and result in severe wear and fractures of all teeth. The condition is passed down directly through each generation with variable expressivity. In cases of severe expressivity, death will occur because of multiple fractures during birth. With mild expressivity, the adult patient may give a history of three or four bone fractures, and the teeth may appear normal.

Autosomal Recessive Disease

Autosomal recessive diseases are typically transmitted through nonaffected carriers. Affected families who are consanguineous (intermarried) have a markedly increased chance that two carriers will produce offspring who will be homozygous for the recessive defect (see the chart). Most recessive disorders produce biochemical defects rather than structural defects; therefore, metabolic diseases are the result. Cystic fibrosis is an autosomal recessive disorder that typically is fatal before age 20. The homozygous recessive proband demonstrates recessive genes on chromosome 7 responsible for a biochemical deficiency resulting in abnormal and excessive secretions of sweat glands, other exocrine glands, and connective tissues. The end result is mucous plugging of pancreatic ducts, bronchi, and salivary glands. Resultant infections and fibrosis of these organs frequently occur, with death usually from pulmonary disease. Treatment and prevention include mucus vacuuming and dislodgment, and use of mucus-dissolving solutions. It is estimated that one in 20 individuals is a cystic fibrosis carrier. Most carriers cannot be detected by biochemical analysis of the mucus-secreting system, but can be detected by DNA analysis. Prevention includes genetic counseling and experimental genetic engineering.

Sex-Linked Recessive Disorders

Occasionally, genetic disorders are carried and coded by the X sex chromosomes rather than by the 22 paired autosomes. Remember that the female genotype is XX, and the male is XY. In most cases, the Y chromosome plays little role in phenotypic expression of genetic diseases. Therefore, male subjects who have a defective recessive gene on the single X chromosome will phenotypically express the condition (see the chart). Only rare female subjects who are homozygous for the recessive gene on both X chromosomes will be similarly affected. Such disorders are called sex-linked recessive conditions and are expressed almost exclusively in male subjects. Several types of hemophilia, color blindness, and ectodermal dysplasia are usually sex-linked recessive conditions. The woman is always the carrier of these conditions and passes the genotype on to her sons.

Hemophilia A is a sex-linked recessive disease in which there is a deficiency of clotting factor VIII. Lack of this factor delays fibrin formation in clotting (see Chapter 10) and results in both posttraumatic hemorrhage and spontaneous bleeding. This condition is well known historically because the mutation occurred in the families of European nobility during the eighteenth and nineteenth centuries. The condition was prevalent among the kings and princes in many European countries and was perpetuated because of the practice of intermarriage. Hemophilia A still occurs in the United States and can now be controlled by administration of concentrated factor VIII.

Codominant Disorders

Occasionally, genetic disorders and traits show a codominant pattern of expression. These disorders allow for expression from both members of the gene pair rather than total dominance of one gene over the other. Sickle cell disease is a good example of a codominant disorder. A recessive genetic defect allows for substitution of a single amino acid (valine) for another amino acid (glutamic acid) on the hemoglobin A molecule of red blood cells. This simple substitution changes the function of the hemoglobin molecule considerably. The changed hemoglobin is now known as hemoglobin S rather than hemoglobin A. Hemoglobin S is very sensitive to lowered oxygen conditions, causing the red blood cells to change configuration to a sickle shape—thus the term sickle cell disease. Sickled red blood cells become hemolytic, lose their ability to transport oxygen (causing anemia), and clog blood vessels. This condition seldom is activated in heterozygotes (for the sickle cell trait) except in instances of extreme hypoxic stress. On the other hand, homozygotes experience severe symptoms and frequently fatal consequences. The homozygous disease is referred to as sickle cell anemia (Fig. 11-4). This codominant condition is much more prevalent in black populations. Symptoms (sickle cell crisis) can be complications of stress secondary to dental treatment.

Polygenic Disease

Finally, many diseases and disorders involve numerous genes on single and perhaps multiple chromosomes. Mutations or defects in combinations of these genes (polygenic combinations) allow for tissue injury or dysfunction. In many instances these disorders are not phenotypically apparent, and mathematical prediction of occurrence is very difficult. Frequently, environmental factors such as viral infections, medications, obesity, or aging trigger expression of these diseases. Such common conditions as diabetes, cleft lip, cleft palate, hepatitis B, and adenocarcinoma of the breast may fall into this category of disease.

The disorder cleft palate serves as a good example of a polygenic disease. This condition involves failure of the processes of the

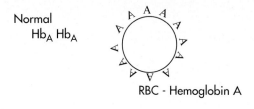

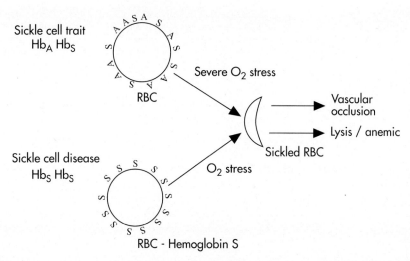

Fig. 11-4 In sickle cell trait the heterozygous hemoglobin genes code for both hemoglobin A and hemoglobin S; therefore sickling can occur under extreme conditions. In sickle cell disease most of the hemoglobin is coded by the homozygous gene for hemoglobin S. Therefore, the cells are readily sickled, resulting in disease.

palate to close during embryogenesis. The condition tends to occur in families; however, multiple generations are skipped. In laboratory animal models, a very susceptible strain of mice has been discovered. This susceptible strain exhibits 25% incidence of cleft palate formation under normal conditions. When pregnant mice are stressed with cortisone, vitamin antagonists, or environmental stress, the rate of clefting doubles and may approach 100%. If mice of different strains are subjected to similar teratogens, clefting only rarely occurs. Therefore, it is concluded that polygenic factors in combination with environmental agents are responsible for defects such as cleft palate (Fig. 11-5).

DEVELOPMENTAL DISTURBANCES OF THE JAWS

A wide variation in jaw size occurs among normal individuals, and this variation is frequently genetically determined. The variation from normal can produce numerous dental problems. The condition of having very small jaws is termed *micrognathia.* Either the mandible or the maxilla, or both jaws may be involved. This condition can give rise to numerous dental problems including impaction and crowding of teeth, and misalignment of the jaws. A pronounced micrognathia often produces facial deformity that is considered nonesthetic. Treatment includes surgical correction of tooth crowding, orthodontic tooth

Strain A = Susceptible strain
Strain B = Nonsusceptible strain

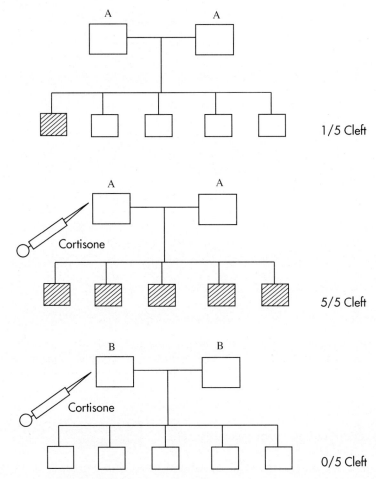

Fig.   11-5   Strain A mice are susceptible to spontaneous developmental cleft palate formation. Strain B mice are not susceptible to cleft palate. When Strain A mice are injected during pregnancy with cortisone, clefting of progeny is markedly increased. However, similar cortisone injections will not induce clefting in Strain B mice.

movement, and in more severe cases, orthognathic surgery to extend, expand, or realign the jaws to a more functional and esthetic position. In some cases, micrognathia is associated with other developmental disturbances (diminished midface area, short stature) and is thus a component of a syndrome. In rare instances, micrognathia results from another developmental disturbance. For example, patients with cleft palate usually demonstrate maxillary micrognathia. Individuals with childhood ankylosis of the condyles may develop mandibular micrognathia.

Macrognathia (large jaws) is uncommon

and is rarely developmental in origin. Again, inheritance is sometimes the cause of large jaws, and either or both jaws may be affected. Problems result from malocclusion, dental spacing, and esthetic consideration. Treatment is usually orthodontic and orthognathic surgery. The majority of instances of macrognathia involve acquired changes secondary to local or systemic disease. Local diseases such as fibrous dysplasia of bone, reactive and neoplastic bone tumors, and odontogenic cysts and tumors frequently result in macrognathia. Systemic diseases such as acromegaly and Paget's disease of bone also frequently are manifest as macrognathia. Of course, most developmental macrognathia occurs during jaw development (childhood), and most acquired conditions occur in adult life and are signaled by postpubescent growth of the jawbones.

DISEASES OF THE TONGUE

Benign Migratory Glossitis

Benign migratory glossitis is a common condition of the tongue that affects approximately 2% of the population. In most cases this condition is idiopathic and is considered developmental, even though lesions are less common in children than in adults. Rarely the tongue lesions are caused by allergy, respiratory tract infection, or iron or vitamin deficiency. Hereditary cases have been reported. The lesions appear as large, red, atrophic patches of the tongue with white, slightly raised, often C-shaped borders. Usually lesions are multiple and occur on the dorsal surface of the tongue. The red areas are void of filiform papillae, whereas the white areas show hypertrophy of papillae. The lesions often resemble the map of the world—therefore, the term geographic tongue is frequently used and is synonymous. Lesions occasionally burn or are irritated; however, most lesions are usually nonpainful. These patches resolve in days to weeks, and papillae regenerate (Fig. 11-6). The condition is recurrent, and therefore the lesions appear to

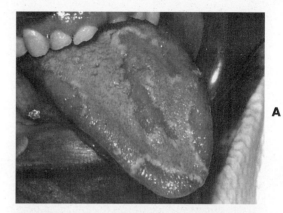

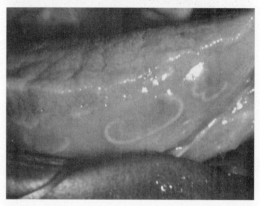

Fig. 11-6 Benign migratory glossitis. **A,** Red atrophic lesions with white borders on the dorsal surface of the tongue. **B,** C-shaped white periphery surrounds red areas on the ventral surface of the tongue.

migrate from area to area. Migration of lesions probably does not actually occur; however, enlargement of lesions is considered normal. Stress may play a factor in stimulating lesion formation. This condition is considered important because it is so common, and its lesions can be confused with more serious forms of glossitis and even premalignant or malignant lesions. There are no major sequelae to migratory glossitis. Diagnosis is usually made based on location, recurrence, and the appearance of lesions. Interestingly, biopsy reveals microscopic changes resembling those of psoriasis of the skin; however, no link between psoriasis and migratory glossitis seems to exist. Treatment consists of proper diagnosis and patient reassurance. Occasionally, topical anesthetics are used for severely symptomatic cases.

Fissured Tongue

This rather common condition occurs in about 5% of the adult population. Because childhood manifestations of fissured tongue are rare, this condition might better be considered an aging phenomenon than a developmental disease. Clinically, furrows, grooves, and clefts develop on the dorsal surface of the tongue. The depth and extent of these fissures and clefts may be striking (Fig. 11-7). Lesions develop over long periods of time and are usually asymptomatic. The patient may become alarmed on noticing the furrows and claim that the lesions arose suddenly; however, this is seldom the case. Careful oral inspection and documentation in the records usually contradict this patient observation. There are no major sequelae to fissured tongue, although burning, impaction of food and debris, and bacterial infections within the fissures are infrequent complaints. Treatment consists of reassurance about the benign nature of the condition, and a regimen of home care irrigation and tongue hygiene for those with symptoms. Patients with fissured tongue have an increased incidence of benign migratory glossitis. Rarely, fissured tongue has been reported as a component of other systemic diseases (pernicious anemia, Melkersson-Rosenthal syndrome).

Varices

Varicose veins (varices) of the ventral surface of the tongue are very common in the aging population. Since lesions are rare before age 40 and are seen in almost everyone over age 60, these lesions probably represent aging, rather than developmental disturbances. The lesions appear clinically as purple, black, or red raised, soft swellings measuring 2 to 5 mm in size. Varices are frequently multiple, with up to 50 blue-black areas becoming apparent (Fig. 11-8). These multiple areas appear as

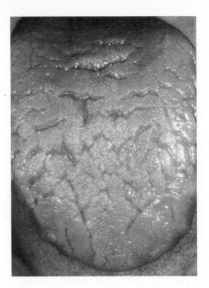

Fig. 11-7   Fissured tongue. This adult patient has a history of associated benign migratory glossitis.

"black caviar" and are sometimes termed caviar spots of the tongue. The soft varices will blanch with pressure, indicating that blood is pushed to another area of the vessel. Occasionally, varicose veins occur on other mucosal surfaces and must be differentiated from other pigmented lesions. Varicose veins are dilated, sometimes tortuous segments of normal veins. They tend to occur as a predictable consequence of aging, or less commonly, secondary to trauma. Thrombi sometimes form within varicose veins—giving the impression of rapid, solid, tumorlike growths. In most instances, diagnosis is based on location, appearance, blanching, and history. Biopsy may be necessary to aid in diagnosis when lesions occur at unusual locations (labial mucosa, buccal mucosa) or when rapid growth (indicating thrombi) occurs. There are no serious sequelae and treatment is unnecessary. Accurate diagnosis is the key to a successful outcome.

Lingual Tonsils and Lymphoid Aggregates

The posterior dorsal and posterior lateral surfaces of the tongue normally contain lym-

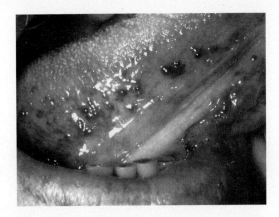

Fig. 11-8 Varices. The lesions of the ventral surface of the tongue in this 70-year-old man are asymptomatic.

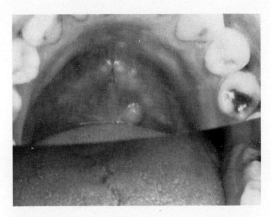

Fig. 11-9 Lymphoid aggregates. The intraoral mirror reflects a lymph nodule of the floor of the mouth.

phoid aggregates admixed with vallate papillae (on the posterior dorsal surface) and foliate papillae (on the posterior lateral surface). These aggregates are occasionally enlarged or may become hyperplastic, and consequently resemble growths or tumors. The enlarged lingual tonsils clinically appear as raised, yellow-pink submucosal swellings that are painless and soft. Enlargement is most commonly noted in the lateral posterior area of the tongue and is frequently bilateral. Sometimes a red, irritated foliate papillitis may accompany the swelling. Diagnosis is often based on location, duration, and appearance of the lesions; however, very large, long-term, and unilateral swellings may be subjected to biopsy to rule out other more serious conditions. There are no major sequelae from lingual tonsils.

Lymphoid aggregates can occur within other submucosal locations of the oral cavity. These also appear as pink to yellow, soft, raised, movable submucosal swellings. These lymphoid aggregates are most commonly located in the pharyngeal tonsillar, uvular, and soft palatal areas, and less commonly in the buccal mucosa, mandibular vestibule, and floor of the mouth (Fig. 11-9). Lesions may become enlarged and hyperplastic when stimulated by an oral or upper respiratory tract infection. When this occurs, the swelling may exceed 1 cm in diameter and biopsy for a definitive diagnosis is usually necessary. There are no serious sequelae from untreated lesions.

Macroglossia

Macroglossia or enlarged tongue is rarely developmental and more commonly an acquired condition secondary to local or systemic factors. Primary macroglossia may be inherited or may be the manifestation of some developmental disorder (mongolism, cretinism). Hamartomatous congenital defects such as lymphangioma (Fig. 11-10) and hemangioma are the usual cause of developmental macroglossia. The enlarged tongue may be an impediment to speech and mastication. Malocclusion and malalignment of teeth result if the macroglossia is left uncorrected during jaw and tooth development. Treatment includes correction of the systemic disturbance or hamartoma and surgical removal of bulk from the tongue.

Acquired macroglossia may arise from a multitude of local and systemic factors, including

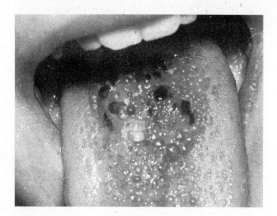

Fig. 11-10 Lymphangioma. This tongue mass was present at birth and was twice surgically reduced in size by age 12.

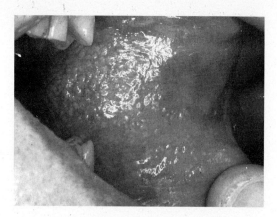

Fig. 11-11 Fordyce's granules. The multiple raised, soft, yellow granules of the buccal mucosa are bilateral.

tongue abscess, infection, lymphedema, neurofibroma, neurilemoma, vascular neoplasms, oral cancer, amyloidosis, and many other diseases. In addition, the tongue tends to enlarge and become flabby in edentulous patients who do not wear dentures. In general, the source of acquired macroglossia must be thoroughly evaluated and diagnosed since several of the conditions that produce it are quite pathogenic and even fatal.

LESIONS OF THE ORAL MUCOSA

Fordyce's Granules

Fordyce's granules are raised, soft, 1- to 3-mm, yellow submucosal lumps that are very common bilaterally on the buccal mucosa. Fordyce's granules are sebaceous gland choristomas that have developed in the submucosa in the absence of hair follicles. In many instances, hundreds of granules may be present and give the appearance of cottage cheese (Fig. 11-11). The maxillary vermilion border and labial mucosa also frequently are involved. Occasionally other mucosal surfaces exhibit Fordyce's granules—where they must be differentiated from other yellow-white lesions. Biopsy at these sites is sometimes necessary to

make this distinction. Fordyce's granules are normal in the buccal and labial mucosal areas and are present in at least 85% of patients. You will be able to readily recognize them by appearance and location. Patients rarely note their presence, nor do they become concerned. Since Fordyce's granules are normal and there are no sequelae, no treatment is necessary.

Leukoedema

The very common condition leukoedema is usually clinically apparent as milky, white-blue, somewhat folded or striated lesions of the buccal mucosa. The lesions are typically diffuse and bilateral (Fig. 11-12). If the lesions are stretched, the mucosa assumes a more normal pink, flat appearance. As the name implies, this developmental condition results from normal intracellular edema of the mucosal epithelial cells, imparting the slightly white, raised appearance. Leukoedema is very common in the black population, with 80% of black individuals estimated to have some degree of change. There are no sequelae, and no treatment is necessary. Occasionally, marked leukoedema must be differentiated from several other clinical white lesions. The term

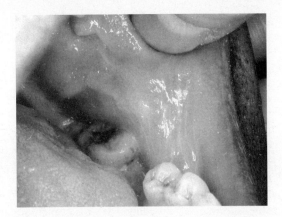

Fig. 11-12 Leukoedema. The buccal mucosa appears bilaterally white and folded.

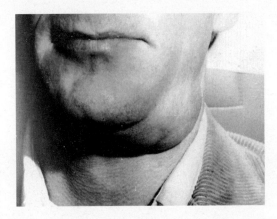

Fig. 11-13 Lymphoepithelial cyst. This large lateral neck cyst has been present for 4 years.

leukoedema should be used judiciously around patients, who may confuse it with the term leukemia—with its more serious consequences.

Lymphoepithelial Cysts

Lymphoepithelial cysts are common lesions that occur when epithelial cells are entrapped developmentally within lymph nodes or lymphoid aggregates. The epithelial component can become hyperplastic and produce an epithelium-lined fluid-filled cavity (cyst) surrounded by lymphoid tissue. A common location for this developmental phenomenon is in the cervical lymph nodes of the side of the neck. This lateral neck cyst appears as a soft, movable swelling that may achieve a large size (comparable to a golf ball) (Fig. 11-13). It must be distinguished from hyperplastic, infectious, and neoplastic lymph node disease. Occasionally the cyst drains externally and decreases in size. Intraoral lymphoepithelial cysts are usually located in the tonsillar areas (Fig. 11-14). However, any site of ectopic lymphoid tissue formation may be involved. These lesions consist of soft, yellow-white, movable, slow-growing submucosal masses. Lesions are usually excised in order to verify

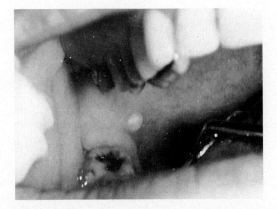

Fig. 11-14 Lymphoepithelial cyst. This small yellow cyst is located on the soft palate.

diagnosis and limit growth. There are no common major sequelae.

Gingival Fibromatosis

Hereditary gingival fibromatosis is a rare developmental lesion causing generalized fibrosis of the gingiva. This autosomal dominant condition causes fibrous proliferation of the free and attached gingiva, often resulting in tumor-like masses and sometimes completely obscuring the teeth (Fig. 11-15). At times the teeth remain impacted because they are unable to

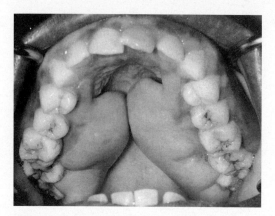

Fig. 11-15 Gingival fibromatosis. This patient is not taking any medicine.

penetrate the dense fibrous gingiva during eruption. Malocclusion is also a common sequela. Hereditary gingival fibromatosis must be differentiated from acquired hyperplastic fibromatosis (caused by drugs, irritation) by careful evaluation of the medical and genetic history and by examination. In chapters 13 and 17 we will discuss hyperplastic fibrous lesions of the gingiva. Surgical gingivectomy is usually necessary to control the condition.

Developmental Cysts

Cysts in the oral cavity develop from epithelial cells entrapped within developing bone, gingiva, or the submucosa of mucous membranes. The source of this epithelium may be entrapped components of tooth development (odontogenic), salivary glands, or embryonic fissures or sutures. A known or unknown stimulus causes these entrapped remnants to hyperplastically proliferate. Serum and cell products within the proliferative mass form a fluid-filled center that is lined by epithelium. A fibrous connective tissue capsule is almost always present. These cysts are slow growing and tend to expand the tissue of origin—be it submucosa or bone (Fig. 11-16). We will discuss the most common developmental cysts

for the remainder of this section. Cysts of odontogenic origin will be described in Chapter 14.

Fissural cysts develop from entrapped epithelium in the fissures and folds of embryonic closure of the face, maxilla, and palate, and from remnants of nasopalatine ducts of the palate. The *nasolabial cyst* is a soft tissue cyst of the upper lip at the ala of the nose. This area of the upper lip is the location of a developmental facial suture line. The cystic lesion is a slow-growing, somewhat soft, movable submucosal swelling that may push up the floor of the nose (Fig. 11-17). The *nasopalatine* (incisive canal) *cyst* occurs in the anterior area of the palate near the midline. This cyst forms from remnants of the embryonic nasopalatine duct. The cyst is frequently found within bone, where it appears radiographically as a well-demarcated radiolucency between teeth No. 8 and 9 (Fig. 11-18). It must therefore be distinguished from the common periapical cyst of odontogenic origin (Chapter 14). Rarely the nasopalatine cyst is confined to soft tissue as a swelling of the incisive papillae, or involves both bone and soft tissue together. Patients may complain of swelling, drainage, and bad taste from such a cyst.

Rare bony developmental cysts are reported in the midline palatal suture area (*median palatal cyst*) and the anterior midline mandibular fold area (*median mandibular cyst*). In addition, a developmental cyst of the maxillary fold between the lateral incisor and canine (*globulomaxillary cyst*) is controversial since the majority of these cysts are now determined to be odontogenic in origin. Since fissural cysts are uncommon, can be destructive, and must be distinguished from more pathogenic cysts and tumors, diagnostic aspiration of fluid and surgical excision (total removal) are often necessary. Sequelae include jaw expansion, tooth movement, and disfigurement. Surgical treatment usually results in a cure.

CYST	ETIOLOGY	COMMON LOCATION
Nasolabial cyst	Nasolabial suture Soft Tissue	Floor of nose Upper lip
Nasopalatine cyst	Nasopalatine duct remnants	Incisive canal area
Median palatine cyst	Palatal suture	Midline hard palate
Median mandibular cyst?	Mandibular fold?	Midline mandible
Globulomaxillary cyst?	Odontogenic?	Maxilla between lateral incisor and canine
Dentigerous cyst	Reduced enamel epithelium	Impacted tooth
Lateral periodontal cyst	Epithelial rests	Mandibular bicuspid area
Odontogenic keratocyst	Reduced enamel epithelium Epithelial rests	Mandible & maxilla
Thyroglossal duct cyst	Remnants of forming thyroid	Midline neck
Lymphoepithelial cyst	Epithelium in lymph nodule	Tonsil, lateral neck, mucosa
Dermoid/epidermoid cyst	Epithelium in dermis	Skin, floor of mouth

Fig. 11-16 Developmental cysts.

The *thyroglossal duct cyst* is a developmental cyst that originates from hyperplastic remnants of the embryonic thyroglossal duct. This duct occurs as a precursor to the thyroid gland and extends from the dorsal posterior surface of the tongue via the midline area of the neck to the thyroid area. Normally the duct degenerates; however, at times remnants can develop into movable, soft, cystic swelling of the midline area of the neck (Fig. 11-19). The cyst wall frequently contains remnants of thyroid gland. Rarely this duct does not fully develop—resulting in a mass of thyroid tissue forming in the posterior dorsal area of the tongue (*lingual thyroid gland*). Thyroglossal duct cyst is excised for diagnosis and to prevent further growth. Care must be taken by the physician to determine the presence of a

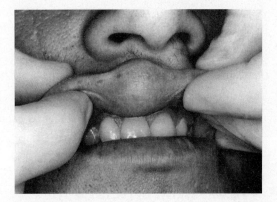

Fig. 11-17 Nasolabial cyst. This freely movable cyst was present for more than 3 years.

normal gland before a lingual thyroid or duct-associated thyroid tissue is removed.

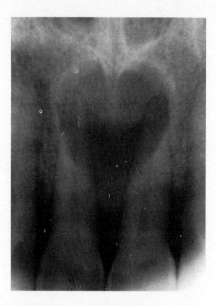

Fig. 11-18 Nasopalatine cyst. The lesion was discovered on a routine radiograph.

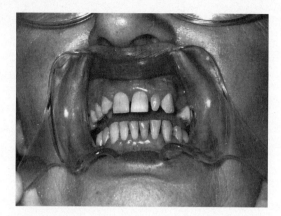

Fig. 11-20 Peg lateral incisor. The patient's parent has similar microdontia of the maxillary lateral incisors.

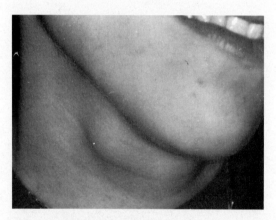

Fig. 11-19 Thyroglossal duct cyst. The origin of this neck cyst was confirmed by biopsy. (Courtesy of Dr. N.H. Rowe)

DEVELOPMENTAL DEFECTS OF THE TEETH

Patients often have improperly developed dentitions. Common defects include developmentally missing teeth, hypoplastic teeth, extra teeth, malformed teeth, and teeth that are impacted or delayed in eruption. These de-fects often result from hereditary influence; however, environmental factors also may cause specific problems with development.

Tooth size is variable within the general population. There is a range of normal tooth size. The development of small teeth that fall below this range is termed *microdontia*. Microdontia most frequently affects a limited number of teeth and only rarely exists within the entire dentition. The most common instances of microdontia occur in the third molar and maxillary lateral incisor region. These exceptionally small teeth are frequently misshapen and are usually nonfunctional. In the anterior areas, microdontia causes esthetic concerns. Peg lateral incisors are maxillary lateral incisors affected by microdontia (Fig. 11-20). These teeth and affected third molars are frequently bilateral and usually familial. Third molars affected by microdontia are usually extracted, while other affected teeth are frequently restored to meet esthetic and functional needs.

Less commonly, teeth may develop that are unusually large. This is termed *macrodontia*. This condition usually involves the entire dentition and results in crowding and malocclusion. Rarely, pituitary giantism or developmental facial hypertrophy is responsible for macrodontia; however, the condition is usually familial or idiopathic. When the condition affects individual teeth, molars are most commonly involved. Treatment often involves tooth extraction or crowning and orthodontic therapy.

Anodontia (absence of all teeth) and *oligodontia* (absence of some teeth) are developmental defects characterized by reduced numbers of teeth and should be distinguished by history and radiography from results of extraction or impaction. Partial anodontia involving third molars and maxillary lateral incisors is a common finding and is frequently familial. Developmental absence of other teeth is less common (Fig. 11-21). Correction ranges from no therapy in some instances (third molars), to prosthetic replacement for esthetics and function. Total anodontia and severe oligodontia are extremely rare and usually indicate a metabolic condition (rickets) or syndrome (ectodermal dysplasia).

Supernumerary teeth are extra teeth. This is a common developmental defect usually occurring in the midline maxillary area (mesiodens), the third molar area (fourth molars), and the maxillary canine areas. These fully formed teeth frequently remain impacted, or if erupted, invariably cause crowding of the adjacent dentition (Fig. 11-22). Supernumerary teeth may cause adjacent root resorption as a consequence of impaction or eruption. Impacted supernumerary teeth can develop odontogenic cysts or tumors. Usually, supernumerary teeth are familial or idiopathic. Some systemic conditions (cleidocranial dysplasia) can result in multiple supernumerary teeth. Therefore, patients with multiple supernumerary teeth must be thoroughly evaluated for other signs and symptoms of systemic disease. Extraction with orthodontic correction of crowding is the common mode of therapy.

Disturbances can also occur in tooth formation with resultant morphologic malformations and defects of the roots, crowns, or pulps. In addition, abnormalities in the texture and composition of enamel or dentin occur. Common morphologic defects include fusion, concrescence, and gemination. *Fusion* occurs when two individual tooth buds join during development. If the teeth are joined by the cementum only, the process is termed *concrescence.* The term *fusion* is used when adjacent teeth are joined by enamel, dentin, and cementum—resulting in formation of a giant tooth (Fig. 11-23). Impaction or esthetic disfigurement may be the consequence of either condition. Special care must be taken with

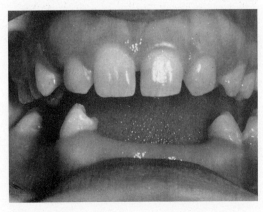

Fig. 11-21 Oligodontia. The missing teeth were never present.

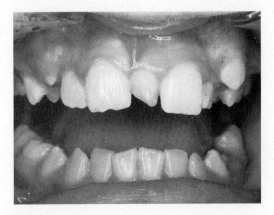

Fig. 11-22 Mesiodens. This supernumerary tooth is causing crowding of the adjacent maxillary teeth.

surgical removal of teeth that may be joined to adjacent teeth. Surgery in such cases is difficult and may result in inadvertent loosening or extraction of the associated tooth or teeth. Occasionally, developing tooth buds will divide and form Siamese twins—termed *gemination*. The end result is a large, malformed tooth with the morphology of two teeth (Fig. 11-24). Both esthetic and orthodontic considerations often warrant extraction of geminated teeth.

Individual teeth often develop with sharp angular defects of the roots, termed *dilaceration*. These angles may be multiple and are sometimes secondary to trauma during development. The secondary dentition is most frequently involved. Crowns of the teeth appear normal and function normally. The dilaceration is usually detected with dental radiographs (Fig. 11-25). Dilaceration may provide a contraindication to root canal therapy and may complicate tooth extraction; therefore, the detection of dilaceration is essential to adequate planning for these procedures.

Taurodontism is the developmental enlargement of molar tooth midbody and pulp components. This asymptomatic condition often affects multiple molars in all quadrants and is an incidental finding on radiographs (Fig. 11-26). The molar teeth show elongated midroot structure with short or absent root tips and long pulp chambers. The cause is usually idiopathic, although rare cases are components of systemic or oral syndromes. No treatment is necessary. Endodontic proce-

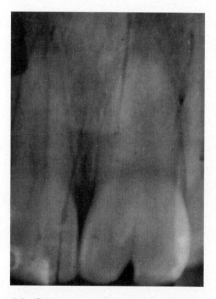

Fig. 11-24 Gemination. This central incisor partially split during development.

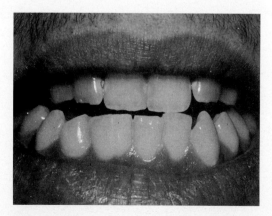

Fig. 11-23 Fusion. The mandibular right lateral and central incisors were fused during formation.

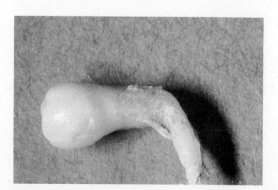

Fig. 11-25 Dilaceration. The root of this extracted canine is bent at a right angle.

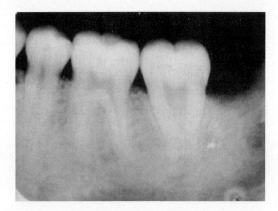

Fig. 11-26 Taurodontism. Note the elongation of the waist of the lower second molar.

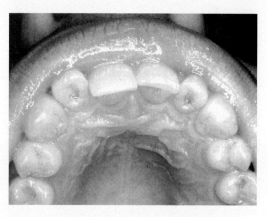

Fig. 11-27 Dens in dente. Bilateral invaginations of the maxillary lateral incisors.

dures can be somewhat complicated by taurodontism.

A rather common developmental morphologic defect of the tooth crown is termed *dens in dente*. This "tooth in a tooth" occurs when there is deep invagination of a developmental pit or fissure forming a pouch within the crown and even the root of the tooth. Maxillary lateral incisors are most often affected, with the pouch formed at the area of the lingual pit (Fig. 11-27). Bilateral occurrence is common. The crown of the tooth often appears normal visually and the defect may only be noted with a radiograph (Fig. 11-28). Frequently dens in dente results in pulp necrosis with chronic periapical infection (granuloma, cyst) that must be treated. Restorative procedures can usually prevent periapical infection if the dens in dente is detected and diagnosed prior to the infection.

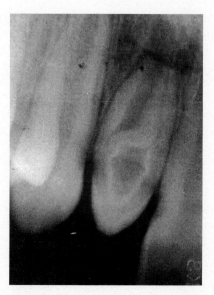

Fig. 11-28 Dens in dente. A radiograph of a maxillary incisor shows a tooth in a tooth.

Enamel Disturbances

Enamel hypoplasia results from diminished development of the enamel rods, or incomplete mineralization of the calcifying enamel. Enamel hypoplasia is usually environmental in origin and is less commonly a hereditary disturbance. *Environmental enamel hypoplasia* results from an environmental insult such as trauma, fever, exanthematous viral or bacterial disease, or ingestion of certain drugs during tooth development. Usually, all teeth developing during the times of exposure will show degrees of hypoplasia. The clinical appearance reflects the chronologic nature of the condition. The teeth show discoloration, roughness, pitting, and absence of enamel affecting all the teeth developing during the time of insult. For example, if the patient developed chickenpox at age 2, we will see a timeline of enamel hypoplasia of the cervical portions of the upper and lower incisors and upper and lower first molars corresponding to the enamel forming during the course of the disease (Fig. 11-29). The cusps of the canines may be hypoplastic as well. Other teeth should be unaffected (review the chronology of tooth development). When the cause of enamel hypoplasia is localized, as with trauma, only the teeth in the area of trauma will be involved. Restorative dentistry is usually adequate to correct the esthetic problems caused by the condition.

Hereditary enamel hypoplasia is termed *amelogenesis imperfecta* (AI). Several variants of this condition occur, with the most common being autosomal dominant. Since the genetic defects dictate hypoplastic enamel formation, all teeth in both dentitions are generally involved. One type of amelogenesis imperfecta (hypoplastic type) usually results in the complete or partial absence of enamel (Fig. 11-30). Teeth develop with crowns that are mostly void of enamel clinically and radiographically. The exposed dentin appears smooth and yellow, and is highly sensitive. Crown coverage constitutes adequate treatment. A second type of AI results in hypocalcified enamel. The enamel is present but is soft, rough, pitted, stained, and thin (Fig. 11-31). The teeth are unsightly, and restorative esthetic coverage is indicated. Finally, a third form of AI results in hypomaturation of calcified enamel (Fig. 11-32). The enamel is formed and of normal thickness; however, it appears white, chalky, and mottled. The enamel may feel rough and flake with a dental explorer. Many variants of these three forms of AI exist. Diagnosis is made based on the appearance, diffuse involvement of dentitions, and family history.

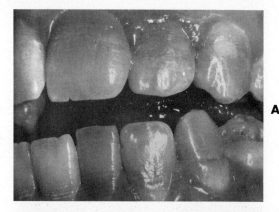

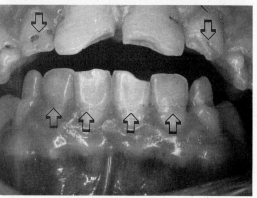

Fig. 11-29 **A,** Enamel hypoplasia—environmental. This patient was treated for multiple infections during tooth development. The linear pitting represents enamel hypoplasia. Tetracycline stains are also apparent. **B,** Severe linear enamel hypoplasia.

Discoloration of Teeth

Some environmental substances can cause developmental discoloration of teeth, with or without enamel hypoplasia. *Tetracycline* is a commonly used, broad-spectrum antibiotic used to treat a multitude of childhood infections. Individuals with long-term infectious diseases (cystic fibrosis–associated diseases, acne, recurrent pneumonia) may take tetracycline for years. The tetracycline is usually incorporated into enamel formation during tooth development, and rarely after eruption.

The enamel appears gray to yellow, depending on the chemical configuration of the antibiotic and the dosage (Fig. 11-29). These "stains" follow the expected incremental chronologic pattern of tooth development correlated to the time the drug was taken. With long-term tetracycline therapy, the entire dentition might be affected. When taken by the pregnant mother, these drugs can traverse the placenta and cause staining of the primary dentition of the infant. Children under the age of 10 and pregnant women should not be given tetracycline therapy if possible in order to prevent this condition. Since the stains are not esthetically pleasing, dental treatment such as vital bleaching of teeth, veneering, or crowning of teeth is frequently required.

Fluorosis is an uncommon condition of teeth characterized by mottled enamel. Fluoride in high concentrations may be ingested, usually from the water supply. Since the fluoride content of most public water supplies is controlled, private well water is usually the culprit. When children with developing teeth are exposed to high levels of fluoride in water,

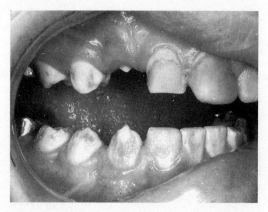

Fig. 11-31 Amelogenesis imperfecta—hypocalcified. The enamel is pitted and stained. The maxillary anterior teeth have been crowned.

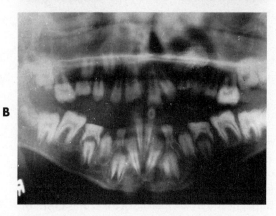

A

B

Fig. 11-30 Amelogenesis imperfecta—hypoplastic. **A,** The teeth are small and the enamel is thin. **B,** A radiograph shows deficient enamel thickness in both dentitions.

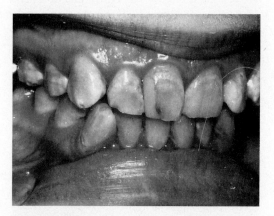

Fig. 11-32 Amelogenesis imperfecta—hypomaturation. The enamel is fully formed but appears chalky white.

discoloration and mottling of the teeth may be the manifestation of the incorporation of fluorohydroxyapatite into the developing enamel. Teeth exposed systemically during development have either brown-stained, brown-pitted, or white-mottled enamel—depending on the concentration of fluoride (Fig. 11-33). These stains may occur as lines on developmentally associated teeth or involve all teeth, again depending on the amount of time the individual drank water with high fluoride concentration. Diffuse dental fluorosis often clinically resembles the hypomaturation type of amelogenesis imperfecta. Since the stain is intrinsic and not attractive, treatment consists of vital bleaching, veneering, or crowning of teeth. Neither fluorosis nor tetracycline staining can be polished from teeth.

Dentinal Disturbances

Several developmental disturbances involve dentin formation. Dentin is the product of odontoblasts that are of connective tissue origin. The organic component of dentin is collagen, and the inorganic component is calcium hydroxyapatite. *Dentinogenesis imperfecta* (DI) is an uncommon developmental disturbance in which excessive imperfect dentin is formed and deposited in the pulp chamber. The disease usually has an autosomal dominant

etiology, and affects both dentitions and all teeth within dentitions. Characteristically the dentin is poorly mineralized and the architecture is distorted. The dentin tends to occlude the pulp chambers imparting a rather characteristic radiographic appearance. The teeth are vital; however, pulp chambers are obliterated on radiographs. Roots often appear somewhat foreshortened. The dento-enamel junction is also deformed in a way that causes the enamel to readily fracture, shear, or wear away. Patients with DI have discolored, opalescent crowns that show marked wear and fracture (Fig. 11-34). Subtypes of dentinogenesis imperfecta occur, differing by clinical appearance and etiology. Dentinogenesis imperfecta may occur in association with *osteogenesis imperfecta* (OI). This systemic bone and connective tissue disease, which we have previously discussed, is also autosomal dominant. The defect in collagen synthesis results in thin, brittle bones that fracture readily. In addition, you will remember that patients often have blue sclera and opalescent teeth similar to those of DI because of the collagen defect. In extreme cases, spontaneous abortion or stillborn infants can occur with this disease. The condition can lead to severely deforming multiple bone fractures, as well as the associated dental problems. The dental treatment for DI and opalescent dentin associated with OI is usually prosthetic crowning of the teeth, often prophylactically to prevent fracture and wear.

Disturbances in Eruption

Disturbances in tooth eruption may be of developmental nature. *Impacted teeth* are very common and usually occur in the third molar region. Maxillary and mandibular permanent canines are also frequently impacted. Impaction may be partial with some eruption of the tooth, or complete with no eruption apparent. The teeth can be prevented from erupting by bone, adjacent teeth, or dense gingival tissues. The cause of most dental impaction is inadequate jaw size or relatively large tooth size resulting in insufficient space

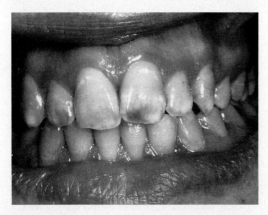

Fig. 11-33 Mottled enamel. This patient drank well water during tooth development.

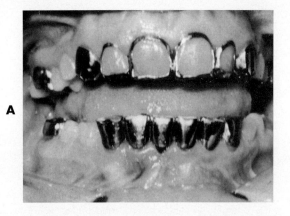

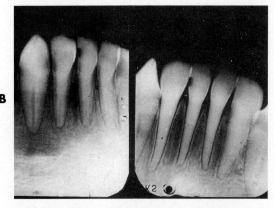

Fig. 11-34 Dentinogenesis imperfecta. **A,** Note the discolored teeth and the crowns to protect from excessive wear and fracture. **B,** Radiographs show sclerosed pulp chambers.

for eruption. Surgical extraction or surgical orthodontic eruption procedures are most commonly used to correct impaction. Impacted teeth are predisposed to develop dentigerous cysts and certain odontogenic tumors, and should therefore not be ignored. Patients with multiple impactions of teeth other than third molars should be evaluated by their dentists and physicians for several rare syndromes.

The chronology of tooth formation and eruption varies within a predictable range from individual to individual. Several condi-

tions exist that can produce either premature eruption or delayed eruption—outside the limits of this range. The concurrent presence of any of several endocrine disturbances or developmental syndromes, gingival fibromatosis, or morbid systemic and local conditions might result in delayed eruption or premature eruption of teeth. We should be cognizant of patient age and progression of tooth eruption. Delayed eruption or premature eruption should be thoroughly investigated to rule out underlying serious conditions.

DEVELOPMENTAL LESIONS OF THE BONES

Tori and Exostoses

Tori are developmental dense bony growths that usually occur in conjunction with jaw formation and growth. The *palatal torus* forms as a dense bony growth of the midline of the hard palate. The lesion is raised, often lobular, and covered with palatal mucosa (Fig. 11-35). These lesions are apparent to some degree in about 25% of the population. *Mandibular tori* are usually bilateral, lobular bony

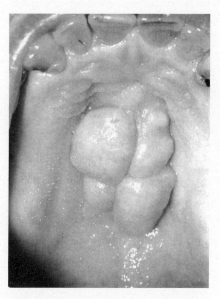

Fig. 11-35 Palatal torus.

nodules that develop in a position inferior and lingual to the lower premolars (Fig. 11-36). These lesions occur in approximately 8% of the population. Individuals with mandibular tori also frequently exhibit palatal tori. Since tori are slow-growing developmental conditions, patients are seldom aware of their existence. Occasionally the mucosa covering a torus will become ulcerated. Sometimes, following a dental procedure, the patient will discover a torus when checking the dental work that has been accomplished. As a result, patients who were not aware of the condition might become concerned about a "tumor" developing and call it to your attention. Reassurance of the patient becomes necessary. Very large tori can pose a physical barrier to prosthetic appliances and occasionally must be surgically chiseled before denture fabrication. Most tori are of no consequence and should simply be noted in the patient's record.

Bony exostoses are uncommon developmental bony growths that can originate as hard nodules from the jaws, alveolus, or palate (Fig. 11-37). Exostoses may be unilateral or bilateral, are slow growing, and grow in coordination with jaw growth. Bony exostoses should be distinguished from jaw cysts and tumors. This is usually easily accomplished by history taking, radiographs, and clinical findings. No treatment is usually necessary; however, the lesions should be recorded in the patient's chart.

Case Studies

Case 1
V.A. is a 12-year-old girl who was referred to her dentist because of brown-stained teeth. Her medical history was normal. Oral examination showed brown-white mottled enamel of the permanent dentition. Radiographs revealed apparently normal thickness and density of the enamel. The enamel felt somewhat soft and flaked when scratched with an explorer. All teeth were vital. A family history revealed that two siblings aged 10 and 14 had similar defects, and two other siblings aged 3 and 2 had no defects of their primary teeth. Neither parent was affected. The family had moved from a farm 5 years previously. A diagnosis of dental fluorosis was rendered, and esthetic dental treatment commenced.

Case 2
R.G. is a 32-year-old woman who complained of a lump of her lower left vestibular mucosa of 2 months' duration. There were no other health or oral problems. Examination revealed a firm, yellowish-pink, 1-cm oval, movable, nonpainful submucosal mass. Clinical diagnosis included be-

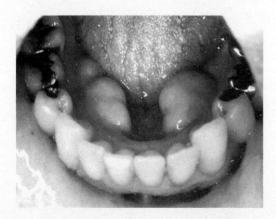
Fig. 11-36 Mandibular tori. These bilateral bony swellings are lobular.

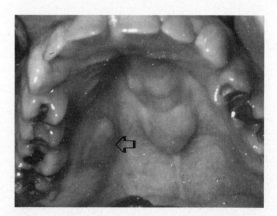
Fig. 11-37 Boney exostosis (*arrow*) and palatal torus. Both lesions have been present for many years without growth. The exostosis has become ulcerated.

nign connective tissue tumor, benign salivary gland tumor, cyst, and ectopic lymphoid tissue. Excisional biopsy revealed a mature lymphoid nodule compatible with ectopic lymphoid nodule. Healing occurred without recurrence.

Case 3

C.K. is a 35-year-old woman referred to the dental office for a red spot on the lateral surface of the tongue. She was otherwise healthy and gave a history of alcohol abuse and 30 pack years of heavy smoking. Oral examination revealed nonpainful red atrophic areas of the anterior lateral and right posterior lateral surfaces of the tongue. Each area measured 1.5 cm and showed a white keratotic border. A moderately fissured tongue was present. The patient feared oral cancer and pledged to stop smoking. When questioned, C.K. thought that similar lesions had been present previously on other areas of the tongue. A provisional diagnosis of benign migratory glossitis was rendered. The patient was placed on multivitamin therapy and scheduled for a return appointment in 3 weeks. Three weeks later the lesions had cleared, although new lesions of similar appearance had developed at the midline dorsal anterior area of the tongue. C.K. was assured that the diagnosis was benign but was warned of the harmful effects of smoking.

Case 4

H.B. is an 8-year-old boy who was missing both permanent maxillary lateral incisors. Radiographs revealed no developing or impacted lateral incisors, and there was no evidence of any other missing teeth. There were no signs of bone disease or ectodermal (hair, sweat gland) malformations. Family history revealed that the father had peg lateral incisors that were capped at age 9. The maternal grandmother—now deceased—had a history of "missing teeth." A diagnosis of congenital partial anodontia was selected, and prosthetic treatment was begun.

Case 5

S.D. is a 12-year-old boy with cystic fibrosis who was referred to the dental office because his permanent teeth were stained. His health history revealed numerous bouts of bronchitis and pneumonia with hospitalization and tetracycline therapy. He was taking medications to reduce secretions and physical therapy to keep his lungs clear. He is 4 feet tall and weighs 67 pounds. There is no history of cystic fibrosis in his parents or the family. One older sibling is not affected. Oral examination revealed gray-stained teeth throughout the dentition. The incisor enamel showed horizontal linear light-to-dark staining. Some linear pits and enamel malformations were noted on the cusps of the canines and cervical areas of all the incisors. A diagnosis of tetracycline stain and mild enamel hypoplasia was rendered. Bleaching reduced much of the stain for a 6-month period.

Case 1

1. Do environmental factors usually cause enamel hypoplasia of both the primary and secondary dentition? When might this occur?
2. If the enamel hypoplasia was autosomal dominant, would you expect this distribution in the siblings?
3. If the enamel hypoplasia was autosomal dominant, would you expect a parent to be affected? Would both parents need to be affected?
4. Explain why the two younger children did not have stained teeth.

Case 2

1. Do benign submucosal tumors appear as such clinically?
2. Which type of soft tissue cysts appear as such clinically?
3. Why was the lesion excised?

Case 3

1. Should a red spot on the lateral surface of C.K.'s tongue be worrisome based on her history of habits?
2. Is this clinical pattern typical of benign migratory glossitis?

3. Is a biopsy mandatory?
4. Is there an association between benign migratory glossitis and fissured tongue?
5. Why was C.K. encouraged to stop smoking?

Case 4

1. Is agenesis of teeth ever associated with syndromes?
2. Is agenesis of teeth ever hereditary?
3. Explain the peg lateral incisors in the proband's father. Do you think they might be related to the partial anodontia?

Case 5

1. Explain the use of tetracycline in S.D. when he was a child. Would you expect stained teeth to form?
2. What is the pathogenesis of bronchitis and pneumonia in this case?
3. Explain why the parents were not affected. Why is there no other family history?
4. Are the changes in the teeth consistent with tetracycline staining? Does tetracycline stain polish off from enamel?

SUMMARY

- Genetic factors play a role in susceptibility and resistance to many diseases.
- Gross chromosomal abnormalities including addition, deletion, and transposition of chromosomal material are implicated in specific diseases.
- Mendelian genetic diseases and characteristics result from expression of gene-derived abnormalities. The genes responsible may be autosomal dominant or recessive, codominant, polygenic, or sex-linked recessive in inheritance pattern.
- Autosomal dominant genotypes are not always expressed phenotypically.
- Polygenic disorders frequently require an environmental trigger for clinical expression of the defect.

- Common conditions of the tongue including benign migratory glossitis, fissured tongue, and tongue varicosities are easily recognized clinically and must be distinguished from more pathologic conditions.
- Macroglossia usually represents an acquired condition rather than a developmental defect.
- Fordyce's granules of the buccal mucosa are common and represent sebaceous choristomas.
- Leukoedema is normal in many patients and is readily recognizable.
- Cysts can develop from entrapped developmental epithelium in embryonic fissures, lymph nodes and nodules, nasopalatine and thyroid ducts, and from remnants of dental development.
- Hereditary or environmental factors may cause enamel hypoplasia.
- Dentinogenesis imperfecta is caused by mendelian gene defects and is often related to osteogenesis imperfecta.
- Morphologic defects in tooth formation such as dilaceration, dens in dente, fusion, and gemination can result from hereditary and environmental influences on development.
- Discoloration of teeth may be extrinsic or intrinsic in nature. Some extrinsic substances taken during development stain teeth permanently.
- Delayed eruption and impaction of teeth may indicate a systemic condition.
- Tori and exostoses are common and recognized by location, clinical, and radiographic features.

Suggested readings

1. Banoczy J, Szaba L, and Csiba A: Migratory glossitis: a clinical-histologic review of seventy cases, Oral Surg Oral Med Oral Pathol 39:113, 1975.
2. Bouchard TJ Jr: Twins reared apart and together: what they tell us about human diversity. In Fox SW, editor: The chemical and biological basis of individuality, New York, 1984, Plenum Publishing, pp 147-178.
3. Cotran RS, Kumar V, and Robbins SL: Robbins pathologic basis of disease, ed 4, Philadelphia, 1989, WB Saunders Co, pp 728-729.

4. Dolan TV Jr: Update: cystic fibrosis, Pedia Ann 15:296, 1986.

5. Kinsey RW, Ballard JB, and Matukas VJ: Sickle cell hemoglobinopathies: a protocol for management, J Oral Surg 37:441, 1979.

6. Leifer C, Chaudhry AP, and Miller RL: Effects of exogenous adrenocorticotropic hormone on palatogenesis in A/Jax mice, J Dent Res 47:843, 1968.

7. Loevy H: Developmental changes in the palate of normal and cortisone treated Strong A mice, Anat Rec 142:375, 1962.

8. Michalowicz BS and others: Periodontal findings in adult twins, J Periodontol 62:293, 1991.

9. Nora JJ and Fraser FC: Medical genetics, principles and practice, ed 3, Philadelphia, 1989, Lea & Febiger, p 202.

10. Sunderland EP and Smith CJ: The teeth in osteogenesis and dentinogenesis imperfecta, Br Dent J 149:287, 1980.

11. Witkop CJ and Stewart RE: Amelogenesis imperfecta. In Stewart RE and others, editors: Pediatric dentistry, St Louis, 1982, Mosby p 110.

12 Dental Caries, Pulpitis, and Apical Inflammation

IN THIS CHAPTER

1. Caries
   - Epidemiology
   - Pathogenesis
   - Etiology
2. Pulpal infection
   - Pulpitis
   - Acute versus chronic pulpitis
   - Reversible versus irreversible pulpitis
3. Periapical diseases
   - Periapical abscess
   - Periapical granuloma
   - Apical periodontal cyst
   - Interrelationships and management
4. Tissue infections subsequent to periapical infection
   - Parulis
   - Acute osteomyelitis
   - Cellulitis—Ludwig's angina
   - Cavernous sinus thrombosis
5. Case studies

After studying this chapter, you should be able to meet the following objectives and define the key terms:

- Explain the decrease in the U.S. caries rate over the past decade.
- List the common etiologic factors that contribute to dental caries.
- Relate the quality of dental plaque and the quantity of dental plaque to the caries process.
- List common preventive procedures and practices that can reduce the caries rate.
- Compare and contrast the pathogenesis of enamel, dentin, and cemental caries.

- Explain the role of saliva in caries control.
- Compare the clinical signs and symptoms of reversible and irreversible pulpitis.
- Describe the pathogenesis of periapical abscesses, cysts, and granulomas.
- List important and pathologic sequelae of periapical infection and inflammation.
- Explain the interrelationship of the periapical diseases to each other.
- Recognize the appearance and significance of a parulis.

CARIES

Dental caries is an infectious disease process that results in localized dissolution and bacterial destruction of hard tissues. The process is caused by endemic bacterial organisms that are found on the surfaces of teeth in most mouths. Teeth of the primary and permanent dentitions may be diseased. In recent years the incidence of dental caries has decreased in children—the age group in which the prevalence of new lesions is the greatest. On the other hand—also in recent years—as adults have begun to retain their dentition longer, the prevalence of new carious lesions in adult teeth seems to have increased. Dental caries continues to be one of the most common diseases to occur in humans. The disease process and its sequelae can cause considerable problems, such as loss of teeth, unsightly dentition, and associated jaw infections. The treatment of dental caries and its sequelae—such as restorative and prosthetic dentistry—still accounts for the majority of all visits to the dentist.

Epidemiology

The epidemiology of dental caries has been studied extensively. We know that certain populations are caries sensitive and that other populations are caries resistant. It has been estimated that 5% of the general population will never develop carious lesions. The incidence of dental caries is greatest in children. Although this incidence has declined dramatically within the past 20 years because of preventive measures, new lesions continue to be most common in the 5- to 15-year age group. Population studies suggest that the following variables play an important role in susceptibility to this disease: diet, geographic variation, access to fluorides, heredity, and access to dental care.

The role of sugars and carbohydrates as cariogenic factors is well known. The rate of caries in westernized populations (the United States, England, Europe) is markedly greater than that in the underdeveloped countries. The direct correlation seen in sugar consumption comparisons between these populations leads one to conclude that sugars, especially the sugar sucrose, are important cofactors in the disease process. Several Scandinavian studies of populations who were sugar deprived during World War II correlate that deprivation with low caries rates in the Scandinavian children. When sucrose was reintroduced subsequent to cessation of hostilities, caries rates returned to prewar levels in children within the endemic Scandinavian populations. Prospective human sucrose studies and animal caries studies support the conclusion that sucrose consumption—and especially frequency of sucrose use—is an important factor in caries activity. Other nutrients seem to play a lesser role in caries incidence. Vitamins A and D, calcium and phosphate ions, fatty foods, and even chocolate may play a role in reduction of caries rates to a minor degree in some populations. Fluoride as a dietary supplement and topical preventive treatment has had a profound effect in reducing caries rates.

Researchers early in the twentieth century observed that there were considerable variations in caries rates across certain geographic areas. When dietary differences were factored into these observations, large variations still existed. Very low caries rates were noted in geographic populations who exhibited tooth malformations (fluorosis) from drinking water highly concentrated with fluoride ions. Subsequent research revealed that geographic populations from areas of high fluoride concentration had lower caries rates than populations from low-fluoride areas—even in the absence of fluorosis. Controlled studies in animals and humans (dealing, for example, with public health fluoridation of water) have confirmed the anticariogenic property of relatively low levels of fluoride added to the oral and systemic environments. It is now estimated that caries rates in children have been reduced 50% in the past 20 years in the United States through fluoride supplementation of public water supplies, and through dentifrices, changes in diet, and prophylactic fluoride treatment.

It has been long known that certain families are caries sensitive (have "soft teeth") and demonstrate especially high caries rates. Other families are identified as caries immune and demonstrate low or null caries rates. Even after such previously discussed variable caries-associated factors as diet (sucrose) and fluoride were controlled, the familial nature of the disease continues to be significant. Large controlled population studies support the concept of caries-prone and caries-resistant families. In general, children born to parents with high caries rates will also develop numerous lesions, whereas children born into families with low caries rates will have a lesser caries prevalence. Identical twin–studies suggest greater similarity of caries rates among identical twins than among siblings. However, separated twin–studies show a greater discrepancy in caries rates among separated monozygotic twins than among monozygotic twins raised within the same environment. This indicates that both familial characteristics and environmental factors play an important role in this disease.

Finally, access to dental care, prophylactic dentistry, and preventive dentistry play a role in reduction of the caries rate. We have already noted that topical fluoride treatment and dietary instruction can have a profound effect on caries rate reduction. The dental office is the best setting for such preventive therapy. The caries activity can be arrested or reduced by caries removal and restorative procedures, application of sealants and coatings to teeth, application of anticariogenic filling materials, and education of the patient by the dental practitioner or assistant concerning plaque removal and prevention.

Pathogenesis

The disease process is primarily one of bacterial (plaque) adherence to exposed dental hard tissues such as enamel and cementum. Acid byproducts generated by bacterial metabolism are concentrated at the hard tissue surface. Calcium hydroxyapatite, the hardening mineral of dental hard tissues is slowly dissolved by the acid, leaving a less mineralized lesion. As more acid seeps from the surface, more mineral is dissolved until finally only a meager protein matrix and a small amount of apatite remain within the enamel. The enamel surface is most resistant to demineralization; however, the largely intact surface allows acids to penetrate to deeper levels. Within the deeper levels of enamel, certain anatomic portions of the microstructure of enamel are more susceptible to the disease process. The result is a focal demineralized area of enamel, which on proximal and cervical smooth surfaces is usually shaped as a cone with its base at the surface of the tooth

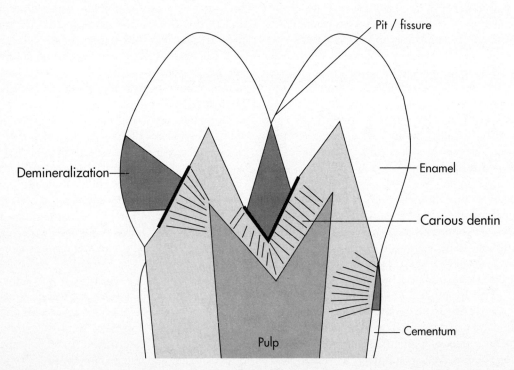

Fig. 12-1 Dental caries. The dark shaded areas represent demineralization of smooth surface enamel, pit and fissure enamel, and cementum. The caries process spreads laterally at the dentinoenamel junction and extends into the dentin along the dentinal tubules.

adjacent to the plaque (Fig. 12-1). The outer 30 to 50 µ of enamel remains relatively mineralized. Clinically, such a lesion appears white and chalky if it can be seen.

Frequently, carious lesions begin within interproximal areas where they cannot be seen. However, radiographs will demonstrate the telltale cone-shaped radiolucency created by the focal demineralized lesion. Once the demineralization advances through the enamel to the dento-enamel junction (DEJ), there is rapid lateral spread and demineralization along the DEJ (Fig. 12-1). Dentin, which is less mineralized than enamel, now begins to demineralize in the presence of seeping acids. The dentinal tubules actually initially become sclerotic because of reactions of the odontogenic processes to the irritation of acids. This reaction, however, is not sufficient to prevent further spread of acid, and the odontogenic processes begin to withdraw, leaving empty, partially sclerosed dentinal tubules. At this stage, the area of demineralized enamel has become so weakened that the surface breaks away and a rough, usually stained surface defect (cavity) begins to develop.

Loss of the intact surface allows for penetration and invasion of the lesion by microorganisms indigenous to the mouth. These organisms readily colonize the base of the cavity and the now demineralizing dentin. Since the lesion base contains open dentinal tubules, microorganisms can easily gain access to these tubules and begin to grow within this environment. Naturally, certain anaerobic organisms will flourish within this environment. Organisms continue to grow and dissolve the adjacent hard tissue by excreting substances that cause acid demineralization, degradation of proteins (proteolysis), and bonding of calcium (chelation) from the dentin with subsequent loss of minerals. Caries in dentin advances more rapidly and the lesion anatomically follows the distribution of the dentinal tubules. The demineralized, liquefied dentin becomes first leathery and stained brown; and subsequently, as more mineral and protein is lost, the tissue

becomes soft and mushy. The end result is a larger void or cavity of enamel and dentin that extends deep into a leathery, stained base. As the infection of microorganisms extends deeply into the dentin, bacteria infect the pulpal tissues and pulpitis occurs.

Carious defects are most easily managed by mechanical removal of the demineralized portions of enamel and infected areas of dentin. This is most frequently accomplished by drilling and excavating soft dentin and by replacement with restorative materials (fillings). Early-stage white enamel lesions can occasionally be arrested or even somewhat reversed by removal of the plaque and recalcification of the lesion with concentrated application of fluoride and calcium salts.

Etiology

Basically, four essential factors must all be present in order for enamel caries to exist. These factors are (1) bacteria, (2) sugars, (3) susceptible dental hard tissues, and (4) time. All four are necessary. If any of the four are inhibited or restricted, the caries process will be prevented or arrested. The dental profession has the primary responsibility to prevent the disease process from occurring and spreading. Methodology for prevention is concentrated on inhibiting or modifying these four factors. We will discuss each factor independently; however, keep in mind that all four are essential in order for the process to occur.

We defined caries as an infectious disease process. The process begins as a series of events caused by numerous indigenous microorganisms. Microorganisms implicated include strains of *Streptococcus mutans, S. salivarius, S. sanguis, Lactobacillus casei,* and strains of *Actinomyces.* Each of these organisms can cause experimental caries when inoculated onto teeth of germ-free animals, given that the other conditions (susceptible surface, sugar diet, time) are present. The degree of cariogenicity varies for different organisms and strains, with *S. mutans* being the most cariogenic for enamel. It is interesting, however, that these microorganisms are indigenous and are found in most mouths—whether caries susceptible or caries free. Therefore, the mere presence (infection) of these organisms is not in itself the cause of dental caries. It has been shown that the quality of microorganisms associated with tooth surfaces has a positive correlation with caries rate. For example, if a bacterial plaque attached to teeth is low in cariogenic bacteria, the caries rate can be expected to be correspondingly low. However, if the same plaque has a higher concentration or cariogenic organisms, the chance of caries activity increases remarkably.

Factors such as amount of sugar in the diet, and length of time of plaque accretion on the teeth affect the quality of the plaque and may select for and promote cariogenic bacterial growth. Plaque that is composed of 1% cariogenic bacteria (noncarious) can become altered to 4% cariogenic bacteria (carious) by multiple exposures to doses of sucrose over a period of time. Of course, if the plaque is removed from the tooth surface, the process of caries development is prevented, or if the sucrose is reduced in the diet, the quality of the plaque may again change. The cariogenic bacteria demonstrate certain properties that account for their participation in the process. Many of these organisms are acidogenic (acid producers), are aciduric (thrive in acid environments), and readily produce the sticky polysaccharide dextran. These properties promote sticking of bacteria to the tooth surface, sticking of cariogenic bacteria to each other (quantity selection), growth of other aciduric organisms (quality selection), and acid dissolution of enamel (early caries).

Once the caries process has proceeded into dentin, other indigenous microorganisms play an important role in the process. Many of these microorganisms are strains of streptococci and actinomyces, and some are anaerobic (live in absence of oxygen). These organisms also tend to produce acids that continue to dissolve the calcium hydroxyapatite of dentin. In addition, these organisms produce to some extent proteolytic enzymes and chelating agents. These byproducts promote destruction of the protein matrix and dissolution of calcium from the dentin, therefore facilitating the spread of the caries process.

Plaque is a necessary ingredient in the carious process. Plaque is defined as a complex composed of microorganisms, polysaccharides, sugars, and salivary proteins that sticks to the enamel or cementum surfaces of teeth. Plaque is soft, usually milky, and very adherent to tooth surfaces. It can form within pits and fissures and on smooth surfaces of teeth. Because it is difficult to locate or reach in some areas (pits, interproximal smooth surfaces), it can be very difficult to remove—even though, once accessed, it is easily removable by mechanical means (brushing, flossing). The greatest majority of plaque is made up of noncariogenic bacteria; therefore, the mere presence of plaque does not predict caries activity. If plaque accumulates over a period of time, it will most likely calcify with salivary salts, and calculus will be the resultant form.

Plaque functions in three ways to promote cariogenicity. Plaque is responsible for adherence of cariogenic organisms to susceptible tooth surfaces, it is responsible for the selective growth of these cariogenic organisms, and it concentrates acids at the tooth surface by being relatively impermeable to the buffering of saliva. Cariogenic bacteria within plaque use sugars as foods and excrete acids as byproducts. In addition, the cariogenic bacteria in plaque have enzymes (glycosyltransferase) that use sucrose to make glucans—long-chain sugars. Since cariogenic bacteria are selectively adherent to each other by means of glucans, the formation of these polysaccharides promotes adhesion of cariogenic bacteria in plaque. Sucrose is the sugar that is most efficiently processed into glucans by *Streptococcus mutans*. When plaque is bathed in sucrose, the percentage of *S. mutans* increases, the amount of glucan production increases, and the amount of acid (low pH) also increases. This initiates the localized acid demineralization of dental caries because the acids produced are isolated adjacent to the enamel surface beneath the relatively impermeable plaque.

Enamel, cementum, and dentin are all dental hard tissues susceptible to the carious process. We have already seen that the streptococci that are adherent by way of glucan receptors and production play a most important role in initiation of enamel caries. Other bacterial populations including *Streptococcus* strains, and *Actinomyces* and *Lactobacillus* play an important role in progression of cemental and dentinal caries because (1) these organisms tend to be aciduric, (2) these organisms can function in low-oxygen environments, and (3) plaque (glucan adherence) plays a lesser role in cemental and dentinal caries. Since the initial event in caries is demineralization of the dental hard tissues, caries can best be controlled by either strengthening the calcium hydroxyapatite bonds or by remineralization of demineralized hard tissue. We know that enamel that is high in fluoride concentration is more resistant to demineralization. The fluoride ions can bond with apatite to form fluorohydroxyapatite both during tooth formation and, later, by cnamcl surface exchange of ions with the fluoride concentrated in saliva or applied to the teeth. Fluorohydroxyapatite is acid resistant. For these reasons, caries rates are reduced both in children who drink fluoridated water during formative years and in adults who receive topical applications of fluoride in water, dentifrices, mouth rinses, gums, etc. The caries resistance of the outer 30 to 50μ of enamel is probably associated with the high fluoride content of this area provided by such topical applications. Other substances such as calcium salts and phosphates have had some limited success in providing remineralization of early carious lesions and caries resistance when incorporated into the dental hard tissues. The dental

hard tissues can be protected from plaque adherence or acids by application of a barrier on the tooth surface. Numerous surface agents have been tested, and certain coatings and sealants are now routinely used to protect some dental hard tissues from plaque and acid.

The process of caries takes time. Although acute caries exists occasionally, the usual process of cavity formation takes months to years before the pulp is threatened. This means that multiple surface plaques contribute to the process and that long-term subsurface infections continue the process. This phenomenon allows the dental practitioner to arrest the process by plaque removal, caries removal, and patient motivation toward better diet, hygiene, fluoride therapy, and other forms of caries prevention.

Saliva plays an important role in caries control. Individuals who have reduced salivary flow resulting from irradiation, salivary gland surgery, medications, salivary disease, or other causes usually have a corresponding increase in caries rate. The term *radiation caries* is often applied to such cases. Radiation caries is characterized by acute caries, frequently in Class V locations (Fig. 12-2). Rapid dental breakdown can readily lead to pulpitis, periapical infection, and subsequent tooth extraction.

Saliva contains a number of anticariogenic substances. Secretory antibodies (IgA) to cariogenic strains of bacteria have been demonstrated in saliva. Numerous products in saliva such as peroxidase, apoferritin, urea, and lysozymes have antibacterial and presumably anticariogenic effects. Saliva itself is a salt solution that has a great neutralizing (buffering) effect on acids; therefore, saliva can help prevent acid demineralization—if the saliva and acids mix. Finally, saliva contains concentrations of both calcium and fluoride salts. These ions are readily absorbed into saliva-exposed tooth surfaces, where they may impart acid resistance to intact enamel and remineralize early-stage carious white lesions. Both the quality and quantity of saliva play an

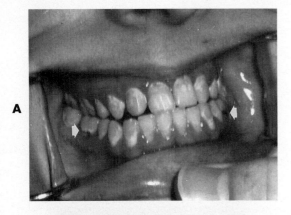

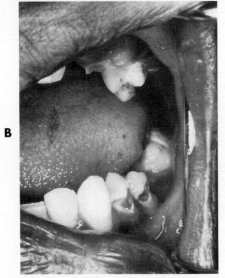

Fig. 12-2 Dental caries. **A,** numerous chalky white lesions of the smooth surfaces are noted. The buccal surfaces of the mandibular first molars show brown stained cavities where the surface enamel has fractured away. **B,** This 14-year-old male was irradiated for pharyngeal cancer. His caries rate increased remarkably after he developed xerostomia.

important role in caries management. This author believes that the familial characteristics of caries susceptibility or caries resistance may be in part a manifestation of differences in the quality of saliva.

Many resources have been and continue to be committed to caries research. A caries vaccine designed to enhance secretory antibodies to cariogenic bacteria is being investigated. Genetic engineering of bacteria to create organisms competitive with cariogenic bacteria seems promising. Mouth rinses, and foods incorporating antibacterial, antibiotic, antiglucan, and buffering systems are being developed and tested. New coatings, sealants, and filling materials are being developed that better adhere to teeth and incorporate anticariogenic substances. Finally, improvements in fluoride delivery and access, dental care, home dental care, and diet should continue to reduce caries rates and allow retention of the dentition.

PULPAL INFECTION

Pulpitis

Pulpitis represents inflammation of the dental pulp. The primary etiologic agents responsible for most pulpitis are carious bacterial infections and trauma. In order for bacteria to produce pulpal inflammation, they must either come in proximity to the pulp and affect the pulp via odontoblastic processes and dental tubules (as in deep caries, severe abrasion, or erosion), or come into direct contact with the pulp via exposure of the pulp to the oral environment. Bacteria may directly enter the pulp through carious exposure, through mechanical exposure during dental procedures, or through coronal fracture following direct trauma to the teeth. This form of pulpitis is classified as septic, because the inflammation is the direct result of bacterial infection.

Aseptic pulpitis represents forms of pulpal inflammation that can result from trauma in the absence of a significant contribution by infectious microorganisms. One of the most common forms of pulpitis is that seen following the routine placement of dental fillings. Subjection of the tooth to mechanical instrumentation (such as drilling) may produce damage to pulpal tissues. The degree of pulpal tissue injury is related to the extent and depth of instrumentation, use of effective tooth coolants during drilling, and degree of tooth desiccation prior to placement of the restoration. Some restoration materials may irritate and injure the pulp chemically. Placement of large, metallic restorations permits rapid pulpal hypothermia following consumption of a cold food or beverage, producing mild pulpal damage and resultant inflammation. Direct physical trauma may also produce aseptic pulpitis. Such trauma may result in superficial coronal fracture (such as chipped incisal edges) or leave the tooth intact while nonetheless producing pulpal damage and inflammation. Of course, severe trauma that may displace teeth in the alveolus may also result in aseptic pulpitis.

Acute versus Chronic Pulpitis

The character of pulpitis can be described generally as acute or chronic. On a clinical level, acute pulpitis is characterized by severe dental pain and is generally abrupt in onset. The duration of pain is usually short, and the intensity of symptoms is often such as to keep the patient awake at night. In contrast, chronic pulpitis usually produces a milder, duller pain that may be somewhat more difficult for the patient to trace to a specific tooth. The duration of pain is typically long, and the patient may report that the intensity of pain varies from time to time. Episodes of pain may be interrupted by relatively pain-free periods.

Strictly speaking, acute and chronic pulpitis may also be distinguished on a histologic basis. In this regard, acute pulpitis would show acute inflammatory cell infiltrates with plentiful neutrophils, vascular congestion, and edema; whereas chronic pulpitis would exhibit chronic cellular infiltrates (see Chapter 3).

Reversible versus Irreversible Pulpitis

The concepts of reversible and irreversible pulpitis have been developed to enable the clinician to make accurate prognostic assessment concerning pulpitis. The dentist's primary goal in assessing clinical pulpitis is to, in so much as it is possible, accurately predict which cases of pulpitis are likely to improve with little or no clinical intervention (reversible pulpitis), and which are destined to end in pulpal necrosis (irreversible pulpitis) and thus require endodontic therapy. Through careful evaluation of patient history and clinical signs and symptoms, it is usually possible to determine whether pulpitis is reversible or irreversible. In this manner the most appropriate therapy may be selected for the patient, and unnecessary endodontic procedures and considerable expense may be avoided.

Patients with reversible pulpitis usually provide a history of mild dental pain that is often diffuse, and usually is not radiating or stabbing in character. The duration of pain is generally short, measured in hours rather than days. Patients describe a pain-eliciting factor (such as cold or heat), and thus the pain is not spontaneous. Such patients will usually not state that the pain is keeping them from sleeping; nor do they say that changes in posture affect the nature and intensity of the pain. It should be pointed out that this type of historical clinical information is only available upon astute questioning by the clinician. Disorganized and/or unfocused patient interviews will usually fail to disclose the needed information.

The typical clinical features of *reversible pulpitis* include pain following thermal tooth stimulation. The pain will not persist following removal of the stimulus. In most other respects the clinical findings will be unremarkable, and noteworthy by the absence of percussion sensitivity, tooth mobility, and radiographic evidence of periapical disease. Clinical examination is likely to disclose some evidence as to the etiologic basis of the pulpitis, be it a recently placed restoration, an old leaky restoration, an unrestored carious lesion, or other relevant factor.

In general, the historical features and clinical signs and symptoms of *irreversible pulpitis* contrast with those of reversible pulpitis in their severity and character. With proper questioning, patients with irreversible pulpitis are likely to describe severe, often radiating pain of long duration and varying intensity. The pain is often spontaneous, and may be affected by changes in posture. The patient will often report that the pain may be induced by hot or cold foods, but that the pain will persist following removal of the stimulus. Clinical examination typically reveals hyperreactive response on electric pulp testing, with continued pain after the stimulus is removed. As with reversible pulpitis, there should be no evidence of percussion sensitivity or increased tooth mobility, or radiographic evidence of periapical disease.

Management of reversible pulpitis is typically conservative, and usually entails alleviating any causative factors that are present. Thus a restoration in hyperocclusion (one that is high) may be adjusted or a sedative dressing may be placed; or, in many cases, patients may merely be assured that the postoperative thermal sensitivity they are experiencing in connection with a recently placed filling will be temporary and will likely resolve without further intervention. Irreversible pulpitis does not offer a similarly positive prognosis. Symptoms indicative of this condition are a clear signal that patient relief will come only through removal of the pulp, followed by appropriate endodontic therapy.

PERIAPICAL DISEASES

The most common diseases of the periapical tissues are the result of pulpal necrosis, with extension of the inflammatory disease process beyond the tooth apex into the surrounding jaw (Fig. 12-3). As pulpal necrosis may occur under septic and aseptic conditions, we observe that some common periapical diseases show a significant infectious component, whereas others do not.

Periapical Abscess

A periapical abscess is an area of liquefaction necrosis and purulent exudation occurring at the apex of a nonvital tooth. In most cases the acute inflammation and necrosis are the result of the presence of a pyogenic bacterial infection, usually originating from the oral flora. The bacteria typically gain access to the apical tissues via the pulp chamber and canal, entering through carious lesions or through fractured teeth. It is important to emphasize that in virtually all cases the pulp is necrotic.

Clinical historical features commonly include a complaint of severe pain, often with fever, malaise, and a history of local facial swelling. Because of the apical inflammation the tooth may be slightly extruded in the socket, leading the patient to indicate problems with chewing on the affected side. The most characteristic clinical finding is extreme percussion sensitivity. Such sensitivity occurs because of the edema and pain-inducing acute inflammatory mediators present at the apex. Physical pressure on this tissue, as through light tapping on the tooth, can literally bring the patient out of the dental chair. The finding of percussion sensitivity serves to clearly distinguish periapical abscess from irreversible pulpitis. Given the nonvital pulp in periapical abscess, pulp tests are usually negative. Extension of the infectious and inflammatory process beyond the immediate area of the tooth apex may produce varying degrees of facial swelling and tooth mobility (Fig. 12-4). Sinus formation and drainage of pus through the gingiva into the mouth may be observed. Radiographic findings usually include an area of ill-defined radiolucency around the apex of the involved tooth. These radiographic changes may be as minimal as a slightly thickened periodontal ligament space, or as pronounced as a well-defined radiolucency. The usual location

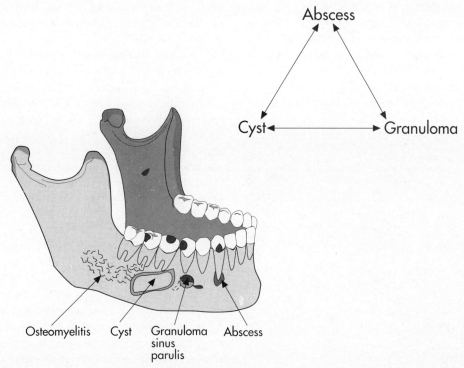

Fig. 12-3 Pulpitis may spread to the jawbone and result in acute localized periapical infection (abscess), chronic localized periapical infection (granuloma), apical cyst formation, or diffuse spread into bone (osteomyelitis). Periapical abscess, granuloma, and cyst evolve into each other depending on patient resistance, severity of infection and virulence of microorganisms.

for these radiographic changes is at the tooth apex, corresponding to the common exit point of pulpal nerves and vessels, and thus a point of communication between the pulp canal and periapical tissues for infectious bacteria and necrotic pulp tissue breakdown products. The presence of accessory canals extending laterally from the pulp to the lateral peridontium or the furcation in multirooted teeth provides an explanation for the occasional finding of periapical abscess in these lateral locations ("lateral" dental abscess). The radiolucent changes are attributable to local liquefaction necrosis of bone and connective tissue, leaving behind a radiolucent pathologic cavity filled with pus.

Periapical Granuloma

The etiology of periapical disease often includes a significant direct contribution of bacterial infection at the tooth apex. However, in many cases periapical disease may develop either in the presence of bacteria of low virulence, or entirely in the absence of apical bacterial infection. It was stated earlier in this chapter that in many instances pulpitis may occur without direct bacterial infection (aseptic pulpitis), and frequently such cases are irreversible and thus lead to pulpal necrosis. It is generally true that following necrosis, irritating tissue breakdown products derived from the pulp exit the dental apex and enter the periapical tissues (Fig.12-3). These substances are potent mediators of inflammation and further necrosis (see Chapter 3), and the resultant chronic inflammatory response produces local destruction of periapical bone with replacement by nonspecific chronically inflamed granulation tissue and scar tissue.

Upon appropriate questioning, the patient usually indicates either no symptoms associated with the tooth, or such mild symptoms as

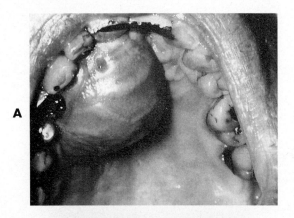

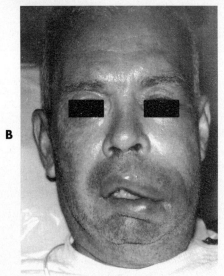

Fig. 12-4 Dental infections. **A,** This palatal infection and swelling represents spread from a carious maxillary lateral incisor. **B,** This cellulitis of the face and upper lip is caused by an infected maxillary anterior tooth.

discomfort on chewing. The tooth is usually percussion sensitive, though significantly less so than in the case of periapical abscess. Pulp vitality testing is usually negative, and slightly increased tooth mobility and presence of draining sinuses are variable findings. The usual radiographic appearance is that of a relatively well defined radiolucency situated around the root apex (Fig. 12-5). Again, the presence of lateral or furcational communications between the pulp and periodontium allow for the development of "lateral" granulomas.

Apical Periodontal Cyst

In nearly every significant respect, the apical periodontal cyst (periapical cyst) closely resembles the periapical granuloma. The condition usually develops as a result of the influence of an adjacent necrotic pulp, and chronic periapical inflammation (Fig. 12-3). Symptoms are typically mild or absent, although percussion sensitivity is usually detectable. Radio-

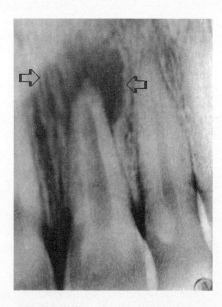

Fig. 12-5 Periapical granuloma. The well-demarcated radiolucency above the maxillary central incisor was determined by biopsy (apical surgery) to be chronic inflammation.

graphic changes are indistinguishable from those of periapical granuloma, with a well-defined apical radiolucency most commonly apparent on dental radiographs (Fig. 12-6). The essential distinction from periapical granuloma concerns histologic appearance. Whereas the periapical granuloma consists of a mass of chronically inflamed granulation tissue, apical periodontal cyst is manifest as a pathologic cavity lined by stratified squamous epithelium that is often surrounded by chronically inflamed granulation tissue. The epithelium lining the cyst is considered to be of odontogenic origin, derived from small remnants (rests) of odontogenic epithelium that persist in the periodontal ligament (rests of Malassez) following completion of tooth formation. It is speculated that under the influence of necrotic pulp–induced apical chronic inflammation, these rests of epithelium may undergo a reactive, hyperplastic proliferation, with central fluid accumulation, ultimately assuming the configuration of an epithelium-lined cavity (cyst).

Interrelationships and Management

It is apparent, based on the preceding discussions, that the periapical abscess, periapical granuloma, and apical periodontal cyst are closely related lesions (Fig. 12-3). All are etiologically related to pulpal necrosis and generally produce periapical radiolucent changes. Development of an abscess can be ascribed to the presence of virulent bacteria. Were the bacteria in a periapical abscess to be eliminated (as may occur through a course of antibiotic therapy or as a result of effective inflammation), the abscess might well become a periapical granuloma through a process of organization and connective tissue substitution (see Chapter 3). The stimulation of odontogenic epithelial rests might lead to development of an apical periodontal cyst. Alternatively, introduction of virulent infective organisms into a previously existent chronic periapical granuloma or cyst could lead to development of an abscess. Causative bacteria might gain access to the apex through pulp chambers and canals exposed by caries. It should also be recognized that host resistance may not remain constant throughout life. Reduction in the effectiveness of the immune system and inflammatory responses could allow a longstanding low-grade bacterial infection in a largely asymptomatic periapical granuloma to surge into a severe dental abscess. Development of diabetes mellitus or disseminated cancer, exposure to antineoplastic radiation or chemotherapy, and immune suppression related to organ transplantation antirejection drugs or HIV infection are the types of events that can severely impair immunity and inflammation.

Management of these periapical diseases is primarily based on elimination of the necrotic pulp. This may be accomplished either through various endodontic procedures, or via dental extraction. In cases where significant infection is suspected (such as periapical abscess), appropriate antibiotic therapy is indicated. Patient progress should be followed after therapy to assure radiographic and clinical resolution of apical disease. Persistence of signs and symptoms of apical disease is an indication for further diagnostic evaluation.

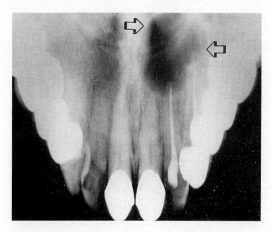

Fig. 12-6 Periapical cyst. This painless lesion (arrow) caused buccal expansion of the maxilla.

TISSUE INFECTIONS SUBSEQUENT TO PERIAPICAL INFECTION

We have observed that bacterial infection may make a significant contribution to the eventual development of periapical disease, be it through the development of caries, septic pulpitis, or periapical abscess. Virulent bacteria may spread beyond the periapical abscess to involve a wider area of bone, soft tissue, and contiguous structures. It should be emphasized that significant infectious organisms also may gain entry into these tissues via periodontal pockets, traumatic injuries (jaw fracture, gunshot wound), sinus infections, and skin infections (abscess, boil). We will complete this chapter with a consideration of several of the more common and important forms of orofacial infection.

Parulis

A parulis (sinus tract, gum boil) represents the drainage point of pus exiting through the gingiva from an underlying infection in the jaw. The origin of infection may be either periapical (as with periapical abscess) or periodontal (as with periodontal abscess). The parulis is typically raised and nodular, being composed of acutely inflamed granulation tissue (Fig. 12-7). At times the parulis may appear to contain substantial amounts of yellowish pus, giving rise to the synonym "gum boil." (See Chapter 17.) Although the underlying infection may be painful and give rise to a variety of other signs and symptoms, the parulis is typically asymptomatic. The communication between the site of bony infection (abscess) and the surface is termed a sinus tract. Sinus tracts are not limited to the jaws or oral cavity, and may extend to the skin surface, or occur in many other infected anatomic sites.

Acute Osteomyelitis

Acute osteomyelitis is a severe, usually bacterial infection of medullary bone that is capable

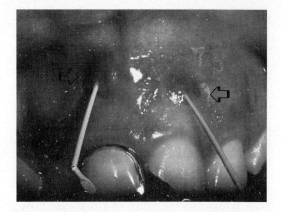

Fig. 12-7 Parulis. The two draining sinus tracts are demonstrated with gutta percha points.

of producing extensive bone destruction. The most commonly implicated bacteria in acute osteomyelitis of the jaws are *Staphylococcus aureus* and *S. albus,* followed by various streptococci, actinomyces, and mixed (oral flora) infections. These infectious agents may gain entry to the bone through carious exposures and periapical disease, periodontal disease, or severe traumatic injuries.

The typical case of staphylococcal acute osteomyelitis is characterized by severe bone pain, loose teeth, purulent drainage, fever, and facial swelling. When occurring in the maxilla, the disease tends to remain localized, whereas in the mandible the chances of spreading are greater. Extension of infection in the mandible to the inferior alveolar nerve may produce altered sensation in the lower lip (paresthesia) or a frankly numb lip (anesthesia). Formation of sinus tracts with purulent drainage through the skin is common (Fig. 12-8). Radiographic changes consist of an area of ill-defined, mottled radiolucency, suggesting an aggressive, tissue-destructive process. Often the radiographs may show fragments of seemingly detached bone. This represents necrotic bone in the center of the disease, termed *sequestrum*.

Management of patients with acute osteomyelitis usually involves surgical removal of

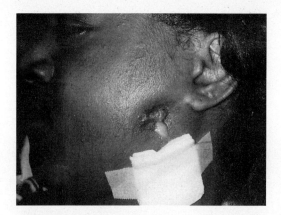

Fig. 12-8 External sinus tracts. There is drainage from a mandibular osteomyelitis, which is caused by an infected mandibular molar. The gauze covers a second drainage site.

infected portions or segments of the jaw, coupled with extended antibiotic therapy. Surgical removal of tissue is necessary, as antibiotic therapy alone will have little impact through much of the lesion. Microorganism culture and antibiotic sensitivity testing are critical in allowing selection of the most effective antibiotics. Hospitalization is usually indicated during the early course of therapy.

Cellulitis—Ludwig's Angina

As discussed in Chapter 3, cellulitis represents a clinical expression of acute inflammation in which there is a prominent degree of edema with marked, diffuse soft tissue swelling. This form of inflammation is acute in nature, with abrupt onset, rapid progression, and accompanying fever. Cellulitis is an important sequela of periapical dental infection. Infection spreading beyond the confines of the jaw and into the surrounding soft tissue can lead to dramatic facial swelling and pain, and may directly interfere with important functions such as chewing (as in trismus), swallowing (as in dysphagia), and breathing (as in dyspnea). Orofacial soft tissue infections of dental origin typically spread along anatomically defined fascial planes that provide boundaries for so-called tissue spaces. The specific tissue spaces that may become infected are in large measure determined by the location of the inciting dental infection. For example, bacterial infection at the apex of a maxillary first premolar may extend from the bone laterally into the tissues immediately adjacent to the maxilla, producing a so-called buccal space infection. Alternatively, infection from a periapical abscess of a mandibular incisor may drain into the soft tissues immediately medial to the chin, involving the submental space.

One of the most important forms of bacterial cellulitis arising from dental periapical infection is Ludwig's angina. Defined as severe cellulitis involving all submaxillary, sublingual, and submental spaces bilaterally, Ludwig's angina usually arises from the medial spread of odontogenic infection from the mandibular molar region. Periapical, periodontal, and pericoronal (that is, pericoronitis) sources of infection have at times been implicated. Culture studies have generally revealed the bacterial infection to be mixed, with streptococcal species common. It is important to emphasize that there is no specific infectious organism that causes Ludwig's angina. Once the infection reaches this anatomic region a rapidly progressive clinical pattern ensues that, if not promptly diagnosed and aggressively managed, can lead to death. Classic clinical features include (1) boardlike swelling of the floor of the mouth; (2) elevation of the tongue; and (3) difficulty in eating, swallowing, and breathing. Fever, rapid pulse (tachycardia), and increased respiration rate are typical. Any patient who has, or who is receiving treatment for, a mandibular dental infection who appears to be exhibiting some of these clinical features should be considered at risk for Ludwig's angina, and managed accordingly.

Extension of infection to the vocal cords (glottis) can occur, resulting in glottal edema and asphyxiation. The goal in management is to either prevent the development of Ludwig's angina, or to achieve early diagnosis and prompt intervention. Patients with this infection are best treated in a hospital environment.

Cavernous Sinus Thrombosis

The cavernous sinus is a paired, anatomically normal venous structure that is located near the base of the brain. Although the cavernous sinus functions in the normal draining of venous blood, it is closely associated with a number of important anatomic structures, including segments of cranial nerves III, IV, V_1, V_2, and VI, and the internal carotid artery. Closely adjacent structures include the optic chiasm, optic nerves, and eyes. Clearly, any aggressive disease process occurring in this region could have wide-ranging effects on vision, ocular motor activity, and upper facial sensory function.

The cavernous sinus receives venous blood from a variety of sources, including anatomically inferior areas such as the maxillary and midface regions. The anterior midface region has venous communication back to the cavernous sinus via facial and angular veins, and the posterior maxilla communicates with the cavernous sinus by way of the pterygoid venous plexus. Thus bacterial infections in the maxilla and skin of the upper lip carry a small but highly significant risk of life-threatening infection in the cavernous sinus. The usual pathogen is *Staphylococcus*. When such bacteria produce infection within vessels, the ensuing retrograde spread and damage to vessel walls results in septic clot formation—thus the name cavernous sinus *thrombosis*.

Patients with cavernous sinus thrombosis, in addition to signs, symptoms, and/or history of recent midfacial or maxillary infection, demonstrate malaise, fever, chills, headache, nausea, and vomiting. Somewhat more specific signs and symptoms include paralysis of external ocular muscles, a variety of visual disturbances (such as blurred or double vision), exophthalmos, and eyelid and conjunctival edema.

The prognosis of cavernous sinus thrombosis is not favorable, and there is a significant mortality rate. The condition represents a dire medical emergency requiring intensive management in the hospital.

Case Studies

Case 1
S.N. is a 14-year-old boy who complained of a toothache of the upper right quadrant. The tooth had been sensitive for 3 weeks to hot and cold and now was painful and throbbing at night. S.N. was otherwise healthy. Oral exam revealed deep interproximal caries on tooth No. 3. The tooth was vital, and there was no obvious radiographic periapical defect. Cold stimulation caused severe throbbing pain for 5 minutes relieved with anesthetic. A diagnosis of acute pulpitis was rendered. The pulp was extirpated and the canal was medicated, and a temporary restoration was put in place in anticipation of root canal therapy. S.N. failed to keep subsequent appointments. Four years later he returned with a bony swelling buccal to the apex of tooth No. 3. The temporary restoration was still in place. Radiographs showed a well-circumscribed, 2-cm radiolucency with a radiopaque border. Apical surgery revealed a periapical cyst and periapical granuloma of tooth No. 3. Root canal therapy and crowning yielded a positive result.

Case 2
A.V. is a 48-year-old alcoholic who came to a mission for the homeless with fever and swelling of the neck and pharynx. He was sent to a dental emergency clinic. Oral exam revealed 13 broken-down, carious teeth, including five in the mandibular posterior regions. Radiographs displayed numerous periapical radiolucencies and revealed focal moth-eaten radiolucent changes of the mandible. The submental, submandibular, and retropharyngeal spaces were red, board-hard, and swollen. A.V. was having some difficulty breathing and was therefore hospitalized. Intravenous antibiotics were begun and the mandibular carious teeth were extracted. Purulent discharge from the extraction sites was cultured.

A diagnosis of early Ludwig's angina secondary to dental osteomyelitis was rendered. A.V. improved steadily and was released 14 days after initial hospitalization and antibiotic therapy. He was scheduled for a follow-up dental appointment 2 weeks later.

Case 3

R.B. is an 18-year-old man who fractured teeth No. 7, 8, 9, and 10 in a bicycle accident. He developed swelling of the anterior maxilla after 24 hours and sought dental treatment for pain. The pulps were extirpated from teeth No. 7 and 8 since they were the most severely fractured. Penicillin to be administered orally was prescribed. The facial swelling continued to enlarge and spread, involving the bridge and ala of the nose. Teeth No. 9 and 10 were extirpated, and intraoral drainage was attempted. The antibiotic was changed. Two weeks later the swelling was slightly greater and now involved the periorbital skin. Some discoloration (black eye) was apparent. R.B. reported several severe headaches. He was hospitalized, and intravenous antibiotic therapy was started. Some pus was drained apical to tooth No. 7, and a culture and drug sensitivity test demonstrated penicillin-resistant organisms that were sensitive to the antibiotic clindamycin. Therapy with clindamycin was initiated and R.B. responded almost immediately. Symptoms cleared in 10 days, and root canal therapy was begun shortly thereafter.

Case 1

1. What does sensitivity to hot and cold indicate?
2. What does persistent pain after exposure to cold indicate?
3. Explain the cause of the periapical cyst.
4. Is it expected that a periapical cyst might take up to 4 years to develop?
5. Can periapical cysts and periapical granulomas appear simultaneously? Why?

Case 2

1. What is the likely cause of the osteomyelitis and Ludwig's angina?

2. Do you think alcoholism had any role in development of this condition?
3. What is purulent discharge? What does it indicate?
4. Why was a culture analysis performed?

Case 3

1. Why did the antibiotics initially fail to control the swelling?
2. Is the location of the fractured teeth significant in development of this condition?
3. Why was the antibiotic changed?
4. What do the symptoms of periorbital swelling and headache suggest?
5. Why was R. B. hospitalized?

SUMMARY

- Dental caries is an infectious disease process that causes the demineralization of dental hard structures by bacterial byproducts.
- The rate of dental caries is affected by a combination of the microorganisms on the surface, the susceptibility of the surface, and the sugar content of the diet.
- Dental plaque allows for adherence of cariogenic bacteria to the tooth surface and concentration of acids adjacent to teeth.
- The pathogenesis of enamel, dentinal, and cemental caries is somewhat related and somewhat different. Acid demineralization, proteolysis, and chelation all play a role in lesion production.
- Saliva is anticariogenic by virtue of its cleansing, antibacterial, buffering, and remineralizing qualities. Reduced salivary flow enhances the caries process.
- Caries prevention is based on interference with plaque maturation, carbohydrate metabolism, bacterial metabolism, and on strengthening of the tooth surface.
- Pulpitis is often the sequela of advanced caries, trauma, or mechanical placement of dental filling materials.
- The distinction of reversible from irreversible pulpitis dictates the treatment necessary.

- Pulpitis and pulpal necrosis can lead to periapical conditions such as abscess, granuloma, and cyst.
- The periapical diseases are interrelated. The type of pathology is dependent on the presence and virulence of infective organisms and the resistance of the patient. Periapical diseases can frequently be distinguished by clinical and radiographic tests.
- Periapical infections may spread and extend as sinus tracts, acute osteomyelitis, and cellulitis.
- Ludwig's angina and cavernous sinus thrombosis are uncommon but potentially life threatening pathologic sequelae of periapical infections.

Suggested readings

1. Menaker L: The biologic basis of dental caries, Hagerstown, Md, 1980, Harper & Row.
2. Muhler JC and others: The effect of stannous fluoride containing dentifrice on caries reduction in children II. Caries experience after 1 year, JADA 50:163, 1955.
3. Rowe NH: Dental caries. In Regezi JA and Sciubba J, editors: Oral pathology, clinical-pathologic correlations, ed 2, Philadelphia, 1993, WB Saunders, pp 521-527.
4. Schachtele CF: Dental caries. In Shuster GS, editor: Oral microbiology and infectious disease, ed 3, Philadelphia, 1990, BC Decker, pp 479-505.
5. Shafer WG, Hine MK, and Levy BM: A textbook of oral pathology, ed 4, Philadelpia, 1983, WB Saunders, chapter 8.
6. Shaw J: Causes and controls of dental caries, N Engl J Med 317:996, 1987.
7. Wood NK, Goaz P, and Jacobs MC: Periapical radiolucencies. In Wood NK and Goaz P, editors: Differential diagnosis of oral lesions, ed 4, St Louis, 1991, Mosby pp 303-325.

Physical and Chemical Oral Injury

IN THIS CHAPTER

1. Physical and chemical injury to teeth
   - Acute injury
   - Chronic injury
   - Resorption of teeth
   - Dental stains
2. Physical and chemical injury to soft tissue
   - Acute physical injury
   - Chronic physical injury
   - Denture-related reactive conditions
3. Chemical injury
   - Chemical burns
   - Phenytoin hyperplasia
   - Amalgam tattoo
   - Exogenous lingual pigmentation
   - Allergic reactions
   - Cancer chemotherapy effects
4. Radiation injury
   - Radiation mucositis
   - Bone necrosis and infection
   - Radiation xerostomia and caries
5. Case studies

After studying this chapter, you should be able to meet the following objectives and define the key terms:

- Define factitial and iatrogenic injury.
- Distinguish attrition, erosion, and abrasion by cause and clinical features.
- Recognize dental injuries suggestive of perimyolysis.
- Discuss common causes of resorption of teeth.
- List common extrinsic and intrinsic stains of teeth.

- Relate common forms of physical injury to the clinical presentation of the conditions.
- Recognize common clinical lesions suggestive of chronic mucosal injury.
- Use appropriate questioning to determine or rule out causes of suspicious injurious lesions.
- Refer lesions that are not readily explainable for further diagnosis.
- Recognize the significance of and describe treatment of pyogenic granuloma, epulis granulomatosum, and fibroma.
- List common denture-related tissue injuries and discuss the etiology and treatment of each.
- Recognize aspirin burn, phenytoin hyperplasia, and amalgam tattoo based on clinical appearance and history.
- Relate certain oral lesions that are caused by allergic reactions to their topical or systemic causes.
- Recognize that cancer chemotherapy and radiotherapy will likely predispose the patient to numerous pathologic oral conditions.
- Help prevent and manage oral lesions in patients undergoing chemotherapy and radiotherapy.
- Help prevent osteoradionecrosis.
- Use special regimens in patients who have radiation xerostomia to prevent caries and periodontal infection.

Physical and chemical assault on the hard and soft tissues of the mouth are among the most

215

common causes of oral lesions. It is important to determine the cause and nature of these lesions for two reasons. First, the lesions must be distinguished from more serious conditions that they may resemble; and second, the cause must be identified so that it can be eliminated. With most acute injuries, diagnosis is relatively simple; there is often pain and the patient is usually aware of the cause. The etiology of chronic physical and chemical injuries may be more difficult to determine. The patient may not be aware of the lesion, much less its cause, if a low-grade, subclinical irritant has been acting over a period of months or years. Diligent inspection and questioning help to determine the nature of chronic irritating lesions. Such lesions usually are hyperplastic or chronic inflammatory or a combined result of both processes.

The circumstances under which injuries are produced are of special concern. Most traumatic lesions are accidental. Many are caused by habits of the patient. Such self-induced lesions produced deliberately or habitually are referred to as *factitial* injuries. These injuries must be recognized as such so that they can be corrected through patient awareness and education. Lesions produced in a patient by a treating health professional are called *iatrogenic.* Such injuries should be documented in records, and the patient should be informed honestly as to their nature. Disorders with no determinable cause are referred to as *idiopathic.* Certain traumatic lesions noted in children may be suggestive of child abuse or neglect. Suspicious nonaccidental injuries must be reported to the proper authorities when detected by health care providers.

PHYSICAL AND CHEMICAL INJURY TO TEETH

The enamel and dentin of the teeth are the hardest tissues of the body and are relatively resistant to damage. However, because teeth are subjected to continual wear and trauma, and because they have limited ability to repair, teeth are susceptible to acute and chronic injury.

Acute Injury

Sudden, forceful mechanical injury to teeth may result in fracture or loss of vitality. Anterior teeth are vulnerable in falls and fights, and in automotive or sports accidents. Posterior teeth can be fractured during chewing of hard materials—particularly if weakened by caries, large restorations, or endodontic treatment. The effect of fractures varies. A small fracture of enamel may be of little consequence but may produce a sharp edge capable of irritating oral tissues. Deeper fractures into dentin cause sensitivity to cold, air, or sweets. Fractures that expose the pulp are destined to devitalize the teeth. Additionally, fractures can make the teeth vulnerable to the process of caries.

Depending on the size and depth of the fracture, treatment can consist of smoothing the surface, restoration of the defect, root canal therapy, or extraction. With coronal fractures, the tooth can usually be retained. Fractures through the root are more difficult to diagnose and treat, and many teeth so damaged require extraction (Fig. 13-1). Evaluation of any dental fracture should occur promptly and include radiographs. Treatment involves protection of any exposed dentin, and stabilization of the tooth if mobile. Following acute trauma, teeth are at great risk of being devitalized even with the slightest manipulation. Air syringes, rotary or hand instruments, and certain medicaments are to be avoided or used with extreme caution.

Chronic Injury

Chronic wearing away of teeth produces shortening or flattening of the crowns with the appearance of shiny, polished surfaces. Such wear occurs under three circumstances. *Attrition* is the result of mechanical wear from years of tooth-to-tooth contact. Although attrition increases with age, it may be accelerated by abnormal habitual tooth grinding (bruxism). Initially, smooth, flat facets are worn into contacting incisal and occlusal surfaces. As attrition continues into dentin, the posterior teeth are worn flat and the crowns are shortened (Fig. 13-2). A brown color may be imparted to the polished dentin. *Abrasion* is also caused by slow mechanical wear, but in this instance, it is produced by a foreign abrasive material. Pipe stems, bobby pins, nails, and other materials held between the front teeth because of habit or occupation may cause selective abrasion of tooth structure (Fig. 13-3). Constant use of toothpicks can abrade and widen interproximal spaces while narrowing the mesiodistal diameter of the teeth. Smokeless tobacco is a particularly destructive abrasive. It causes gingival recession and periodontal destruction along with abrasion of the labial aspects of the crowns and roots it contacts. Vigorous back-and-forth toothbrushing with hard bristles and/or abrasive toothpaste can cause "toothbrush abrasion," appearing as V-shaped divots worn into the labial surfaces at the gingival (cervical) aspect of affected crowns (Fig. 13-4). This cervical abrasion may resemble caries radiographically, but not clinically, since the lesions cannot be penetrated with an explorer point. Frequent dietary intake of gritty foods may produce a pattern of abrasion resembling attrition and that may be differentiated only by patient history. Abrasion and attrition are typically asymptomatic because the process is slow. Therefore, teeth have the opportunity to form a protective layer of reparative dentin under the worn tooth structure. This reparative process prevents pain and pulp exposure as it causes sclerosis of the pulp chamber.

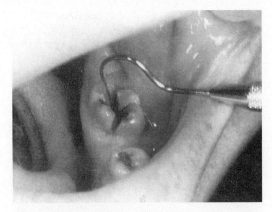

Fig. 13-1 Fracture of crown and root. The fracture is apparent with lateral pressure from an explorer.

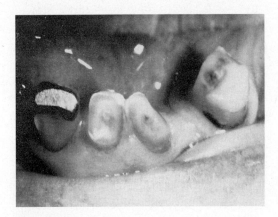

Fig. 13-2 Attrition. This elderly patient had severe bruxism.

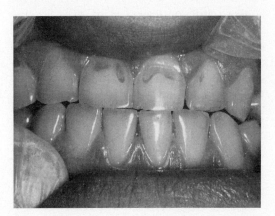

Fig. 13-3 Abrasion. This labial wear is caused by excessive brushing with an abrasive to clean the teeth.

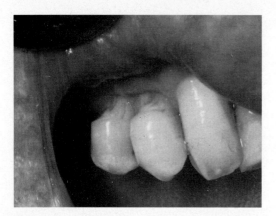

Fig. 13-4 Toothbrush abrasion. Note the cervical grooves of the posterior teeth.

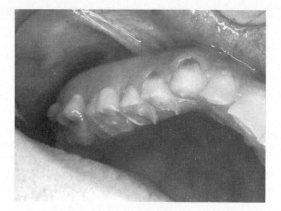

Fig. 13-5 Erosion and attrition. This 14-year-old patient has both gastrointestinal disease and bruxism.

A third process resulting in slow wearing of tooth structure is termed *erosion*. It differs from abrasion and attrition in that erosion is chemically produced, usually by acids. Cervical erosion is most common. It clinically resembles toothbrush abrasion; but instead of having a V-shaped profile, the tooth contour appears dished or is gently curved. The source of the acid is often undetermined, but it may be the result of a lowered pH in the gingival sulcular fluid (Fig. 13-5). Those who habitually ingest large amounts of citrus fruit or apples (citric or maleic acid) may develop erosion. A peculiar form of erosion called *perimyolysis* is sometimes seen on the palatal surfaces of maxillary teeth. It is caused by constant bathing of those surfaces by acids retained on the dorsal surface of the tongue, and it is seen mostly in individuals who frequently regurgitate or bring up stomach acid (Fig. 13-6). This is typical of people with stomach problems or psychological disorders such as bulimia or anorexia nervosa. Erosion may be asymptomatic or cause the patient to complain of tooth sensitivity to cold, air, or sweets—complaints that mimic the symptoms of caries. When a patient complains of a cavity and none can be found, an explorer may discover a sensitive area of cervical erosion that is the source of the patient's symptoms.

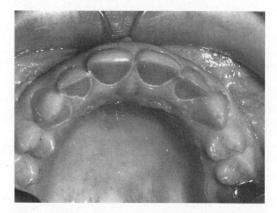

Fig. 13-6 Erosion from perimyolysis. This female patient admitted to bulimia after questioning. Note the smooth dissolution of the lingual surfaces of the upper teeth.

Resorption of Teeth

The dental root can be damaged by chronic physical forces. Pressure on roots caused by adjacent impacted teeth, cysts, and tumors may cause *external resorption*. Inflammation, infection, or previous trauma may also lead to root resorption. Root resorption frequently results in shortening of the root and blunting of the apex. Occasionally, irregular destruction of the root surface occurs. Excessive orthodontic force is an iatrogenic cause of resorption often seen radiographically as blunting of anterior root apices (Fig. 13-7). Completely impacted teeth may resorb spontaneously as a natural occurrence. A rare type of resorption affecting multiple teeth is seen in young women. Here, the cervical portions of the roots resorb, leaving only unsupported crowns that must then be extracted (Fig. 13-8). The cause of this disorder is unknown—thus the name *idiopathic external resorption*.

Dental Stains

Not all dental injuries involve the loss of tooth substance. Certain factors cause discoloration either by adding a layer of stained material to the tooth surface (*extrinsic stains*) or by discoloring the internal portions of the teeth (*intrinsic stains*). Accretions of stained calculus account for much of the extrinsic staining of teeth (Fig. 13-9). Colored food substances such as coffee, tea, cola, and tobacco products account for the largest segment of brown extrinsic stains. Some black, brown, green, and orange stains are caused by chromogenic bacteria or blood substances. Orange and green stains are closely related to poor oral hygiene. The use of chlorhexidine mouth rinse frequently causes brown adherent staining of residual plaque (Fig. 13-10). With varying degrees of difficulty, most extrinsic stains can be removed with scalers and dental abrasive pastes and polishes.

The most prevalent cause of intrinsic stains is the use of tetracycline antibiotics. The drugs bond with calcium hydroxyapatite and incorporate into the dentin and enamel of developing teeth. The teeth erupt with a yellow, gray, brown, or purplish discoloration (Fig. 13-11). The severity and extent are determined by the type, amount, and duration of tetracycline therapy. This unsightly stain cannot be removed with polishing, and other techniques such as vital bleaching, veneers, or crowns may be needed to restore a cosmetic dentition. It is much easier to prevent tetracycline stain than to treat it. Tetracycline should not be administered to pregnant women or children younger than 8 years—the age at which most coronal tooth development has been completed. Minocycline is a synthetic tetracycline that can actually cause intrinsic staining of previously fully formed and erupted adult teeth. Fluoride causes intrinsic staining of developing teeth when ingested in drinking water. In geographic locations where the fluoride content of the drinking water exceeds one part per million, *dental fluorosis* may occur. As the teeth erupt, they show brown, tan, and opaque white areas of mottling of the enamel surface. Since both tetracycline and fluoride act systemically, all teeth forming during administration will be affected. (Review Chapter 11.)

PHYSICAL AND CHEMICAL INJURY TO SOFT TISSUE

The mucosa of the oral cavity is covered by stratified squamous epithelium, a resistant lining well equipped to protect against the physical

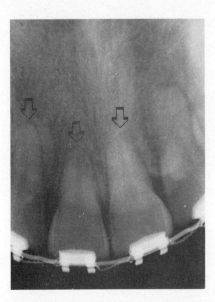

Fig. 13-7 External resorption. Blunting of the lower anterior roots was secondary to orthodontic treatment. (Courtesy of Dr. B.E. Johnson)

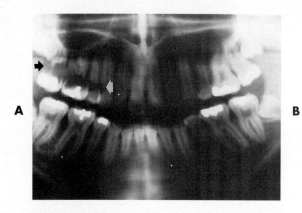
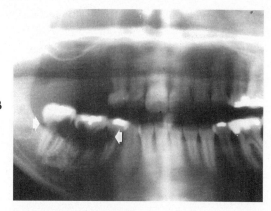

Fig. 13-8 **A,** Idiopathic external resorption. **B,** Note the progression of the cervical resorption over a 2-year time.

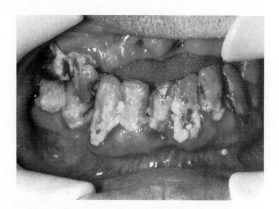

Fig. 13-9 Stains and calculus. These accretions result from poor hygiene and exogenous agents.

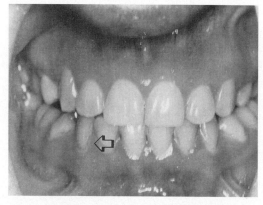

Fig. 13-10 Chlorhexidine staining. Note the brown stains adherent to the cervical portions of the crowns (*arrow*).

and chemical agents that enter the mouth. Aided by the lubricating effect of saliva and the underlying strength and elasticity of the submucosa, the integrity of the mucosa is maintained against most ingested substances. These barriers can be overwhelmed and the mucosa acutely traumatized by mechanical force, electromagnetic energy, cautery, or caustic chemicals. Mucosa can also be chronically damaged by low-grade irritants acting over a long time span.

Acute Physical Injury

Several terms are used to describe patterns of injury caused by acute mechanical trauma:

1. *Abrasion* (as it applies to soft tissue) is a superficial scraping that removes portions of the surface epithelium.
2. *Laceration* is a tearing of soft tissue as might be caused by a blunt object.
3. *Incision* is a cut or slice into tissue caused only by a sharp cutting edge like a scalpel blade or knife.

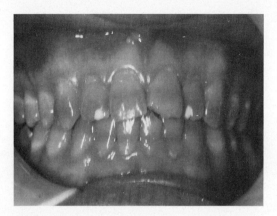

Fig. 13-11 Tetracycline stains. There are incremental lines of staining. The lateral incisors have labial fillings.

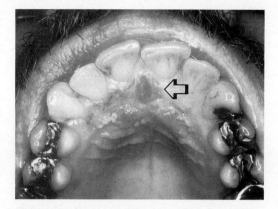

Fig. 13-12 Burn. This location is typical of a pizza burn (*arrow*).

4. *Contusion* is a bruise occurring when a mechanical force breaks capillaries resulting in bleeding into surrounding connective tissue.
5. *Hematoma* is a collection of blood within soft tissues caused when a large vessel is disrupted or broken.

Iatrogenic examples of acute injury include the following: *Cotton roll injury* occurs as an abrasion caused by the rapid removal of a cotton roll that has dried against and become adherent to the mucosa. *Saliva ejector injury* represents a contusion caused by suction of soft tissue of the buccal mucosa or floor of the mouth into a saliva ejector. An *injection hematoma* is an immediate swelling and discoloration of the cheek caused by injection of local anesthetic into the buccal fat-pad or pterygoid plexus of veins.

Factitial examples of acute injury include the following: *Pizza burn* results from eating pizza, allowing the hot cheese and spices to burn the anterior hard palate, leaving a red, raw, peeling area (Fig. 13-12). *Palatal petechiae* represent tiny focal contusions of the soft palate caused by acute physical trauma or forceful sucking. When seen, they call for a careful history to document the etiology, because some serious diseases such as infectious mononucleosis, leukemia, bleeding disorders, and viral infections can also cause palatal petechiae.

When soft tissue is acutely damaged, it responds with acute inflammation followed by healing and restoration of structure and function.

Chronic Physical Injury

Low-grade, chronic irritation has a much different effect on mucosa than does acute injury. The injurious agent may not be sufficient to disrupt and tear tissue. Because there is little actual tissue damage, acute inflammation is not present. Instead, the irritant stimulates adaptive and reparative processes resulting in abnormal and excessive healing. The mucosa thickens in an attempt to protect itself from the irritant. Hyperplastic lesions that develop in response to an irritant and subsequently stabilize or regress when the stimulus is removed are known as *reactive lesions*. Such reactive responses include the following:

1. *Acanthosis* is a hyperplastic thickening of the epithelium.
2. *Hyperkeratosis* is a thickening of the keratinized surface layer of the

epithelium, similar to callus formation on the skin.

3. *Pyogenic granuloma* is an excessive mass of young capillaries and fibroblasts (granulation tissue).
4. *Fibrosis* is a hyperplasia of fibrous connective tissue and collagen.

Mild friction, pressure, chemicals, or heat can stimulate the epithelium to produce a protective layer of keratin on its surface. This hyperkeratosis may also be associated with acanthosis. The affected area appears as a single, defined white patch on the epithelial surface that cannot be removed by rubbing or scraping. It may occur in any oral soft tissue location but is most common in areas that commonly receive continual trauma, such as the buccal mucosa, hard palate, and edentulous ridges. Sometimes the white patch is adjacent to a sharp tooth or irritative dental prosthesis, but often the source of trauma is not apparent. Special patterns of hyperkeratosis can be identified. For instance, patients who knowingly or subconsciously chew on their labial or buccal mucosa develop *cheek-biting injury,* a distinctive pattern of acanthosis and hyperkeratosis occurring along a broad zone of the buccal or labial mucosa bilaterally, adjacent to the occlusal line. Clinically, the tissue appears roughened and white, or red and white. Of course, lesions are located only in areas that can be reached by the teeth. The mucosa of the lateral surface of the tongue may be involved if the habit is severe. Chronic cheek biting can be differentiated from *linea alba,* a bilateral, slightly raised, thin white line running the length of the buccal mucosa at the level of the occlusal line. This common finding is believed to be the result of suction of the buccal mucosa against the occluding surfaces of the posterior teeth (Fig. 13-13). *Nicotinic stomatitis* represents hyperkeratosis secondary to the chronically applied heat of pipe or cigar smoke on the mucosa of the hard palate. The palate appears diffusely white, showing fissuring and small red dots (Fig.

13-14). *Snuff dipper's keratosis* represents hyperkeratosis and acanthosis appearing as a fissured white patch underlying the area where smokeless tobacco is habitually held, usually in the buccal or labial vestibule (Fig. 13-15).

The detection of even the smallest of white lesions is of extreme importance, because cancers of the mouth also begin as white patches. The carcinogens in tobacco frequently

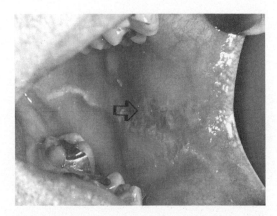

Fig. 13-13 Linea alba and cheek-biting injury. The white horizontal raised line is the linea alba. The red and white roughened area is caused by cheek chewing (*arrow*).

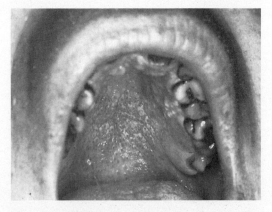

Fig. 13-14 Nicotinic stomatitis. This patient is a long-term pipe smoker.

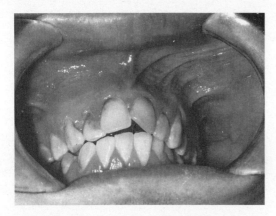

Fig. 13-15 Snuff dipper's keratosis. This patient places his smokeless tobacco in his maxillary buccal vestibule.

cause a white hyperkeratotic lesion as a fore-runner of more detrimental premalignant or malignant lesions (Fig. 13-16). There is no reliable way to clinically differentiate an irritative hyperkeratotic white patch from a white patch destined to evolve into a lethal cancer (dysplasia), although there are some guidelines that help us make this distinction. White patches of the "high risk" areas for oral cancer (see Chapter 19) are more worrisome than white patches of the cheeks, hard palate, or

alveolar ridges. White patches adjacent to or associated with an obvious irritant are less suspicious, although the only assurance of safety is to document the regression of the lesion after removal of the irritant. Otherwise, biopsy should be performed to better establish a diagnosis.

The *pyogenic granuloma* is a reactive lesion composed of granulation tissue. It forms in an area of trauma and is most often seen on the gingiva adjacent to broken, carious, or periodontally involved teeth. It may also be seen on the lips, cheeks, and tongue. A pyogenic granuloma appears as a soft, red to reddish-gray, dull-surfaced, ulcerated protruding mass that is relatively painless but bleeds profusely when lightly touched. The lesion will persist and continue to grow as long as the irritant is present; therefore, treatment of the lesion must include not only its excision but removal of the cause. Pyogenic granulomas are prone to develop on the gingiva of pregnant women because the action of minor irritants is accentuated by hormonal stimulation of granulation tissue (Fig. 13-17). This lesion is now termed a *pregnancy tumor*. A pyogenic granuloma that grows out of a recent tooth extraction site is called an *epulis granulomatosum*. When present, it usually indicates a sharp

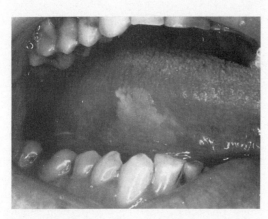

Fig. 13-16 White plaque. Biopsy of this tongue lesion confirmed hyperkeratosis.

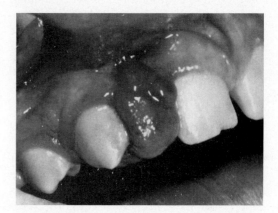

Fig. 13-17 Pyogenic granuloma. This female patient is 7 months pregnant. Tooth No. 7 is missing.

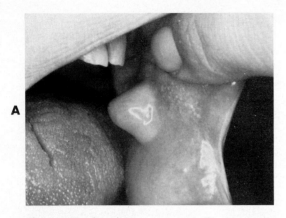 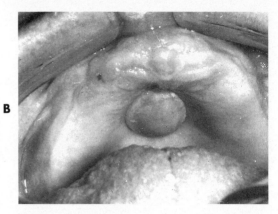

Fig. 13-18 Fibroma. **A,** This soft lesion has been present for many years. **B,** This firm lesion was present beneath a loose denture.

bony margin, bony sequestrum, or foreign body within the socket as the source of irritation.

The *fibroma* is a reactive fibrosis resulting from low-grade, chronic mechanical irritation. It is a common lesion, particularly along the buccal and labial mucosa in areas prone to accidental biting. Like the pyogenic granuloma, the fibroma is an elevated nodule, but it is covered by normal, shiny, pink to white mucosa (Fig. 13-18). It is painless and either soft or firm, and does not bleed. Since it protrudes into the mouth, it is easily retraumatized and should be removed. Other reactive lesions of the gingiva—the peripheral giant cell granuloma and peripheral ossifying fibroma—are discussed along with periodontal diseases in Chapter 17.

Denture-Related Reactive Conditions

Dentures can cause some unique reactive lesions. *Denture sore mouth* is a bright red, relatively painless mucosal lesion underlying a denture base and conforming to its outline (Fig. 13-19). Patients with ill-fitting or unclean dentures are more likely to develop this reaction, as are patients who sleep with their dentures in place. The irritated tissue be-

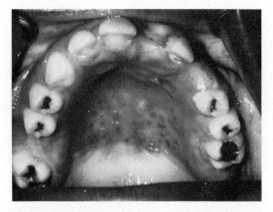

Fig. 13-19 Denture sore mouth. The red painless area of the palate conforms to the shape of an acrylic partial denture.

comes predisposed to opportunistic *Candida* infection, which in turn aggravates the condition. Rarely, acute painful denture sore mouth may represent a reaction to residual acrylic monomer present after delivery of poorly cured dentures or a denture repair. Treatment of denture sore mouth involves removal of the denture, treatment of *Candida* infection if present, and use of a tissue conditioner or fabrication of a new prosthesis. If left untreated, the inflamed palatal and maxillary mucosa can form lobular masses of granulation tissue under the denture. These may later mature into small fibrous bumps that resemble multiple fibromas (Fig. 13-20). This so-called *papillary hyperplasia* occurs almost exclusively on the hard palate and is also commonly associated with *Candida* infection. Because these lesions are composed of mature fibrous tissue, they will not disappear even if the irritant is removed and therefore must be surgically removed.

Epulis fissuratum is another type of denture-induced fibrous hyperplasia related to the fibroma. It develops in the buccal or labial vestibule as a result of pressure and irritation from an overextended denture flange (Fig. 13-21). The construction of the denture itself is not necessarily faulty. Even when a denture is fabricated correctly, ridge resorption may cause the flange to slip deeper into the fold as the denture settles. The lesion appears as flabby, elevated, hyperplastic folds of tissue paralleling the denture border. The denture flange rests in the fissure between the folds of

tissue. Epulis fissuratum requires surgical removal, with construction of a new denture or shortening of the flange.

Fibrous hyperplasia of the ridge is a common sequela of ridge resorption and accompanying poorly fitting dentures. The space between the denture and the resorbed ridge fills with dense, often firm fibrous connective tissue covered by mucosa (Fig. 13-22). The tissue is

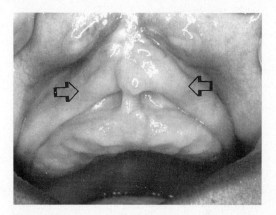

Fig. 13-21 Epulis fissuratum. The denture flange fits between the ridge and the fibrous hyperplasia (*arrows*).

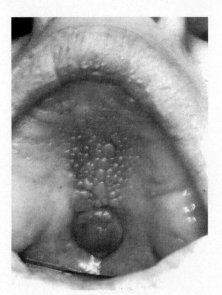

Fig. 13-20 Papillary hyperplasia of the palate. This patient has worn his upper denture for years.

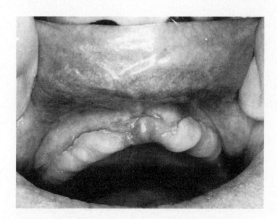

Fig. 13-22 Fibrous hyperplasia. This firm tissue has formed on the ridge beneath a poorly fitting upper denture.

somewhat movable and can become pinched or irritated beneath a loose-fitting denture. The anterior upper and lower ridges are most commonly involved. Treatment includes removal of the hyperplastic tissue and relining or refabrication of the dentures.

CHEMICAL INJURY

Chemicals may act locally or systemically to cause acute or chronic lesions. Many are factitial or iatrogenic.

Chemical Burns

Aspirin burn is the name applied to the white, or red and white lesion caused by contact between mucosa and aspirin. Chemically, aspirin is acetylsalicylic acid, an analgesic that acts systemically. Some patients treat toothaches by placing an aspirin tablet on the nearby mucosa, erroneously believing that it has a topical effect. Instead of relieving the toothache, the acid burns the epithelium, causing coagulation necrosis. The white, sloughing membrane produced by the coagulated protein is similar to the whitening effect produced by boiling eggwhites (Fig. 13-23). The patient is

not usually aware of the lesion, so it takes a clever diagnostician to focus on the clues that would lead to questioning the patient about aspirin use. These clues include the presence of the opaque white, fissured, sloughing membrane on the gingiva or vestibule adjacent to a painful tooth. Other chemicals such as eugenol-containing toothache drops, phenol, silver nitrate, and other over-the-counter medicaments can cause similar chemical burns. A patient with a suspicious lesion should be asked about substances placed on the tooth for relief of pain.

Phenytoin Hyperplasia

Phenytoin (Dilantin), a drug used for epileptic seizures and pain syndromes, has long been known to stimulate diffuse, firm, fibrous hyperplasia of mildly inflamed gingiva (Fig. 13-24). More recently, other medications such as calcium channel blockers (for heart patients) and cyclosporine (for organ transplant patients) have been reported to have a similar effect. The gingival overgrowth can be surgically trimmed, but it tends to recur. Patient education is important, since good oral hygiene can slow down or prevent the return of the hyperplasia.

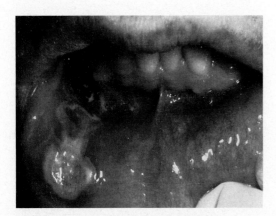

Fig. 13-23 Chemical burn. This burn was caused when aspirin was applied directly to an aphthous ulcer of the labial mucosa.

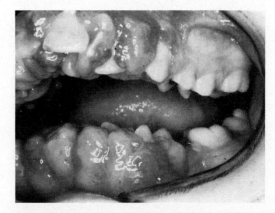

Fig. 13-24 Phenytoin hyperplasia. The patient has taken phenytoin for many years for seizures.

Amalgam Tattoo

The *amalgam tattoo* is a small, blue-gray area of oral pigmentation representing an implantation of silver amalgam fragments into the mucosa. Frequently, amalgam filings enter a mucosal laceration during the placement or removal of an amalgam restoration. Since the laceration is often produced by the bur or matrix band, the tattoo is usually located in the gingiva adjacent to the restoration. However, a mucosal abrasion tear or ulceration in any part of the mouth can retain amalgam particles following manipulation of an amalgam filling. Amalgam tattoos are sometimes seen in the alveolar mucosa overlying a tooth that has been treated endodontically by amalgam restoration (retrofilling) of the surgically exposed root. Amalgam tattoo also frequently occurs when an amalgam restoration shatters during an extraction and some of the fragments enter the open socket. Amalgam does not severely irritate tissue; therefore, the area

heals normally and without symptoms, leaving only the discoloration as evidence of the iatrogenic injury (Fig. 13-25). The presence of amalgam within tissue can sometimes be seen radiographically as a cluster of small opaque particles corresponding to the discoloration. However, since particles may be very small, the absence of radiographic findings does not preclude the diagnosis of amalgam tattoo. Other pigmented lesions resembling amalgam tattoos can be produced by graphite from "lead" pencils that accidentally penetrate oral mucosa. The amalgam tattoo does not require treatment, but pigmented lesions should be brought to the attention of the dentist. Some of them, particularly those located on the hard palate or gingiva, may represent more serious diseases including malignant melanomas.

Exogenous Lingual Pigmentation

Discolorations covering the dorsal surface of the tongue are common and are sometimes

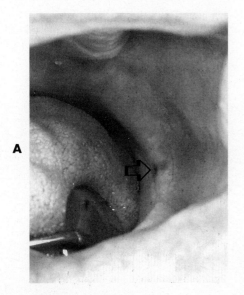
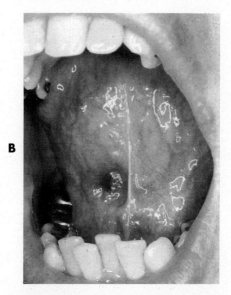

Fig. **13-25** Amalgam tattoo. **A,** A small area of the mandibular ridge (*arrow*). **B,** A large area of the floor of the mouth; a radiograph of this area revealed fine particles.

induced by medications. Licorice, tobacco, coffee, or tea may impart a black or brown coloration to the keratin on the surface of the tongue. Bacterial decomposition of certain heavy metal salts may also cause black tongue (Fig. 13-26). For instance, Pepto Bismol, which contains bismuth, may cause a harmless black coating that appears soon after its use. *Black hairy tongue* refers to marked elongation of the filiform papillae in conjunction with a black discoloration attributed to chromogenic bacteria or tobacco. The cause of black hairy tongue is uncertain, but it usually occurs in heavy smokers and occasionally follows the use of antibiotics that might stimulate an overgrowth of resistant bacteria (Fig. 13-27). The condition is harmless and the thickened dead layer of keratin can be painlessly removed by brisk scraping of the dorsal surface of the tongue with the edge of a spoon or a toothbrush.

Allergic Reactions

Some individuals have unpredictable sensitivities to a wide variety of foods, cosmetics, medications, toothpastes, or mouthwashes. Many of these reactions are allergic, although others are idiosyncratic. Oral lesions resulting from these sensitivities are among the most challenging lesions to diagnose. This is because they are unpredictable. The lesions are varied and nonspecific in appearance. They may be single and small or multiple and confluent. They may appear localized to one area or limited to a specific anatomic location (such as gingiva or lips), or may involve multiple mucosal surfaces. They appear as ulcers, blisters, swelling, or red, white, or pigmented patches. They may occur with or without associated skin or systemic lesions. They may be asymptomatic or cause burning, peeling, bleeding, or severe pain. The number of substances capable of inducing such sensitivities is so extensive as to make identification impossible without elaborate testing. Sensitivity reactions can be divided into two types—*contact stomatitis (stomatitis venenata)*, representing direct oral mucosal contact with the sensitizing agent, and *stomatitis medicamentosa*, representing an oral reaction to a systemically acting medication. Agents commonly implicated in contact stomatitis include dental metals such as gold, nickel, and copper

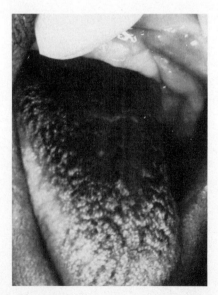

Fig. 13-26 Bismuth-coated tongue. This patient dissolved bismuth antacids on the tongue.

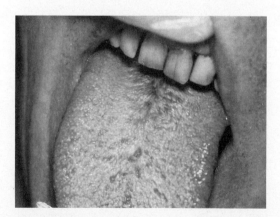

Fig. 13-27 Hairy tongue. This patient is a heavy cigarette smoker.

(Fig. 13-28), and flavoring agents, particularly cinnamon. The first step in determining a possible cause is to look for a contacting material. Next, the patient should be asked about habits and the use of any foods or oral health products that had been taken concurrent to lesion occurrence. All medications listed by the patient should then be looked up, with special note made of their adverse effects and contraindications. If feasible, possible offending agents should be eliminated one by one. Patch testing of the patient's skin or mucosa with possible allergens can sometimes be effective in determination of allergy, but it can cause serious and even fatal reactions and is therefore best left to the allergist.

Cancer Chemotherapy Effects

Medications used systemically to treat cancer may also frequently cause drug-induced injury to the oral mucosa. These drugs are potent poisons that kill cells. The basis of their use is that they preferentially damage rapidly grow-ing cells such as cancer cells. Unfortunately, oral mucosa and many other cells in the body (bone marrow and lymphoid cells, intestinal epithelium, and germ cells) also grow rapidly and are injured by chemotherapy. In the oral cavity, chemotherapy directly causes severe, painful ulcers that can easily become infected (Fig. 13-29). In addition, the chemotherapy patient frequently develops viral, bacterial, and fungal stomatitis secondary to xerostomia and immune suppression. The pain is often so severe as to limit eating and swallowing. Treatment must be both prescriptive (antibiotics, antivirals) and palliative (pain relievers).

RADIATION INJURY

The therapeutic radiation used to destroy cancers of the head and neck often damages normal tissue as well. The penetrating energy of radiation presumably acts by damaging the DNA and altering proteins, enzymes, or other chemicals within the cell. Radiation may cause acute or chronic damage to cells or may cause cancers to develop many years later. The effects of radiation are cumulative. Multiple small doses or a single large dose can

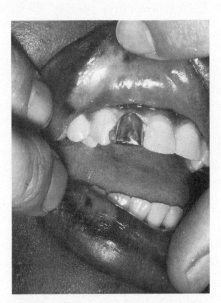

Fig. 13-28 Contact stomatitis reaction to metal. These painful areas developed after placement of the jacket crown on tooth No. 7.

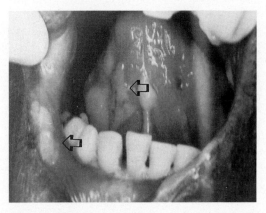

Fig. 13-29 Chemotherapy ulcerations. These painful ulcers developed after chemotherapeutic treatment for lymphosarcoma.

cause injury. Cells that are capable of rapid growth and regeneration are most easily killed by high-dose radiation. As with chemotherapy, this selective advantage allows radiation to destroy fast-growing cancer cells before doing lethal harm to normal cells. But when radiation is delivered in amounts sufficient to kill tumor cells, some damage results to the normal tissue through which it passes.

Radiation Mucositis

Radiation mucositis results from destruction of the mucosa following direct therapeutic irradiation through mucous membranes. Radiation-exposed mucosa becomes red, swollen, and ulcerated and painful approximately 2 weeks after the radiation treatment. The symptoms are severe, and the lesions may resemble those seen following chemotherapy. Healing occurs after several weeks, but tissue may remain reddened, atrophic, or fibrotic.

Bone Necrosis and Infection

Radiation has little effect on mature connective tissue, therefore formed collagen, bones, and teeth remain relatively unaltered. The lining of blood vessels, however, is sensitive to high-dose radiation, and vessels within bone can become damaged. Thus, irradiated bone may be stable and functional as long as it is not injured. If there is a bone infection, fracture, or tooth extraction, the damaged blood vessels may reduce the capacity of bone to respond with inflammation and repair. Massive necrosis and infection of the irradiated bone known as *osteoradionecrosis* may ensue. Osteoradionecrosis most commonly occurs in the mandible, and the risk of occurrence is related to the radiation dose. Importantly, once bone is irradiated, it never returns to its normal vascular state and will always be vulnerable to osteoradionecrosis.

Radiation Xerostomia and Caries

Direct radiation injures salivary gland tissue resulting in temporary or permanent loss of saliva. Dry mouth or *xerostomia* is the unpleasant result. The importance of saliva is underestimated by many individuals until it is no longer present. Without the lubrication of saliva, the oral mucosa becomes irritated as the result of infection and friction. The mucosa becomes red, sore, and atrophic. Opportunistic *Candida* infection frequently results. Taste sensation is altered, swallowing is impaired, and dentures lose retention, making eating difficult. Without the anticariogenic action of saliva, the dentition rapidly succumbs to severe cervical caries that encircles and destroys the crowns (Fig. 13-30). This so-called *radiation caries* is, therefore, not due to any direct effect of radiation but rather the indirect effect of xerostomia.

The management, care, and treatment of a previously irradiated patient is complicated and risky. Xerostomia predisposes the patient to caries. However, the needed extractions can cause osteoradionecrosis. To avoid these complications, it is recommended that some patients undergoing radiation treatment have extractions performed prior to therapy. Patients with severe periodontitis or inability to maintain oral hygiene are at the greatest risk and may have to sacrifice their teeth if the mandible and salivary glands are going to receive high-dose radiation. Following radiotherapy, simple procedures like denture construction, dental prophylaxis, and extractions can all result in severe and life-threatening osteoradionecrosis. Irradiated patients who retain teeth must be placed on a regimen of meticulous oral hygiene to prevent periodontal disease and caries. This regimen includes daily topical fluoride. Artificial saliva helps lubricate the mouth, and antimicrobial mouth rinse (chlorhexidine) helps reduce oral microorganisms involved in caries, periodontal disease, and candidiasis. Furthermore, because these patients are predisposed to developing new oral cancers, periodic and careful oral exams must be performed for the remainder of the patient's life.

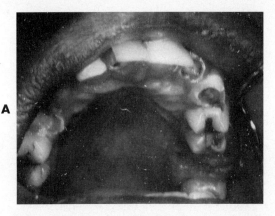 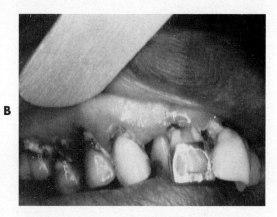

Fig. 13-30 Radiation caries. **A,** This 14-year-old has been treated with therapeutic radiation for nasopharyngeal cancer. **B,** Note the cervical caries in this adult oral cancer patient.

It should be obvious from the foregoing discussion that radiation can cause serious damage to body tissues. Thus, even though diagnostic dental radiography is safe when administered according to standard techniques, great respect must be paid to radiation safety.

Case Studies

Case 1
W.B. is a 40-year-old woman who went to her dentist with a painless, pink, slightly firm raised mass of the right buccal mucosa. She was missing tooth No. 29, and the mass fit into the space when her mouth was closed. She had been aware of the lesion for at least 7 years. Recently W.B. had been irritating the lesion, and she requested its removal. Simple excisional biopsy revealed a fibroma. A bridge was constructed to replace tooth No. 29. There was no recurrence of the fibroma.

Case 2
N.K. is a 35-year-old woman who is 7 months pregnant with her fourth child. The dental hygienist noted a 0.8 cm raised, red, soft, painless growth of her buccal gingiva between teeth No. 3 and 4. N.K. thought that the area had been bleeding with toothbrushing for at least the past 4 months. After a provisional diagnosis of preg-

nancy tumor, the lesion was excised and calculus was removed from the adjacent teeth. The biopsy confirmed pyogenic granuloma. The healing was uneventful, and N.K. delivered a healthy baby boy 6 weeks later.

Case 3
G.G. is a 58-year-old man who wears a lower partial denture and upper complete denture. He made his first dental appointment in 6 years. On oral examination, the hygienist noted red, slightly papillary changes of the palate beneath the upper denture. In addition, a large 2.5 x 0.8 cm pink, nonpainful mass of the right maxillary buccal vestibule was noted that encased the posterior denture flange in that area. G.G. admitted that the upper denture was 23 years old and he wore it constantly. It fit poorly and rocked with lateral pressure. A smear test of the palate was positive for candidiasis. Following 14 days of antifungal therapy, the palatal redness cleared. Surgical removal of the vestibular mass was performed, and it was diagnosed as epulis fissuratum. Biopsy of two of the larger palatal papillae resulted in a diagnosis of fibrosis. New upper and lower dentures were fabricated, and the mucosa now appears healthy and lesion free.

Case 4
On routine examination, the dentist noted a 0.5 cm pigmented macule of the palate on

patient E.B., a 55-year-old woman. The lesion had not been noted at the time of a previous visit, when two upper amalgams had been replaced. A radiograph of the area was negative. Excisional biopsy of the lesion was performed to rule out nevus or melanoma. Biopsy revealed an amalgam tattoo with minimal inflammatory response. The patient was assured that the lesion was benign.

Case 1

1. Does the 7-year history indicate benign or malignant growth?
2. What is the association of the fibroma with the missing tooth No. 29?
3. Give two reasons for removal of the fibroma.
4. Would you consider this fibroma neoplastic or reactive?

Case 2

1. What caused the pyogenic granuloma?
2. What promoted growth of the pyogenic granuloma?
3. Is a pyogenic granuloma the same lesion as a pregnancy tumor?
4. Are pregnancy tumors usually painful?

Case 3

1. What tissues form the papillary hyperplasia and epulis fissuratum?
2. What infection frequently complicates papillary hyperplasia?
3. What are the causes of papillary hyperplasia?
4. What is the cause of the epulis fissuratum?
5. What is the oral location of epulis fissuratum in most cases?

Case 4

1. Is the palate a worrisome area for melanoma formation?
2. Why might this lesion not have been seen with radiography?

3. Explain the etiology of this lesion in E.B.
4. What are the sequelae of an amalgam tattoo?

SUMMARY

- Physical injuries to the oral hard and soft tissues are common and may be acute or chronic in duration. They may be accidental, factitial or iatrogenic in etiology.
- Teeth can show abnormal wear from attrition, erosion, or abrasion. The cause can frequently be distinguished by careful analysis and questioning.
- Oral soft tissues usually respond to chronic physical and chemical irritants with fibrous hyperplasia and epithelial thickening. These hyperplasias are frequently diagnosed by location, appearance, and history of irritation.
- Specific recognizable hyperplastic lesions are associated with tobacco use, medications, dentures, and pregnancy.
- Acute chemical burns are usually factitial or iatrogenic and are frequently related to application of preparations to the oral mucous membrane.
- Phenytoin therapy induces inflammatory hyperplasia of the gingiva. Other medications can facilitate similar hyperplasia.
- Amalgam particles are frequently deposited in oral mucosa and bone during dental procedures. The resultant tattoo might be confused with other pigmented oral lesions.
- Exogenous pigments from tobacco tars, bismuth, bacterial pigments, and beverages can impart a black or black hairy appearance to the dorsal surface of the tongue.
- Allergic reactions and contact allergies to medicine, dental products, foods, and flavoring agents can cause acute and chronic lesions of the oral mucosa. Some of these lesions may be ulcerative, blistering, lichenoid, or white and are readily confused with more serious pathologic conditions.
- Cancer chemotherapy predisposes patients to oral ulcers, and to bacterial, viral, and fungal infection.

- Possible side effects of therapeutic radiation include mucositis, xerostomia, and osteoradionecrosis. Careful planning and management can help reduce or prevent these sequelae.

Suggested readings

1. Bhaskar SN, Beasley JD, and Cutwright DE: Inflammatory papillary hyperplasia of the oral mucosa: report of 341 cases, JADA 81:949, 1970.
2. Buchner A and Hansen LS: Amalgam pigmentation (amalgam tattoo) of the oral mucosa, Oral Surg Oral Med Oral Pathol 49:139, 1980.
3. Carl W, Schaaf NG, and Chen TY: Oral care of patients irradiated for cancer of the head and neck, Cancer 30:448, 1972.
4. Ferretti G and others: Chlorhexidine prophylaxis for chemotherapy- and radiotherapy-induced stomatitis: a randomized double-blind trial, Oral Surg Oral Med Oral Pathol 69:331, 1990.
5. Fischman S: The patient with cancer, in symposium on patient with increased medical risks, Dent Clin North Am 27:235, 1983.
6. George DL and Miller RL: Idiopathic resorption of teeth, Am J Orthod 89:13, 1986.
7. Greer RO and Poulson TC: Oral tissue alterations associated with the use of smokeless tobacco by teenagers, Oral Surg Oral Med Oral Pathol 56:275, 1983.
8. Marx RE and Johnson RP: Studies in the radiobiology of osteoradionecrosis and their clinical significance, Oral Surg Oral Med Oral Pathol 64:379, 1987.
9. Miller RL, Gould AR, and Bernstein ML: Cinnamon induced stomatitis venenata—clinical and characteristic histiopathologic features, Oral Surg Oral Med Oral Pathol 73:708, 1992.
10. Rossie KM and Gugenheimer J: Thermally-induced nicotine stomatitis: a case report, Oral Surg Oral Med Oral Pathol 70:597, 1990.

14 Odontogenic Cysts and Tumors and Other Bony Lesions

IN THIS CHAPTER

1. Review of normal tooth development
2. Odontogenic cysts
   - Periapical cyst
   - Dentigerous cyst
   - Lateral periodontal cyst
   - Gingival cyst of the adult
   - Residual cyst
   - Odontogenic keratocyst
3. Odontogenic tumors
   - Ameloblastoma
   - Other epithelial odontogenic tumors
   - Odontogenic myxoma
   - Cemento-ossifying fibroma
   - Cementoma
   - Ameloblastic fibroma
   - Odontoma
4. Pseudocysts
   - Traumatic bone cyst
   - Central giant cell granuloma
   - Stafne bone cyst
5. Other bony lesions
   - Fibrous dysplasia
   - Idiopathic histiocytosis
   - Paget's disease
6. Differential diagnosis of bony lesions
7. Case studies

After studying this chapter, you should be able to meet the following objectives and define the key terms:

- Explain the origin and etiology of common odontogenic cysts
- Discuss normal tooth development
- Draw a typical dentigerous cyst and indicate its position in approximation to teeth
- Identify lateral periodontal cysts based on radiographic interpretation and clinical tests
- Explain the significance of the odontogenic keratocyst
- Recognize the significance of adenomatoid odontogenic tumors, calcifying epithelial odontogenic tumors, and calcifying odontogenic cysts
- Compare and contrast the behavior of a meloblastoma with that of odontogenic myxoma
- Discuss the clinical and radiographic signs of ameloblastoma
- Recognize the terms cemento-ossifying fibroma and cementoma
- Distinguish clinically and radiographically the compound and complex odontoma
- Draw and describe a typical traumatic bone cyst and Stafne bone cyst
- Discuss the presentation, treatment, and course of fibrous dysplasia
- Define idiopathic histiocytosis and categorize it by age of appearance, location, and prognosis
- Recognize important features of Paget's disease

The cysts and tumors derived from teeth are of unique interest to the dental profession. The intensive training received by dental professionals in dental anatomy, embryology, and radiographic interpretation best prepares us to understand the pathogenesis, behavior, diagnosis, and treatment of these disorders. Most of these lesions are discovered radiographically; therefore, the radiograph becomes the focal point around which a diagnosis is pursued. Other information such as history and clinical findings assist in the diagnosis, which may be ultimately confirmed by biopsy. Many odontogenic cysts and several benign odontogenic tumors are diagnosed exclusively by assimilation and correlation of clinical findings. Treatment is based on the clinical or the microscopic diagnosis.

REVIEW OF NORMAL TOOTH DEVELOPMENT

The behavior of an odontogenic cyst or tumor depends, in part, on the degree of differentiation and histopathologic appearance of cells and tissues. A review of normal tooth development is essential to the understanding of the natural history of these lesions.

In the 6-week embryo, the future jaws consist of two horseshoe-shaped ridges covered by oral ectodermal epithelium. Strands of this epithelium called *dental lamina* grow downward at each point destined to become a tooth (Fig. 14-1*A*). At its deepest penetration, each dental lamina buds to form an *epithelial cap,* which induces formation of a central core of mesenchyme known as the *dental papilla,* and a peripheral capsule of mesenchyme, the *dental follicle,* which surrounds the epithelial cap (Fig. 14- 1*B*).

As the cap enlarges, it forms three distinct layers: *inner enamel epithelium* (IEE), *outer enamel epithelium* (OEE), and a middle zone called the *stellate reticulum* (SR). The epithelial component of these cells is now known as the *enamel organ,* and the entire structure including the enamel organ, dentinal papilla, and dental follicle is called the *tooth bud* (Fig. 14-1*C*). The inner enamel epithelium rests against the dentinal papilla and induces the dentinal papilla to form a layer of *odontoblasts,* which then secretes dentin (Fig. 14-2). The dentin causes the inner enamel epithelium to transform into elongated *ameloblasts,* which

secrete a layer of enamel on top of the dentin (Fig. 14-2). As the enamel and dentin layers grow and incrementally thicken, the ameloblasts and odontoblasts move farther away from each other. A resulting dental crown forms around a core of dental papilla that will ultimately become the pulp (Fig. 14-2). When crown formation is completed, the ameloblasts and other epithelial cells of the enamel organ fuse to form a thin membrane, the *reduced enamel epithelium* (REE), which encloses the crown of the dental follicle (Fig. 14-3). When the tooth erupts, the REE fuses with the gingival epithelium and remains as the epithelial collar that surrounds the neck of the tooth (Fig. 14-3).

Root development begins at the lower margin of the formed crown. From here, a column of epithelial cells called *Hertwig's sheath* proliferates downward, inducing and stimulating odontoblasts to form root dentin. As the root forms and elongates, it is accompanied by an extension of the dental follicle that forms the periodontal ligament (Fig. 14-2). Cementoblasts made in this periodontal tissue penetrate through Hertwig's sheath and deposit cementum on the outer root surface (Fig. 14-3). When Hertwig's sheath finally degenerates, small nests of its cells persist within the periodontal membrane as *rests of Malassez* (Fig. 14-3).

ODONTOGENIC CYSTS

As defined for the oral regions, a cyst is a pathologic cavity lined by epithelium and surrounded by a fibrous cyst wall. The cyst originates from entrapped odontogenic epithelium that begin to grow, accumulate fluid, and induce peripheral reactive fibrous connective tissue formation. For odontogenic cysts, this epithelium can come from four sources: the developing enamel organ, the reduced enamel epithelium of the dental follicle, rests of Malassez, or residual nests of dental lamina remaining within the bone or gingiva.

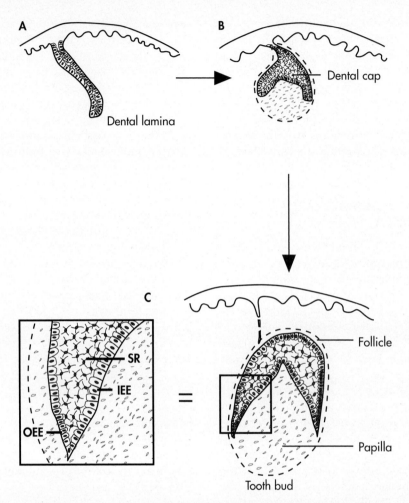

Fig. 14-1 Tooth development. The dental lamina buds from the surface epithelium of the developing jaws (**A**). The dental lamina develops into a dental cap (**B**). The cap stage continues to differentiate into the tooth bud with a papilla and follicle (**C**). Note that the inner enamel epithelium (**IEE**), the outer enamel epithelium (**IEE**), and the stellate reticulum (**SR**) are now formed.

Historically, odontogenic cysts have been reported for over 100 years. The earliest classification was based on their relationship with teeth. Such terminology as periapical cyst, lateral periodontal cyst, dentigerous cyst, and gingival cyst reflect this. Histology was considered unimportant because all these cysts are lined by a somewhat similar appearing stratified squamous odontogenic epithelium. As our knowledge of these cysts progressed, it was realized that subtle histologic differences in the epithelium could predict the behavior of some of these cysts. The result is that the old classification has been modified to delete certain cysts and to accommodate new ones.

Periapical Cyst

By far the most common odontogenic cyst is the periapical (radicular) cyst. It represents a

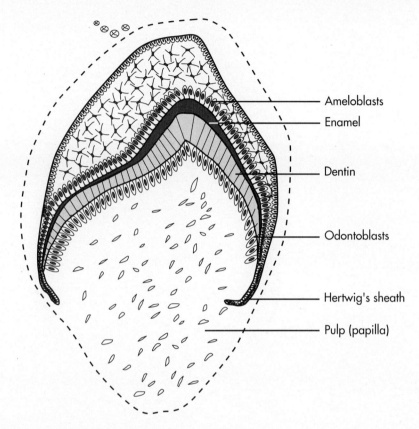

Fig. 14-2 As the tooth bud further develops, the odontoblasts are formed from the papilla and lay down dentin. Ameloblasts form from the inner enamel epithelium and begin to make enamel. The Hertwig's sheath proliferates from the dental cap.

reactive, inflammatory cyst that occurs in association with a nonvital tooth. It develops from inflammatory stimulation of rests of Malassez contained within a periapical granuloma (discussed in Chapter 12). The necrotic pulp is the source of the irritant that escapes into surrounding bone through the apical foramen. Most of these cysts, then, develop around the apex of teeth. As with other hyperplastic reactive lesions, periapical cysts may continue to enlarge as long as the irritant remains. Progressive fluid accumulation within the cyst lumen causes the cyst to expand. Because it is nonpainful, the periapical cyst is usually unnoticed until a radio-graph discloses its presence. When symptomatic, there may be swelling of the jaw or mild discomfort of the associated tooth during biting. If the cyst becomes secondarily infected, abscess formation, severe pain and drainage may ensue. Development of cancer within a periapical cyst is not expected, but this complication has occurred in rare instances.

Radiographically, the typical appearance of a periapical cyst is that of a well-demarcated, round to oval radiolucency symmetrically placed around the apex of the dead tooth (Fig. 14-4). The lamina dura around the involved tooth's apex is missing. A thin radio-paque rim usually surrounds the cyst. The

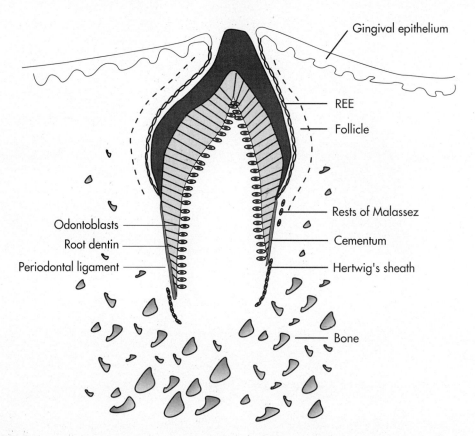

Fig. 14-3 As the tooth further develops, the reduced enamel epithelium (**REE**) fuses with the gingival epithelium. The Hertwig's sheath guides the formation of root dentin and cementum. Remnants of Hertwig's sheath are entrapped as rests of Malassez in the periodontal ligament.

periapical cyst cannot be distinguished radiographically from the periapical granuloma from which it develops. However, the larger the periapical lesion, the more likely it is to be a cyst. Certain variations in the radiographic appearance may occur. Some periapical cysts, particularly those of the maxillary lateral incisor, may not be situated directly over the apex, but may shift slightly distally to form a pear-shaped radiolucency wedged in between the roots of the lateral incisor and canine. Conversely, not every periapical radiolucency represents a cyst or granuloma; it may be a completely different lesion. Before making the diagnosis of periapical cyst or granuloma and instituting therapy, one should be certain that the associated tooth is nonvital.

The preferred treatment for a periapical cyst is either endodontic therapy or extraction if the tooth cannot be salvaged. Following endodontic therapy, the cyst will usually disappear. Occasionally, the cyst will persist. If the cyst does not disappear after a suitable length of time, removal with biopsy of the lesion is often necessary, since other less common lesions can give a similar clinical presentation.

Dentigerous Cyst

The follicle around the unerupted tooth provides the site for development of the dentigerous cyst. When teeth are impacted, the follicle does not fuse with the surface. The reduced enamel epithelium lining the follicle can

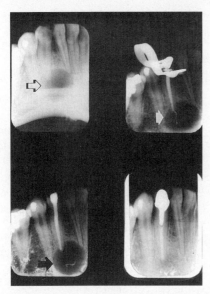

Fig. 14-4 Periapical cyst. This slow-growing expansile, well-demarcated radiolucency (upper left) is treated endodontically (upper right). Excess cement falls into the base of the cyst (lower left). One year later (lower right) the bone has filled the defect.

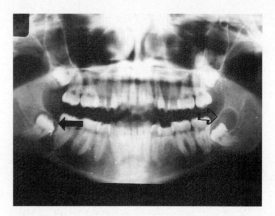

Fig. 14-5 Dentigerous cyst. Compare the cystic space (open arrow) to the opposite dental follicle (dark arrow).

develop squamous metaplasia and separate from the enamel. Fluid then accumulates centrally. The resulting cyst forms around the crown of the tooth (Fig. 14-5). Although most dentigerous cysts are noted as incidental radiographic findings, some can grow large and cause bony swelling, tooth displacement, pain, or infection, or lead to pathologic jaw fracture. Rare cysts can transform into tumors capable of considerable growth and destruction. Any impacted or unerupted tooth can develop a dentigerous cyst. Since mandibular third molars are the teeth most frequently impacted, they are associated with the greatest number of dentigerous cysts. Maxillary third molars and impacted permanent canines are less commonly affected.

Radiographically, a dentigerous cyst shows a well-demarcated, single, oval radiolucency surrounding the crown of an impacted tooth. It attaches at the neck of the tooth and resembles an enlarged dental follicle. An exact diagnosis of dentigerous cysts cannot be made radiographically because there are other cysts and tumors that share the same features. The radiograph merely suggests a diagnosis, which must then be proven by biopsy. Any pathologic pericoronal radiolucency should be an indication for biopsy. If the diagnosis turns out to be dentigerous cyst, the cyst will not likely recur.

Lateral Periodontal Cyst

The lateral periodontal cyst is one of the cysts that was caught in the crossfire when the classification of cysts was modified. Originally, this cyst was defined radiographically, as a cyst appearing in between the roots of two adjacent teeth. The etiology was thought to involve epithelial inflammation from either a periodontal pocket or a lateral root canal of a nonvital tooth. However, the inflammatory etiology does not hold up because the cyst wall usually fails to show inflammation and the adjacent teeth do not show periodontal or pulpal disease. It is now felt that this cyst develops from rests of dental lamina in the interradicular bone and that it is unrelated to an inflammatory process.

These cysts are rare and are seen mostly in men over the age of 50. The vast majority are found in the mandibular premolar area, and the rest are seen in the maxillary anterior area. They are almost always small and asymptomatic; they seldom enlarge. The radiograph discloses a small, round, well-demarcated radiolucency within alveolar bone between the roots of the teeth specified earlier (Fig. 14-6). When discovered, these cysts should be removed for biopsy to differentiate them from more significant conditions they may resemble.

Gingival Cyst of the Adult

The gingival cyst appears as a small bump or blister on the buccal surface of the gingiva in the mandibular premolar area of a middle-aged person. Because it develops within soft tissue rather than bone, it is not seen radiographically. The gingival cyst is considered to be the soft tissue equivalent of the lateral periodontal cyst because of the similarity in location, behavior, and histology. Its histogenesis is thought to involve hyperplasia of the rests of Serres—which represent residual dental lamina within the gingiva. There are no major clinical sequelae.

Residual Cyst

When teeth are removed, cysts that might have been present in the area may persist. Years later, such a cyst may be detected clinically or during a routine radiographic series as a radiolucency unassociated with a tooth (Fig. 14-7). Since it is improper to label a cyst as dentigerous or radicular if the relationship to the tooth is unknown, the term residual cyst is used as a convenience. Most residual cysts do indeed represent a previous periapical or dentigerous cyst. Once surgically removed, residual cysts seldom recur. Rarely, long-standing residual cysts have been known to become cancerous.

Odontogenic Keratocyst

In 1962, a new odontogenic cyst was described. It did not fit well into the preexisting classification of cysts because its cause, histogenesis, and relationship to teeth were uncertain. What was certain was that this cyst was the most aggressive of the odontogenic cysts. Radiographically, it could not be characterized because it could assume any size or shape and

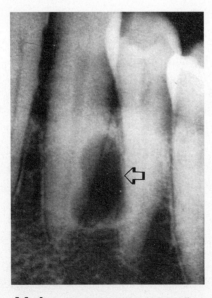

Fig. 14-6 Lateral periodontal cyst. This asymptomatic radiolucency is between the canine and first premolar. The adjacent teeth are vital.

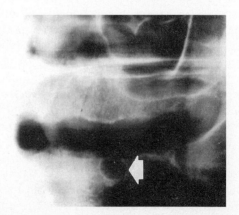

Fig. 14-7 Residual cyst. This well-demarcated radiolucency of the edentulous mandible (arrow) represents the residual growth from a periapical cyst removed 6 years previously.

could occur anywhere within the jaws. In fact, the only way a diagnosis could be made was on the basis of a biopsy, in which the squamous cyst lining showed subtle microscopic differences that could distinguish it from all other odontogenic cysts. Obviously, odontogenic keratocysts existed prior to their discovery in 1962, but the importance of their special histology in determining their behavior had not yet been recognized. And because keratocysts could mimic any other cyst radiographically, they were misinterpreted as variants of dentigerous cysts, residual cysts, or lateral periodontal cysts. For those keratocysts that did not conform radiographically to any of these, there was a previous designation known as primordial cyst. The primordial cyst was considered to be a cyst that developed instead of a tooth. This term has been deleted from modern classifications of odontogenic cysts now that the keratocyst has been documented and is well recognized.

The odontogenic keratocyst is relatively common. Radiographically, it often is a radiolucent lesion that may appear around the crown of an impacted tooth in a dentigerous relationship. Alternatively, it may be found between teeth, like a lateral periodontal cyst, in an edentulous area, like a residual cyst, or bear no relationship to teeth. It may be small or large; and it may appear as a well-demarcated round or oval lesion, or as a huge "soap bubble" multilocular radiolucency resembling an ameloblastoma (see the discussion of odontogenic tumors later in this chapter). In fact, almost any radiolucent lesion of the jaws may turn out to be an odontogenic keratocyst when diagnosed by biopsy. The keratocyst may, rarely, even mimic a periapical cyst. In this situation, the correct diagnosis is usually not discovered until the "periapical cyst" fails to heal following root canal therapy and a subsequent biopsy reveals its true nature.

The odontogenic keratocyst is slow but persistent in its growth, and it is capable of hollowing out large areas of the jaw, causing swelling, secondary infection, and possible fracture (Fig. 14-8). Even after attempted surgical removal, 25% of these cysts redevelop, requiring additional surgery. Patients who have had surgery for this condition must be monitored for years for possible recurrence.

The proposed histogenesis of odontogenic keratocysts explains its aggressiveness and range of appearances. This cyst is thought to arise from embryonic remnants of dental lamina. Since this epithelium is widely distributed throughout the jaws, that explains the variable locations of the keratocyst. Dental lamina is also a primitive tissue with great growth potential. The odontogenic keratocyst does not grow like other cysts that enlarge primarily from fluid pressure. Expansion of the keratocyst is most likely due to active proliferation of the epithelium and therefore somewhat resembles the growth of a benign neoplasm.

One important consideration regarding the odontogenic keratocyst is that it is sometimes associated with the *basal cell nevus syndrome,* a genetic condition running in families and characterized by multiple keratocysts, multiple basal cell carcinomas of the

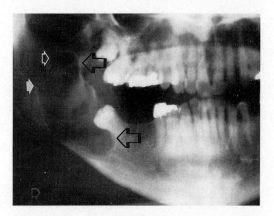

Fig. 14-8 Odontogenic keratocyst. This large expansile multiocular cyst of the mandible (arrows) was proven to be a keratocyst at biopsy. Note the impacted molar associated with the cyst.

skin, and a facial profile showing a broad forehead, flat nasal bridge, widely spaced eyes, and protruding lower jaw. Affected individuals may develop multiple destructive odontogenic keratocysts in all areas of the jaw. Identification of the syndrome early in life through detection of the keratocysts can help these people get genetic counseling and early treatment for their skin cancers and help prevent massive jaw destruction by the cysts.

ODONTOGENIC TUMORS

A wide variety of neoplasms and hamartomas can originate from the tissues that form the teeth. Since teeth are derived from both epithelium and mesenchyme, epithelial, mesenchymal, and mixed neoplasms are possible.

Ameloblastoma

The ameloblastoma is the most common epithelial odontogenic neoplasm. It is derived from dental lamina or reduced enamel epithelium and, as it grows, reproduces the histology of the enamel organ. The cells proliferate as nests and islands of enamel epithelium but are unable to produce enamel or induce formation of dentin or cementum. Although the ameloblastoma may occur anywhere in the jaws, its favorite location is in the posterior mandible where it is frequently associated with an impacted molar. Some ameloblastomas develop in teenagers, but most are discovered between the ages of 30 and 50.

You have learned about benign and malignant tumors and the features that characterize each. The ameloblastoma is peculiar in that it shares features of both benign and malignant tumors. It is slow-growing and unlikely to metastasize, like a benign tumor. However, it is also unencapsulated and invasive and it infiltrates through bone, destroying tissue locally like a malignancy. Maxillary ameloblastomas can extend into the brain and face and cause death. Because there are only two cat-egories of tumors to choose from, the ameloblastoma has been designated as benign because it is usually curable. However, it should be understood that the tumor acts in a manner that is intermediate between benign and malignant. Perhaps it should be given its own category of "benignant."

Radiographically, the typical ameloblastoma appears as a large multilocular radiolucency that expands and thins the bony cortex. Smaller ones may resemble dentigerous cysts (Fig. 14-9).

The aggressive behavior of these tumors dictates their treatment. Ameloblastomas continue to grow and destroy bone. The larger they become, the more difficult and destructive the surgical removal. Even following attempted removal, the recurrence rate approaches 50%. Since ameloblastomas are not sensitive to radiation or chemotherapy, surgery is the only choice, and it requires removal of large segments of jaw bone and associated teeth. A generous border of normal bone must also be sacrificed as a margin around the tumor in order to prevent recurrence.

Other Epithelial Odontogenic Tumors

There are three other epithelial odontogenic tumors that are all too rare to merit more than a few sentences highlighting their key features. The *adenomatoid odontogenic tumor* (AOT) is a benign, nonaggressive tumor occurring in children. Most cases occur in the anterior maxilla. The tumor surrounds the crown of an unerupted tooth, resembling a dentigerous cyst. Diagnosis is based on the histopathologic appearance of this tumor. Once removed, the tumor never recurs.

The *calcifying epithelial odontogenic tumor* (CEOT), also known as Pindborg tumor, is a benign, aggressive tumor whose behavior resembles that of an ameloblastoma. Diagnosis is based on its histopathologic appearance.

The *calcifying odontogenic cyst* (COC), also known as Gorlin cyst, is a cystic neoplasm

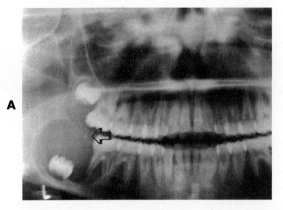

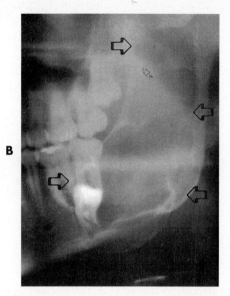

Fig. 14-9 Ameloblastoma. **A,** This unicystic ameloblastoma appears as a dentigerous cyst. Biopsy, however, proved ameloblastoma. **B,** This multilocular expansile radiolucency extends from an impacted third molar to the coronoid notch.

capable of obtaining a large size but rarely recurring following removal.

All three of these neoplasms present radiolucencies that may calcify and therefore frequently contain irregular radiopacities within.

Odontogenic Myxoma

The odontogenic myxoma is an uncommon odontogenic tumor derived from the mesenchymal component of a developing tooth. It is composed of a soft, gelatinous, pulplike tissue containing no epithelium. Even though the histology is completely different from that of the ameloblastoma, the tumor behaves like an ameloblastoma. It appears as an expansile, multilocular radiolucency that grows slowly (Fig. 14-10), infiltrates bone, and destroys normal tissue. The age of occurrence and preferred location also mimic those of the ameloblastoma. Myxomas usually require rather aggressive treatment including surgical removal of the tumor mass and surrounding normal bone. The possibility of recurrence necessitates careful patient follow-up.

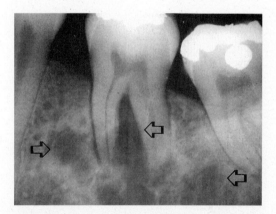

Fig. 14-10 Odontogenic myoxoma. A multiocular radiolucency (arrows) of the mandible proved to be a myxoma at biopsy.

Cemento-Ossifying Fibroma

Bony neoplasms of the jaws can be influenced by the presence of teeth to produce neoplastic cementum, as well as bone. The cemento-ossifying fibroma is such a benign neoplasm composed of a combination of fibroblasts, bone, and cementum. It is an uncommon but not rare tumor seen mostly in the mandible of young women.

Radiographically, it begins as a well-defined circular radiolucency that becomes progressively more radiopaque as the cementum and bone content increases (Fig. 14-11). Since it is benign and encapsulated, it grows by expansion rather than infiltration. When the tumor encounters dental roots, it often pushes them out of the way, causing them to spread apart. Following complete removal, these lesions seldom recur.

Cementoma

The name cementoma suggests a benign neoplasm of cementum; however, the lesion designated by this name is, in reality, a reactive disturbance in periapical bone. The condition is better termed *periapical cemental dysplasia.* These lesions usually occur in the anterior mandibular region of middle-aged black women. Lesions are totally asymptomatic and are discovered on routine dental radiographs. In the early stages, periapical cemental dysplasia resembles a periapical granuloma or cyst, appearing as a periapical radiolucency usually adjacent to lower incisors. As the lesion matures, it acquires calcification and appears as a

mixed radiolucency with opaque areas (Fig. 14-12). Older lesions may be predominately radiopaque. The lesions do not cause symptoms and require no treatment. It is of critical importance to differentiate the early radiolucent stage of cementoma from a periapical cyst or granuloma, which it resembles radiographically and clinically, in order to avoid unnecessary endodontic treatment. The key clue in differentiation of the lesions is that the tooth associated with the cementoma is vital, whereas the teeth associated with cysts and granulomas are nonvital. Whenever a healthy-appearing tooth shows a periapical radiolucency, vitality and percussion sensitivity must be assessed before root canal treatment is performed. When multiple expansive cementomas are present as numerous radiolucencies, mixed lesions, or radiopacities throughout the jaws, the condition is called *florid osseous dysplasia* (Fig. 14-13).

Ameloblastic Fibroma

Although the ameloblastic fibroma is a rare odontogenic tumor of children, its role among odontogenic neoplasms is considered important because of its histogenesis. It is derived from both germ layers (epithelial and connective tissue) of the tooth bud.

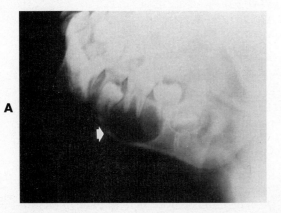 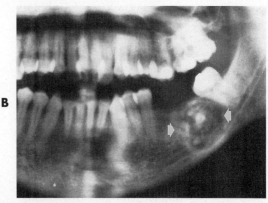

Fig. 14-11 Cemento-ossifying fibroma. **A,** A well-defined expansile radiolucency expands and thins the mandibular inferior cortical plate. **B,** This lesion appears more radiopaque.

Its epithelial component microscopically resembles the enamel organ, somewhat like ameloblastoma. But unlike ameloblastoma, the epithelium can activate the mesenchyme into producing a pulplike tissue that accompanies the epithelial proliferation. These two tissues grow side by side in the ameloblastic fibroma.

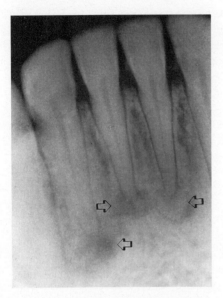

Fig. 14-12 Periapical cemental dysplasia. Radiolucent, mixed, and radiopaque lesions appear simultaneously.

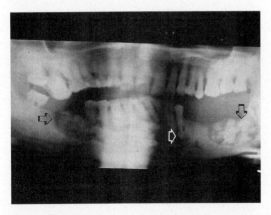

Fig. 14-13 Florid osseous dysplasia. These radiopaque masses are especially notable in the mandible.

This tumor is seldom mature enough to produce enamel or dentin. Radiographically, most cases resemble a dentigerous cyst, growing around an unerupted tooth, usually of the posterior mandible.

Odontoma

The odontomas, like ameloblastic fibromas, form from the interaction between dental epithelium and mesenchyme. In fact, in the odontoma, the two tissues carry the maturation process much further, including the formation of enamel, dentin, and cementum. In the *complex odontoma,* the dental hard tissues are randomly distributed, and in the *compound odontoma,* they are more orderly and form a conglomeration of multiple tiny toothlike structures. Odontomas are the most common of the odontogenic tumors. Because they consist of excessive developmental tissue, they must be considered hamartomas. Odontomas appear most commonly in children and are usually asymptomatic. However, they may cause slight swelling or pain. Since they occur in the same areas where teeth form, they often act as physical barriers to normal tooth eruption and are therefore discovered when radiographs are made to determine the status of an impacted tooth.

Radiographically, the complex odontoma appears as a spherical opaque mass surrounded by a thin radiolucent border. It is often seen overlying the crown of a tooth that it has blocked from erupting (Fig. 14-14). The compound odontoma appears as multiple tiny radiopacities contained within a well-demarcated oval radiolucency (Fig. 14-15). The treatment for an odontoma is excision. This surgery may be similar to the extraction of an impacted tooth.

PSEUDOCYSTS

There are several bony lesions of the jaws that resemble odontogenic cysts radiographically but are neither true cysts nor of odontogenic

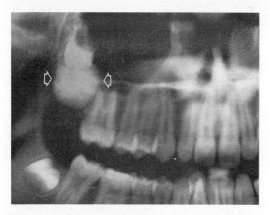

Fig. 14-14 Compound odontoma. This lesion causes impaction of the maxillary lateral incisor. Note the toothlike structures within the demarcated lesion (arrow).

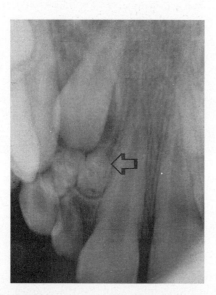

Fig. 14-15 Complex odontoma. The odontoma may have formed from the maxillary second molar tooth bud.

origin. These lesions are sometimes termed pseudocysts (false cysts).

Traumatic Bone Cyst

The simple bone cyst or traumatic bone cyst is a large cystlike lesion of the mandible seen mostly in children and adolescents. In spite of its name, a history of trauma to the area is mentioned in only half of the cases. This false cyst is not lined by epithelium and may represent an area of bony degeneration that has failed to heal. It is usually asymptomatic or occasionally may cause mild swelling. Radiographs often reveal a large radiolucent lesion with the upper border frequently scalloped in between dental roots (Fig. 14-16). The associated teeth are vital. When the lesion is explored surgically, the surgeon discovers a large cavity unlined by any epithelium. The hole may be empty or contain some clear or bloody fluid. The diagnosis becomes apparent once this observation is made. The traumatic bone cyst usually will heal spontaneously, although the surgical procedure necessary to make the diagnosis hastens the healing process.

Central Giant Cell Granuloma

Another lesion seen mostly in children and adolescents is the central giant cell granuloma. It usually appears as a radiolucency of either jaw. It may be found in all locations but is most common anterior to the molars. Radiographically, it may assume many sizes and shapes, from a small, well-demarcated, single circular radiolucent area to a large, expansile multilocular radiolucency mimicking an ameloblastoma. It usually causes painless, progressive swelling (Fig. 14-17). At surgery, solid, soft, reddish brown, hemorrhagic tissue is curetted out. Healing after conservative surgery is the rule, but some cases recur and require surgical resection to include neighboring teeth and normal bone. As the name implies, this tumor may be reactive in origin; however, the exact cause is unknown. Rare cases are related to systemic hyperparathyroidism (see Chapter 19). Diagnosis is based on the histopathology of the lesion.

Stafne Bone Cyst

An occasional panorex radiograph may disclose a small, very well demarcated radiolucency located in the posterior area of the mandible below the mandibular canal (Fig. 14-18).

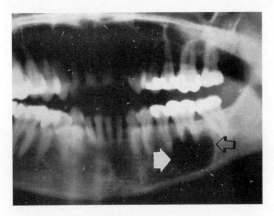

Fig. 14-16 Traumatic bone cyst. This asymptomatic radiolucency scallops the roots of the mandibular second premolar and first molar (arrows). Biopsy revealed an empty cavity and was consistent with traumatic bone cyst.

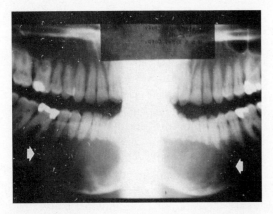

Fig. 14-17 Central giant cell granuloma. This large multiocular lesion (arrows) has been causing painless swelling of the anterior mandible. The teeth are vital.

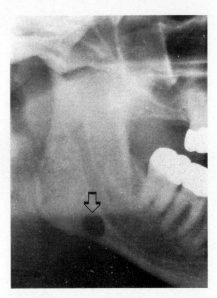

Fig. 14-18 Stafne bone cyst. This is the classical location and configuration of this mandibular defect.

Such a finding is most likely to represent a Stafne bone cyst. This is not a true cyst but usually represents a depression in the lingual cortical surface of the mandible. It is often filled with normal salivary gland tissue. Since this represents an anatomic variation rather than a pathologic lesion, it does not grow or expand and does not require treatment. When such a lesion is observed radio-

graphically, it should be noted and then followed on subsequent radiographs to ensure that it has not increased in size.

OTHER BONY LESIONS

Several other lesions of bone are notable because they are somewhat common and can cause considerable disease or even death. These lesions are not of odontogenic origin but may clinically resemble odontogenic tumors and are therefore discussed in this chapter.

Fibrous Dysplasia

Fibrous dysplasia is a benign fibroosseous overgrowth of tissue that occur centrally within the jaws as well as within other bones of the body. The lesion is usually singular and may occur as a slow-growing, painless expansile, fusiform swelling of either jaw. The lesion may move or impact erupting teeth, but only occasionally causes root resorption. Children are almost exclusively affected, with growth beginning during childhood and stabilizing

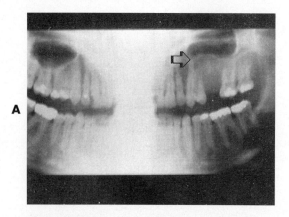 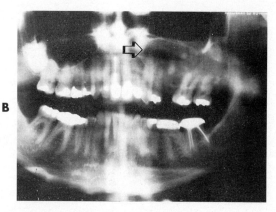

Fig. 14-19 Fibrous dysplasia. **A,** The "ground glass" radiopacity is expanding the left antrum (arrows). **B,** Eight years' lateral minimal growth and further opacity has occurred.

around the time of puberty. The etiology is unknown. The lesion therefore might be best characterized as an aggressive hamartoma of fibroblasts that form bone. Histologically the lesion consists of proliferating fibroblasts that are forming spicules of bone or cementum metaplastically. Microscopically the lesion is similar to the cemento-ossifying fibroma and cementoma. Radiographically, the lesions appear as expansile with either a multilocular radiolucent appearance or a mixed radiolucent and radiopaque presentation. Unlike cemento-ossifying fibroma, fibrous dysplasia is poorly delineated. It frequently demonstrates fine diffuse calcifications imparting a so-called ground-glass (bathroom window) radiographic appearance to the lesion (Fig. 14-19). Although somewhat disfiguring and initially frightening, these tumors are usually controllable with cosmetic surgery. Excision is difficult since the lesion is so poorly demarcated. Because the lesion is usually self-limiting and ceases growth at puberty, pathologic consequences are not serious and treatment is conservative.

Idiopathic Histiocytosis

Idiopathic histiocytosis is also termed *histiocytosis X* and is characterized by proliferations of antigen-processing cells (histiocytes) in multiple areas of the body. The distribution of lesions frequently includes jaw lesions. As the name implies, the cause is unknown. The disease is most common in infants and children. The behavior of the histiocytic proliferation varies considerably, and the disease is often subtyped accordingly. The acute disseminated form (Letterer-Siwe disease) occurs as widespread proliferation involving skin, middle ear regions, bones, and visceral organs. The chronic disseminated form (Hand-Schüller-Christian disease) usually involves the posterior orbital space (causing exophthalmos), pituitary gland (causing diabetes insipidus), and jawbones. Chronic localized disease (eosinophilic granuloma) also frequently involves the jaw. Bony lesions are radiolucent and destructive, and frequently involve teeth, giving a "tooth floating in air" appearance (Fig. 14-20). These lesions may be easily confused with periapical and periodontal infection, inflammation, and even neoplastic lesions of the jaws. The diagnosis is made when histologic examination of material removed by biopsy reveals proliferation of Langerhans-type histiocytes. The acute disseminated form usually occurs in infants and is frequently fatal. The chronic disseminated form most frequently occurs in young children, and the localized forms occur in adolescents, where the lesion is controlled with radiation therapy and chemotherapy. The prognosis for the chronic disseminated form is excellent.

Paget's Disease

Paget's disease (osteitis deformans) is an idiopathic bone disease characterized by increased formation of bone, in excess of the bone that is physiologically resorbed. As a result of this process, many bones become thickened both endosteally and periosteally, with impingement on cranial nerves. The patients develop subsequent auditory and visual disturbances, hip pain when walking, and noticeable growth of the maxilla and skull. The patients may complain that their upper denture does not fit or that their upper teeth are spreading and their jaw bone is expanding. When questioned they may note an increasing hat size reflecting calvarial growth. This condition occurs almost exclusively in the sixth generation and above. Oral radiographs taken at advanced stages of the disease reveal multiple "cotton wool" radiopacities that may resemble multiple cementomas (as in florid osseous dysplasia) (Fig. 14-21). Skull radiographs also show calvarial thickening and cotton wool appearance of bone. Diagnosis can be verified with biopsy and blood tests for alkaline phosphatase—an enzyme of bone formation. The disease is of a very chronic nature, and treatment is usually directed at symptoms. Although the sequelae can be serious, Paget's disease is seldom fatal.

DIFFERENTIAL DIAGNOSIS OF BONY LESIONS

Having reviewed most of the bony lesions, it is appropriate to consider the approach to making a radiographic diagnosis of pathology. At this point in the text, we have studied numerous lesions that may appear on a dental radiograph. These lesions can assume only a few forms—a radiolucency, an opacity, or a combination of both. Therefore, many lesions share similar radiographic appearances. To further confuse the issue, some lesions can assume a variety of shapes and sizes. Thus, when a lesion is noted on a radiographic film, it is not appropriate to simply make a diagnosis. One should combine information from the

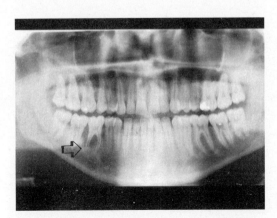

Fig. 14-20 Idiopathic histiocystosis. The mandibular first molar (arrow) is suspended in a dense infiltration of histiocytes and eosinophils. The patient has the chronic localized form and has developed several other oral bony lesions.

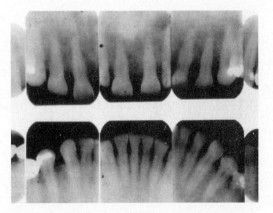

Fig. 14-21 Paget's disease. This 60-year-old patient has noted thickening of the bone and spreading of the teeth for several years. The maxillary bone appears mottled and "cotton wool" in appearance, and the lamina dura is obscured.

radiograph with the patient's history and clinical symptoms and then systematically consider all the possibilities, listing them in order of likelihood of occurrence. This is known as formulating a differential diagnosis. It allows for a safe and organized plan of treatment.

Table 14-1 divides bony lesions into three categories depending on their appearance. They are listed roughly in the order of their incidence. This list enables the diagnostician to select appropriate diagnoses when a certain type of radiographic appearance is seen and provides a listing so the practitioner can consider all possibilities. The diagnostician can then refer back to the text for each lesion in determining the proper patient management.

It can be seen from Table 14-1 that a multilocular radiolucency is always of concern because all conditions within that category are aggressive lesions. Conversely, lesions with radiopacities are usually nonaggressive with the exception of CEOT, which is rare, and osteosarcoma, which would be accompanied by worrisome clinical signs of pain, paresthesia rapid growth, or tooth movement. Single radiolucencies are the most difficult to

evaluate because they contain the largest numbers of diverse lesions ranging from insignificant conditions to significant diseases that can kill the patient. This is where evaluation of radiographic features, clinical signs, and patient history is most useful to develop a differential diagnosis and treatment plan.

Case Studies

Case 1
R.B. is a 28-year-old man who noticed a swelling of the angle of the left side of his mandible of 6 months' duration. He was otherwise healthy, and there was no pain associated with the swelling. His dentist confirmed buccal plate expansion in the area and noted a well-demarcated 2 cm unilocular radiolucency about the crown of distally impacted tooth No. 17. The provisional dentigerous cyst and impacted tooth were removed and submitted for histopathologic study. A diagnosis of odontogenic keratocyst was rendered. One year later, follow-up examination revealed that R.B. had developed a 0.5 cm radiolucency in the same area. Biopsy and histologic examination of the excised lesion revealed recurrent odontogenic keratocyst. No recurrent lesion has

TABLE 14-1
Categories of bony lesions

Single radiolucency	Multilocular radiolucency	Mixed lucency-opacity
Periapical cyst, granuloma	Odontogenic keratocyst	Odontoma
Dentigerous cyst	Ameloblastoma	Cementoma
Odontogenic keratocyst	Central giant cell granuloma	Ossifying fibroma
Residual cyst	Myxoma	AOT
Early cementoma	Hemangioma	COC
Lateral periodontal cyst		CEOT
Traumatic bone cyst		Osteosarcoma
Cemento-ossifying fibroma		
Central giant cell granuloma		
Stafne bone cyst		
Cancer		
Idiopathic histiocytosis		
Ameloblastic fibroma		

been found at serial 6-month follow-ups over a 3-year period.

Case 2

V.M. is a 50-year-old woman who came to her dentist with swelling and tooth movement in the left anterior region of her mandible that had been present and growing for at least 2 years. The lower incisors had recently become loosened and painful. Oral examination revealed marked labial and lingual plate expansion from tooth No. 24 to tooth No. 19. Radiographs revealed a well-demarcated multilocular radiolucency that was 2.5 cm long and extended from tooth No. 24 to the distal surface of tooth No. 19. A provisional diagnosis of ameloblastoma versus odontogenic keratocyst was rendered. Incisional biopsy led to a diagnosis of odontogenic myxoma based on histopathologic study. A block of the mandible including the entire lesion, teeth No. 24 to 19, and a margin of bone 0.5 cm beyond the periphery of the lesion was excised. The inferior border of the mandible was saved, and bone chips were placed to aid healing. The patient is now tumor free 4 years after excisional surgery. A special fitted partial denture helps fill the bony defect and replace the teeth.

Case 3

T.B. is a 10-year-old girl whose parents were very concerned about a bony growth of the left side of the maxilla. Oral examination showed painless buccal expansion above areas No. 14 and 15. Both teeth were impacted. Radiographs showed displacement of forming teeth No. 14 and 15 and a 1.5 cm poorly demarcated ground-glass radiolucency with radiopacity. Incisional biopsy confirmed a diagnosis of fibrous dysplasia. T.B. was closely monitored by her dentist for the next 11 years, and twice surgery was performed to reduce the size of the lesion. The lesion has become quiescent, and no surgery has been necessary for the past 5 years.

Case 4

J.O. is a 9-year-old child who complained of a toothache about erupted tooth No. 18. Oral exam revealed pain and mobility of tooth No. 18 to

pressure, and radiographs showed substantial bone loss about tooth No. 18. Extraction and biopsy revealed idiopathic histiocytosis. A systemic workup revealed a 2 cm radiolucency of the right hip that was also diagnosed microscopically as histiocytosis. Both lesions were surgically excised. One year later a lesion of the posterior orbital region was discovered and has been irradiated.

Case 1

1. Is the clinical behavior characteristic of malignant growth? Why or why not?
2. Why was a provisional diagnosis of dentigerous cyst made?
3. Does an odontogenic keratocyst behave differently than a dentigerous cyst? Is it a malignant cyst?
4. Do odontogenic keratocysts recur more often than dentigerous cysts?
5. Are odontogenic keratocysts ever associated with other abnormalities? Should R.B. be examined for other components of a syndrome? If so, what should the physician or dentist look for?

Case 2

1. What is the significance of multilocular radiolucency versus unilocular radiolucency?
2. What is the significance of loosened teeth adjacent to a radiolucent lesion?
3. Is an odontogenic myxoma benign or malignant? Is it aggressive?
4. Do odontogenic myxomas frequently behave like ameloblastomas?

Case 3

1. Is T.B. the usual age for appearance of fibrous dysplasia?
2. The lesion was poorly demarcated on radiographs. What impact does this have on the differential diagnosis?

3. What will most likely occur if a fibrous dysplasia is not treated?
4. Why wasn't the lesion totally excised?

Case 4

1. What is meant by "tooth floating in air"? Can this be the result of periodontal diseases?
2. Based on clinical findings, what type of idiopathic histiocytosis does J.O. exhibit?
3. What is the prognosis for this type of histiocytosis in this age group?

SUMMARY

- The tooth is formed from epithelial and mesenchymal components. Completion of tooth development depends on the interaction of these components. Odontogenic cysts and tumors originate from hyperplastic or neoplastic growth of these developmental dental elements.
- Odontogenic cysts form from proliferations of remnants of dental lamina, rests of Malassez, or reduced enamel epithelium.
- Odontogenic cysts can usually be distinguished and classified by location, cause, or clinical behavior.
- Odontogenic keratocysts are aggressive cysts that have a specific histopathologic appearance. They often occur in a dentigerous or lateral periodontal relationship with teeth. These are sometimes a component of basal cell nevus syndrome.
- The ameloblastoma is an aggressive, invasive, benign odontogenic tumor that originates from entrapped odontogenic epithelium.
- Other specific epithelial odontogenic tumors include the very benign AOT and the aggressive CEOT.
- The odontogenic myxoma is a mesenchymal tumor that acts aggressively. This neoplasm is benign.
- The cemento-ossifying fibroma is a slow-growing, circumscribed, benign neoplasm of the periodontal membrane.
- Periapical cemental dysplasia commonly causes bony lesions of the periapical

periodontal membrane. Stages of periapical cemental dysplasia can be radiographically similar to periapical pathoses and must be clinically distinguished for correct treatment. Florid osseous dysplasia causes multiple lesions that frequently become expansile.

- Odontomas represent neoplasms or hamartomas formed of randomly arranged elements of tooth formation. Odontomas frequently cause impaction of associated teeth.
- Several bony lesions resemble cysts radiographically. However, traumatic bone cysts, central giant cell granulomas, or Stafne bone cysts are not true cysts. Clinical and radiographic features are important in diagnosis and differentiation. Histopathologic confirmation is often necessary.
- Fibrous dysplasia represents a hamartomatous overgrowth of benign fibro-osseous tissue in the jaws. These lesions demonstrate a relatively distinctive radiographic appearance and are usually confirmed histopathologically. Although frequently quite expansile and deforming, the growth usually declines at puberty.
- Idiopathic histiocytosis represents a spectrum of disease types characterized by uncontrolled proliferation of histiocytes. The forms most common in infants and children often behave in a malignant manner.
- Paget's disease causes excessive bone to form in the hips, skull, jaws, and about the foramina of some of the cranial nerves. Signs and symptoms reflect this excessive growth. Dental changes include radiographic density, jaw expansion, and spreading of teeth.

Suggested readings

1. Brannon RB: The odontogenic keratocyst—a clinico-pathologic study of 312 cases: part I clinical features, Oral Surg Oral Med Oral Pathol 42:54, 1976.
2. Choung R and others: Central giant cell lesions of the jaws: a clinicopathologic study, J Oral Maxillofac Surg 44:708, 1986.

3. Dahlin DC: Bone tumors, ed 3, Springfield, Ill, 1978, Charles C Thomas, pp 420-438.
4. Gold L. Biologic behavior of ameloblastoma. In Asseal LA, editor: Benign lesions of the jaws, Oral and Maxillofac Surg Clin North Am 2:21, 1991.
5. Jaffe HL: Giant cell reparative granuloma, traumatic bone cyst and fibrous (fibro-osseous) dysplasia of the jaw bones, Oral Surg Oral Med Oral Pathol 6:159, 1953.
6. Kaugars GE and Cale AE: Traumatic bone cyst, Oral Surg Oral Med Oral Pathol 63:318, 1987.
7. McDonald JS and others: Histocytosis X: a clinical presentation, J Oral Pathol 9:342, 1980.
8. Regezi JA and Sciubba J: Oral pathology clinical-pathologic correlations, ed 2, Philadelphia, 1993, WB Saunders, chapters 10, 11.
9. Shear M: Cysts of the jaws: recent advances, J Oral Pathol 14:43, 1985.

15

Diseases of the Salivary Glands

IN THIS CHAPTER

After studying this chapter, you should be able to meet the following objectives and define the key terms:

- Describe the location of major and minor salivary glands.
- List the common causes and sequelae of xerostomia.
- Relate acute and chronic sialadenitis to obstruction of flow.
- Recognize the signs and symptoms of epidemic parotiditis.
- Explain autoimmune sialadenitis and Sjögren's syndrome.
- List common causes of bilateral parotid swelling.
- Explain the pathogenesis and rationale for treatment of mucoceles.
- Define ranula.

- Recognize mucoceles based on clinical presentation, history, and location.
- Distinguish benign mixed tumors and Warthin's tumors from malignant neoplasms by clinical presentation.
- Recognize the need for extracapsular excision of parotid mixed tumors.
- Differentiate low-grade, intermediate-grade, and high-grade mucoepidermoid carcinoma and recognize the variation in prognosis.
- Explain the signs and symptoms of adenoid cystic carcinoma and relate them to the expected behavior of the tumor.

The salivary glands are tissues that secrete mucopolysaccharides, proteins, antibodies, and minerals into the oral cavity. These secretions are extremely important in maintenance of oral health. Saliva functions to help emulsify and begin digestion of foodstuffs, lubricate the mucosa and upper digestive tracts for swallowing and speech, dissolve substances for taste perception, and provide protection through antibacterial and antimicrobial effects. The oral cavity is a complex ecologic system with interaction, stimulation, and inhibition of microbial flora. Saliva plays a major role in the maintenance of this system.

As you remember, saliva is secreted from both major and minor salivary glands through ducts to their orifices at mucosal surfaces. There are three sets of major salivary glands. The parotid glands are large and bilateral and lie anterior to the ear, inferior to the temporomandibular joint (TMJ) and superficial to the masseter muscle. The facial (VII) nerve radiates through the glands, and a tail may extend well into the cervical (neck) region. The parotid secretion is serous (watery) in content and is discharged from bilateral parotid ducts at orifices of the parotid papillae—a raised area of the buccal mucosa at the level of the maxillary second molars. The submandibular glands (SMGs) are discrete, bilateral, paired glands located lingually and inferior to the mandible at the level of the mandibular first and second molars. They secrete a mixed serous-mucous secretion through paired ducts that discharge from caruncles (papillae) on either side of the lingual frenum at the midline of the floor of the mouth. The sublingual glands are mixed and lie within the submucosa bilaterally in the floor of the mouth. They secrete by multiple small ducts to the floor of the mouth or occasionally to the submandibular gland ducts.

Minor salivary glands are often overlooked as functioning glands and as a source of disease by the dental team. These submucosal glands are found beneath almost all oral mucosal surfaces except those of the free and attached gingiva and bound hard palate, and portions of the dorsal surface of the tongue. The thousands of minor glands provide thick, mucus lubricants to the mucosa through minute individual ducts. You have already seen how minor salivary ducts are accentuated in the midregion of the hard palate and soft palate in nicotinic stomatitis. Pathologic conditions can affect either minor or major salivary tissues. All locations of salivary tissue are within the purview of the dental team and should be examined on a regular basis.

XEROSTOMIA

Individuals may have salivary deficiencies termed xerostomia (xero: dry, stomia: mouth) for numerous reasons. Hundreds of drugs, including common antidepressants, antihypertensive drugs (that reduce blood pressure), and antisialagogues (that reduce secretions), may cause xerostomia as a dose-related effect

or side effect. Surgery, irradiation, or chronic inflammation of salivary tissues may occur fairly commonly and cause xerostomia. Some common systemic diseases such as diabetes, cirrhosis, and endocrine disturbances can decrease saliva production and secretion and contribute to xerostomia. Aging in itself contributes to decreased salivary flow.

The sequelae of dry mouth are those expected when we understand salivary function. Patients have difficulty chewing their food and swallowing because of the dryness. Food loses its taste; therefore, xerostomia patients tend to have decreased desire for food. The mucous membranes become dry, reddened, atrophic, and frequently infected, burning, or painful. The preceding can then contribute to reduced intake and digestion of food and occasionally to anorexia and poor nutrition. Saliva stimulants such as flavoring agents and drugs, or saliva substitutes that are commercially available or prescribed can help reverse these effects.

Patients with chronically dry mouth may have bacterial stomatitis, oral candidiasis, accelerated periodontitis, and the radiation type of dental caries as described in Chapter 13. These infections result from overgrowth of normal oral organisms because of the absence of antimicrobial agents such as peroxidases, lysozymes, and specific antibodies—all constituents of normal saliva. As a result, the patient will be bothered by discomfort, denture intolerance, mucosal changes, and the sequelae of the acute caries process. The dental team must intervene with lubricants, salivary stimulants, special hygienic protocol, fluoride supplementation, and educational support.

INFECTION

Infections of major and minor salivary tissues are commonly encountered by the dental practitioner and may have profound impact on the patient. Acute infections tend to be painful and swollen, whereas chronic infections tend to be firm, tumorous, and only slightly irritative. Infections may be specific and contagious in nature or nonspecific and obstructive in etiology.

Epidemic Parotiditis

Epidemic parotiditis (viral mumps) is a specific acute infection of the parotid glands caused by a highly contagious *Paramyxovirus* organism. This once-common childhood infection is now rarely encountered because of the effectiveness of a vaccine and mandatory public health measures. Occasional outbreaks occur in populations of unvaccinated individuals or as a result of vaccination failure. The droplet-spread infection causes fever, malaise, swelling, and pain of the parotid glands after approximately 2 to 3 weeks' incubation. Bilateral parotid swelling and pain is usual, and pharyngitis and xerostomia may accompany the chipmunklike facial appearance (Fig. 15-1). Acute febrile pancreatitis, orchitis (inflammation of the testes), and meningoencephalitis may accompany the more obvious clinical acute parotiditis. The infection persists for several weeks, is treated by bed rest and support, and usually resolves with resumption of normal parotid flow rates. Occasional adult

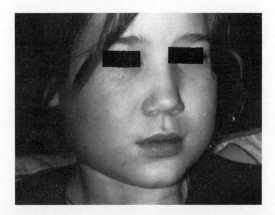

Fig. 15-1 Epidemic parotiditis. Bilateral acute swelling of the parotid glands of 4 days' duration. The patient's sister has similar lesions.

men develop testicular atrophy and sterility secondary to the orchitis.

Nonspecific Sialadenitis

Acute and chronic *sialadenitis* are commonly encountered in dental patients. These infections are usually caused by endemic oral bacterial flora such as staphylococci and streptococci. Normally, salivary glands are sterile and self-cleansing—that is, the flow and pressure of secreted saliva washes bacteria from ducts and prevents retrograde (reverse) infection of glands. Any obstruction, impedance of flow, or gross reduction in flow negates this cleansing effect and allows for ascending infection by oral flora. Therefore, most cases of suppurative sialadenitis are secondary to obstruction (caused by plugs, stones), impedance (caused by scars, edema of ducts), or reduced flow (dryness). For example, acute suppurative parotiditis is an occasional sequela of acute dehydration secondary to general anesthesia. The surgery patient develops dryness of the glands and ducts as a result of the anesthetic, antisecretory surgical drugs, and the lack of salivary stimulation during lengthy surgical procedures. Ascending infection via the parotid ducts results in acute suppurative parotiditis with parotid abscesses. Prophylaxis and treatment for this condition called "postsurgical mumps" include antibiotic therapy.

Chronic suppurative and subacute recurrent suppurative sialadenitis are not uncommon infections. They can occur in either the major or minor salivary glands. These low-grade infections cause enlargement, firmness, and reduced flow from the affected gland (Fig. 15-2). The lesions are usually not very painful, although the patient may complain of acute pain while eating when there is accompanying obstruction. The pain is more a product of obstruction, salivary retention, and capsule (parotid, SMG) stretching than of infection or inflammation. Therefore, some painless chronic lesions are often clinically similar to certain salivary tumors. As previously explained, obstruction of the parotid ductal system often contributes to the cause of these lesions. Furthermore, since there is a low-grade infection (inflammation), obstruction may result from the inflammation. As reviewed in Chapter 3, inflammation of salivary ducts can change pH, initiate exudation (fibrin, pus), and cause sloughing of ductal cells. These changes can result in a cellular or exudative plug or initiate stone formation—which in turn further obstructs and allows for retrograde infection. This may become a vicious circle. Treatment for chronic and subacute sialadenitis of the major glands usually involves removal of the obstruction by sialolithectomy (stone removal), or ductal probing and dilation to remove plugs and dilate constrictions. Frequently in minor glands and less commonly in major glands, the entire chronically scarred and inflamed gland must be surgically excised.

Sialolithiasis

Salivary stone formation (*sialolithiasis*) is a rather common source of salivary gland ob-

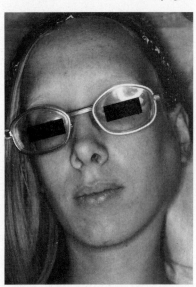

Fig. 15-2 Recurrent subacute parotiditis. Here, the partially obstructed parotid gland is infected. The parotid gland was subsequently removed because of the ductal constriction and recurrent infection.

struction. The SMG is most often affected, although other major and minor glands may be involved. Stones are composed of salivary calcium salts that precipitate within ducts at sites of infection, inflammation, or plugging. Since the SMG saliva is very concentrated in calcium salts (hence the calculus on lingual lower anterior teeth), these stones are most often present in the submandibular glands. The obstruction frequently leads to chronic suppurative sialadenitis of the affected gland and occasionally to acute obstructive sialadenitis with associated acute pain. Many sialoliths are asymptomatic or manifest as painless firm swellings (Fig. 15-3). Clinically, stones can be detected by the history and/or manifestation of pain and swelling of the gland upon stimulation (as in tasting, eating) and by radiography (Fig. 15-4). Most sialoliths will appear radiopaque if soft tissue radiographs are properly positioned and exposed. Surgical removal is indicated and usually gives relief. Chronically inflamed salivary tissues regenerate when the cause of inflammation is removed.

Autoimmune Sialadenitis

Autoimmune chronic sialadenitis (benign lymphoepithelial lesion) is a condition that may be encountered within a general dental practice. These lesions may involve all of the salivary glands but usually are most pronounced in the parotid region. Although the etiology is unknown, we are aware of several important features. Most lesions occur in women (85%) after menopause. The disease is frequently associated with other autoimmune disorders like rheumatoid arthritis, systemic lupus erythematosus, and other mixed connective tissue diseases. We have discussed some of these in Chapter 4. In the benign lymphoepithelial lesions there is atrophy of the affected salivary tissue and infiltration of dense aggregates of lymphocytes. As a result, several clinical features almost always accompany

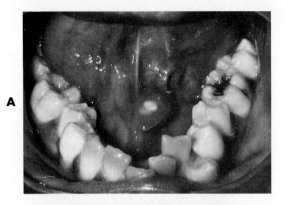

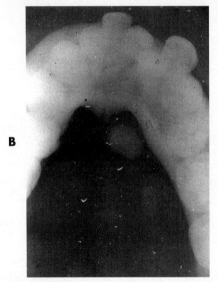

Fig. 15-3 **A,** Sialolithiasis of the SMG duct. **B,** An occlusal radiograph demonstrates two stones within the duct.

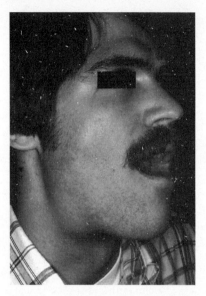

Fig. 15-4 Sialolithiasis. The obstructed right SMG is swollen and painful. Radiography revealed two sialoliths.

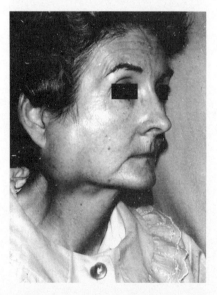

Fig. 15-5 Autoimmune sialadenitis. These bilateral parotid swellings are accompanied by xerostomia and xerophthalmia. (Courtesy of Dr. N. Burzynski)

this condition. Xerostomia results from salivary atrophy, and firm, painless, chronic parotid swelling results from the dense lymphocytic infiltrations (Fig. 15-5). The term *Mikulicz' disease* is often used to denote this relatively minor condition. In some patients the benign lymphoepithelial lesions are more widespread and extend to the lacrimal glands (causing xerophthalmia), pharynx, and esophagus. When this disease extension occurs, it is designated Sjögren's syndrome. These benign lymphoepithelial lesions are important to the dental team because we must treat the xerostomia and its sequelae (caries, mucositis). In addition, the firm, chronic parotid swellings can appear similar to those of benign and malignant salivary neoplasms. Therefore, a thorough history, clinical assessment, and sometimes biopsy are necessary to ensure proper diagnosis. A low rate of malignant transformation to lymphosarcoma (2% to 4%) has been reported from Sjögren's syndrome. Treatment includes special oral hygienic prophylaxis, saliva substitutes, steroids, infection prophylaxis, and, occasionally, surgical removal of large lesions.

Other Parotid Swellings

Benign parotid swellings (sialadenosis) can accompany several systemic conditions and may create the impression of mumps. In most cases the glandular tissue demonstrates hypertrophy—perhaps in response to a defect in the secretory mechanism. Lesions are usually chronic, bilateral, and somewhat soft in consistency (Fig. 15-6). Patients seldom complain of symptoms other than swelling and occasional xerostomia. Such systemic conditions as chronic liver disease (cirrhosis), vitamin A deficiency (nutritional mumps), thyroid mediation (chemical mumps), diabetes, and bulimia can cause sialadenosis. These swellings are best diagnosed based on patient history and a systemic workup. Treatment of the underlying condition is mandatory, although salivary stimulants such as sugarless gum and candy can reduce swelling and increase salivation.

MUCOUS RETENTION

Mucous retention is an extremely common oral salivary lesion that you will encounter on a regular basis in your practice. As the name implies, mucus salivary product is retained

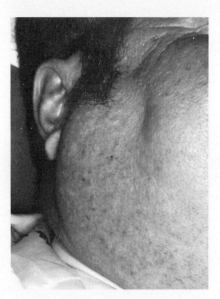

Fig. 15-6 Bilateral parotid swelling and alcoholism. These bilateral swellings are long-standing and nonpainful.

within the mucosal tissues. Most frequently this occurs when a minor salivary duct is ruptured by trauma and the secretory mucin spills into the submucosal connective tissues (Fig. 15-7). The lesion formed is often referred to as a *mucocele* (mucus cavity). The spilled mucin initiates a low-grade inflammatory reaction, with formation of a granulation tissue pseudocapsule at the periphery. These lesions clinically are raised, soft, fluctuant, and blue to pale in color, and appear to grow (swell) rapidly (Fig. 15-8). Very superficial lesions may resemble clear blisters. Patients will be concerned and sometimes complain that the mucocele drains thick, ropy fluid and then recurs. Mucoceles of the floor of the mouth develop rapidly and grow to large size because of the loose nature of the submucosa that does not limit spread and the large output of mucin spilled by the sublingual glands. These large floor-of-the-mouth mucoceles are called *ranulas* because of the resemblance to the belly of a frog (rana)

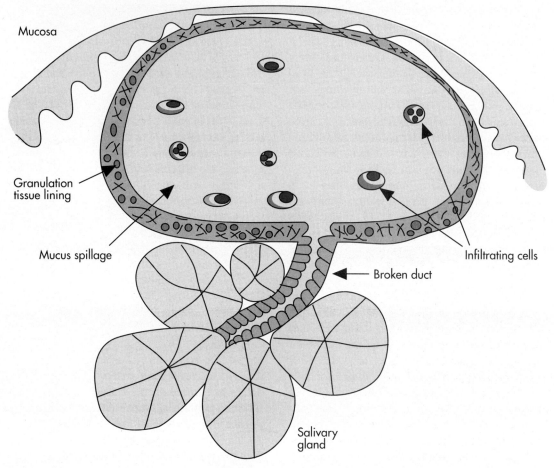

Mucosa

Granulation
tissue lining

Mucus spillage

Infiltrating cells

Broken duct

Salivary
gland

Fig. 15-7 Mucocele.

(Fig. 15-9). Mucoceles are most common in areas of frequent trauma such as lower labial mucosa, buccal mucosa, and the soft palate and are uncommon on the gingiva, anterior area of the hard palate, and upper labial mucosa where salivary gland tissue is rare or trauma is less common. Occasionally, the mucous retention phenomenon is caused by occlusion of excretory salivary ducts. When this occurs the mucus is retained in dilated ducts or cysts and the term *mucous cyst* is appropriate. The treatment for the mucous retention phenomenon is usually surgical excision of the lesion and associated salivary tissue. Recurrence is rare.

SALIVARY NEOPLASMS

Salivary neoplasms can occur in any of the major or minor salivary tissues. In general the parotid glands are the most commonly involved sites extraorally, and the minor glands of the palate are most commonly involved intraorally. Tumors of the sublingual glands and tongue are the most rare. Benign salivary tumors, as a rule, behave according to the general principles for benign neoplastic growth outlined in Chapter 7. This means that these tumors grow very slowly; are encapsulated and readily movable; do not cause tissue destruction, ulceration, or nerve damage; and

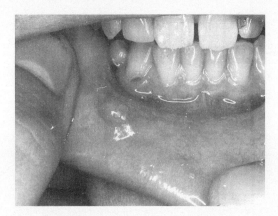

Fig. 15-8 Mucocele. This soft, raised, blue lesion has been present for 2 days.

remain localized. Malignant salivary tumors also act as expected: they grow more rapidly, ulcerate the surface, damage nerves, and metastasize to remote organs or lymph nodes, resulting in considerable disease and even death if left unchecked. Most malignant salivary tumors are adenocarcinomas. They most frequently arise in the parotid glands and minor salivary glands of the mucous membranes. Adenocarcinomas tend to grow rapidly, are poorly defined, ulcerate or destroy adjacent tissue, and damage associated nerves, causing pain, paresthesia, or anesthesia (trigeminal nerve), or paralysis (facial nerve). Numerous histopathologic subtypes of these benign and malignant neoplasms exist, and they present nuances and differences that help the dentist and surgeon select a treatment plan and make a prognosis. We will discuss the two most common and important benign and malignant salivary tumors to illustrate these differences. (See Table 15-1.)

Benign Mixed Tumor

The benign mixed tumor (BMT)—sometimes called *pleomorphic adenoma*—is the most common salivary neoplasm. As the names imply, this benign ductal growth stimulates a mixed connective tissue response within the tumor. As the lesion grows, the nonneoplastic

supportive connective tissue begins to react and form cartilage, fibrous collagen, bone, and other specific connective tissues. This material frequently composes the bulk of the growth and imparts a density or firmness to the tumor clinically. Tumors may arise in the parotid region or SMG, or as submucosal minor gland neoplasms (Fig. 15-10). The cause is unknown. These tumors follow the aforementioned rules of benign behavior. Because of the slow nondestructive growth, patients will frequently disregard the presence of the neoplasm and allow the tumors to attain great size (Fig. 15-11). The tumor is encapsulated in collagen; however, small nests of tumor may extend into the capsule. When removed, this capsule tends to split, and nests of tumor will remain in the retained collagen. It is therefore prudent for the surgeon excising this tumor to remove associated glandular tissue or connective tissue to ensure total capsular excision. This is especially important for tumors of the parotid area because the presence of recurrent tumors and their subsequent removal jeopardizes the integrity of the facial nerve—with the risk of Bell's palsy. BMTs should be excised totally when possible because long-standing tumors may undergo malignant transformation.

Papillary Cystadenoma Lymphomatosum

The *papillary cystadenoma lymphomatosum* (Warthin's tumor) is an aptly named benign neoplasm that occurs only in the parotid region. This tumor grows from salivary tissue that was entrapped developmentally within lymph nodules of the parotid region (Fig. 15-12). As the slow-growing neck tumor develops, it becomes fluid filled (cystic), and when viewed with a microscope, demonstrates fingerlike projections of ductal tumor cells into the cystic spaces. Therefore, the designation papillary cystadenoma lymphomatosum is appropriate. Like the parotid BMT, this tumor is slow growing and encapsulated.

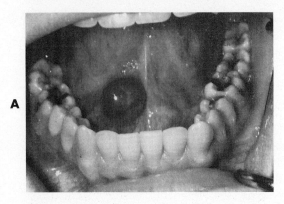
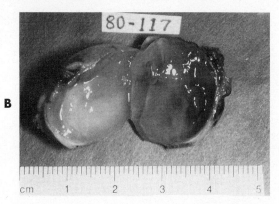

Fig. 15-9 Ranula. **A,** The mucin-filled area of the floor of the mouth appears blue. **B,** The surgical tissue is opened to show the mucus.

TABLE 15-1

Common salivary tumors

Type	Common location	Special characteristics	Prognosis
BMT	Parotid, intraoral	Bone, cartilage, collagen formation	Excellent, some recurrent
Warthin's	Parotid only	Cysts in lymph nodes	Excellent
MEC—low grade	Parotid, intraoral	Predominance of mucous cells	Good, 90% survival rate
MEC—high grade	Parotid, intraoral	Predominance of squamous cells, keratin	Grave, 5% survival rate
ACC	Intraoral, parotid	Swiss cheese appearance, perineural routes	Good—5-year survival rate; poor—20-year survival rate

Unlike BMT, conservative surgical excision almost always results in a cure.

Mucoepidermoid Carcinoma

The *mucoepidermoid carcinoma* (MEC) is the most common salivary adenocarcinoma. This tumor occurs most often in the parotid gland. The epithelial element consists of a mucous gland component and a squamous (epidermoid) component. The degree of malignancy, and therefore the treatment and prognosis of this tumor, is highly dependent upon the microscopic composition of these cells within the neoplasm. A low-grade mucoepidermoid tumor is composed primarily of mucin cells, goblet cells, and mucin-filled cysts, with very little squamous proliferation. We frequently use the designation "tumor" for this low-grade lesion since the survival rate is excellent (90%). Treatment is conservative, wide-marginal surgery. The *high-grade* mucoepidermoid carcinoma has a considerable squamous cell keratinizing histology with only rare mucous cells noted by the pathologist—even when special mucin stains are used. This carcinoma has a very poor prognosis since it metastasizes to both lymph nodes and lungs. Radical surgical treatment and medical workup for metastases are usually mandatory. A 5-year 5% survival rate underscores the grave

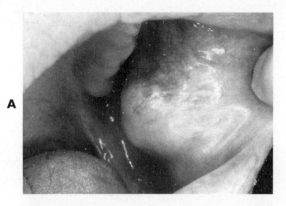

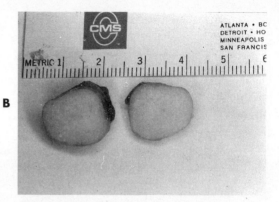

Fig. 15-10 Benign mixed tumor. **A,** This firm, movable tumor of the buccal mucosa has been present for at least 5 years. **B,** Cut section reveals a well-demarcated, solid tumor with a capsule.

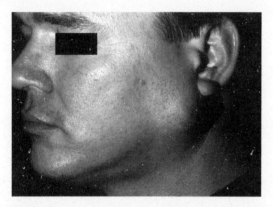

Fig. 15-11 Benign mixed tumor. The parotid tumor was present for many years.

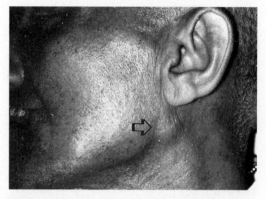

Fig. 15-12 Warthin's tumor. The tumor of the parotid tail is freely movable.

nature of this lesion. Intermediate-grade tumors with mixed histopathology have an intermediate prognosis. The low-grade MEC may clinically resemble a mucocele since it is mucin filled. Since intraoral MEC tends to occur in the palate, retromolar areas, and upper lip, clinical mucoceles in these areas should be especially suspect and should be excised (Fig. 15-13).

Adenoid Cystic Carcinoma

The *adenoid cystic carcinoma* (ACC, or cylindroma) originates within minor salivary glands and, less commonly, in the parotid glands. The palate is the most frequently involved intraoral

area (Fig. 15-14). This adenocarcinoma grows rather slowly for a malignancy but is invariably poorly demarcated. The tumor cells are remarkably neurophilic (nerve loving) and therefore tend to grow into and along perineural spaces. Symptoms therefore include pain, paresthesia, and numbness for intraoral growths and paralysis for parotid lesions. The arrangement of ductal tumor cells microscopically often appears like cysts (thus the term *adenoid cystic*) that are described as cylinders or swiss cheese by pathologists. This slow-growing tumor is very difficult to excise because of perineural extension of the tumor beyond the apparent clinical margins. Because

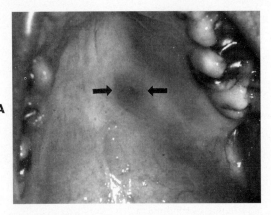

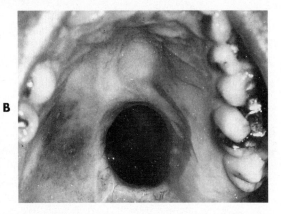

Fig. 15-13 Mucoepidermoid carcinoma. **A,** This small low-grade lesion clinically resembled a mucocele. **B,** Post-surgical defect. The patient exhibited a contact allergy to her metal-based denture (causing ulcers).

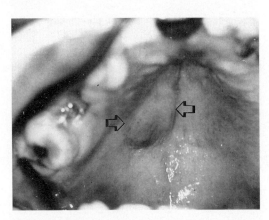

Fig. 15-14 Adenoid cystic carcinoma. A tumor of the palate is invading the bone (*arrows*).

of this, 5-year survival rates are good (75%); however, 10-year (50%) and 20-year (15%) cures are much more sobering. Late metastases are usually widespread and probably by way of hematogenous routes.

Case Studies

Case 1
S.H., a 53-year-old woman, went to her dentist for normal restorations and periodontal care. On examination the hygienist and dentist noted a pea-sized knot of her left parotid area that had not been present 18 months previously at her last dental exam. She noted a recent lag in the blink reflex of her left eye and was able to smile evenly when instructed. Biopsy revealed a mucoepidermoid carcinoma, high grade, of the left parotid area. Although the surgeon and pathologist thought the tumor was excised, a subsequent parotidectomy was performed and Bell's palsy was acquired. A systemic workup showed no tumor metastasis to the neck or other organs. She is examined every 3 months at the university oncology clinic. She returned to the dental office, where she received special fluoride treatment, a regimen for office and home care, and saliva stimulants (gum) for a mild xerostomia.

Case 2
D.G., a 22-year-old college wrestler, complained of a 1-cm growth of his lower labial mucosa of 4 weeks' duration. The soft, blue, raised lesion had almost disappeared 3 weeks previous but has now recurred and enlarged. He gave a noncontributory health history and indicated he was frequently elbowed in that area. Surgical excision of the blue, fluid-filled lesion resulted in a diagnosis of mucous retention phenomenon (mucocele) with associated ruptured salivary duct. The lesion has not recurred in 2 years, and the patient is the conference wrestling champion.

Case 3

M.R. is a 61-year-old alcoholic woman who complained to her dentist of a swelling of the left anterior surface of the soft palate of 18 months' duration. The area was not painful, but M.R. thought it might be an abscess from tooth No. 15. Examination revealed a firm, movable, nonpainful submucosal mass measuring 7 mm in diameter. The mass was not fixed to the mucosa. There was no demonstrable infection or pathologic condition about tooth No. 15. An oral surgeon excised the mass and noted that it was "rolled out" from the adjacent tissue surgically. The biopsy report gave a diagnosis of pleomorphic adenoma and noted that bone and cartilage were present within the tissue. M.R. was tumor free 2 years after surgery.

Case 4

W.K. is a 61-year-old woman who complained to her dentist about progressive dryness of the mouth of almost 10 years' duration. Recently she had been unable to properly chew food and had difficulty with speech because of the dryness. She further complained that her dentures irritated her mouth. Health history revealed an 8-year history of rheumatoid arthritis treated with nonsteroidal antiinflammatory drugs. She used artificial tears frequently for dryness of her eyes. Oral examination revealed atrophic glossitis and mucositis and mild atrophic candidiasis. Biopsy of her lower lip revealed benign autoimmune sialadenitis. With a diagnosis of Sjögren's syndrome, W.K. was given prescriptions for a salivary stimulant, artificial saliva, and an antifungal medication. Her physician was notified of the diagnosis and subsequently prescribed prednisone (cortisone). Her denture irritation resolved, and she became more comfortable and better able to masticate her food.

Case 1

1. What cranial nerve is responsible for innervating the eyelid (controlling blink) and the facial muscles of expression? Does this nerve have any relationship to the salivary glands?

2. What is the significance of the designation "high-grade" mucoepidermoid carcinoma? Can such a designation be made microscopically?
3. If the tumor was excised, why was the entire parotid gland removed?
4. Is S.H. considered cured?
5. Explain the need for special dental care.

Case 2

1. What is the most common location of mucoceles? Why do they occur at this location?
2. What is the significance of the changes in size of the swelling?
3. Why was the lesion excised?

Case 3

1. Is this a common location for a salivary tumor?
2. After clinical examination, did you think this was benign or malignant? Why?
3. What is a benign mixed tumor?
4. What is the significance of bone and cartilage within this tumor?
5. Do you think this tumor might recur? Why? If it does, what treatment will be necessary?
6. What was the tissue of origin of this tumor?

Case 4

1. Which clinical signs and symptoms suggest that W. K. has Sjögren's syndrome?
2. What role does lip biopsy play in the diagnosis of Sjögren's syndrome?
3. What do you think was the source of her denture irritation?
4. Why was W. K. prescribed antifungal medications?

SUMMARY

- Common diseases and disorders of the salivary glands may affect the three major glands or numerous minor glands.

- Xerostomia is a common condition that is most likely secondary to medications that act systemically, aging, autoimmune disease, surgery, or irradiation. Xerostomia patients often develop associated caries, mucositis, and problems with mastication.
- Epidemic parotiditis is an acute viral infection that is usually prevented by vaccination.
- Major and minor salivary glands are susceptible to acute and chronic infection. Patients with reduced salivary flow or obstructed salivary ducts are predisposed to such infections.
- Salivary gland stones most often occur in the submandibular ducts and are related to the calcium saturation of saliva and associated inflammation of the ductal tissues.
- Autoimmune sialadenitis most often occurs in postmenopausal women. Features often include xerostomia, autoimmune parotid swelling, xerophthalmia, and associated autoimmune diseases.
- Systemic conditions such as cirrhosis, diabetes, vitamin A deficiency, effects of certain medications, and bulimia can cause chronic mumpslike swelling of the parotid glands.
- Mucoceles are common submucosal accumulations of mucin that are most frequently formed as a result of breaks in the minor gland ducts with subsequent spillage of mucin into the submucosa. Mucoceles of the floor of the mouth tend to be large and are termed ranulas.
- The benign mixed tumor is the most common salivary gland neoplasm. These slow-growing tumors can occur in the major or minor glands and show evidence of connective tissue metaplasia.
- Papillary cystadenoma lymphomatosum represents a benign neoplasm of salivary

tissues entrapped in lymph nodes in the parotid area.
- The behavior of mucoepidermoid carcinoma ranges from almost benign to extremely malignant and is reflected in the varying histopathology. Some mucoepidermoid carcinomas can clinically mimic mucoceles.
- The adenoid cystic carcinoma is slow growing but tends to invade and grow along nerve bundles. For this reason, long-term cure rates are poor.

Suggested readings

1. Batsakis JG: Lymphoepithelial lesion and Sjögren's syndrome, Ann Otoe Rhinol Laryngol 96:354, 1987.
2. Basatkis JG: Tumors of the head and neck: clinical and pathological considerations, ed 2, Baltimore, 1979, Williams & Wilkins, chapters 1, 3.
3. Chaudhry AP, Vickers RA, and Gorlin RJ: Intraoral minor salivary tumors: an analysis of 1414 cases, Oral Surg Oral Med Oral Pathol 14:1194, 1961.
4. Harrison JD: Salivary mucocoeles, Oral Surg Oral Med Oral Pathol 39:268, 1975.
5. Moutsopoulous H and others: Differences in the clinical manifestations of sicca syndrome in the presence and absence of rheumatoid arthritis, Am J Med 66:733, 1979.
6. Spiro RH: Salivary neoplasms: overview of a 35-year experience with 2807 patients, Head and Neck Surg 8:177, 1986.
7. Waldron CA, El-Mofty SK, and Gnepp DR: Tumors of the intraoral minor salivary glands: a demographic and histologic study of 426 cases, Oral Surg Oral Med Oral Pathol 66:323, 1988.

16   Lesions of Skin and Mucosa

IN THIS CHAPTER

1. Paraoral skin lesions
   - Basal cell carcinoma
   - Squamous cell carcinoma
   - Seborrheic keratosis
   - Nevus
2. Intraoral skin disease
   - Lichen planus
   - Pemphigus
   - Pemphigoid
   - Lupus erythematosus
   - Erythema multiforme
   - Contact stomatitis, medication stomatitis, allergy
3. Case studies

After studying this chapter, you should be able to meet the following objectives and define the key terms:

- Recognize features of squamous cell carcinoma and basal cell carcinoma of the face.
- Recognize common forms of seborrheic keratosis by appearance and location.
- Recognize features of pigmented skin lesions that distinguish between benign and malignant growth.
- Recognize common forms of lichen planus.
- List types of agents that may lead to lichen planus or lichenoid mucositis.
- Demonstrate communication skills acknowledging cancerophobia in lichen planus patients.
- Develop a differential diagnosis for lichenoid lesions.
- Help manage patients with lichen planus.

- Discuss the etiology and clinical course of pemphigus.
- Define Nikolsky's sign.
- Differentiate pemphigus from pemphigoid.
- Differentiate types of lupus erythematosus.
- Recognize characteristics of lupus skin lesions.
- Explain the course and prognosis of systemic lupus erythematosus.
- List the clinical features of erythema multiforme and Stevens-Johnson syndrome.
- Give examples of agents that cause contact stomatitis and medication stomatitis.

Diseases of the skin commonly produce lesions of the oral mucosa. This is often surprising to students. Many of the features and functions of oral mucosa appear to sharply contrast with those of skin. Skin is dry, whereas mucosa is moist. Skin is exposed to the weather, whereas mucosa is exposed to saliva and lubricants. However, on reflection, it is clear that the functions and structures of skin and oral mucosa are more alike than different. Both are composed of stratified squamous epithelium and connective tissue, both have their respective specialized organs (hair and sweat glands versus minor salivary glands), and both fulfill a primary function as a protective barrier against the environment. In these and many other subtle ways, skin and oral mucosa are quite alike. Therefore, disorders commonly associated with skin would be expected to frequently produce disease of the oral mucosa.

The diseases that affect both skin and oral mucosa are numerous, numbering in the hundreds. In many such diseases simultaneous skin and oral involvement is the rule. Attention in this chapter is directed toward diseases of skin and oral mucosa that are common, as well as of sufficient importance to patient health as to be appropriate for study by dental hygienists.

PARAORAL SKIN LESIONS

As a component of routine patient evaluation, the dental team must evaluate the facial skin, with particular emphasis on the skin immediately around the mouth. Although many skin disorders can occur in this and other cutaneous locations, several disorders occur with sufficient frequency in this location as to justify consideration in this section.

Basal Cell Carcinoma

Basal cell carcinoma was extensively discussed in Chapter 9, including consideration of etiology, clinical features, and treatment. This most common form of skin cancer is frequently encountered on paraoral skin, showing a marked predilection for the upper lip. Typically sparing the vermilion border, it has clinical characteristics on hair-bearing paraoral skin that are much the same as its characteristics when occurring on other cutaneous sites. Common features include the development of a pearly, firm, nodular elevation, frequently showing early central ulceration with development of a crusted, depressed center (Fig. 16-1). Telltale dilated vessels typically cross the pearly yellow border.

Squamous Cell Carcinoma

As a major disease of oral mucosa, squamous cell carcinoma is extensively discussed in Chapter 9. SCC of paraoral skin, like its counterpart of the vermilion border, is caused by chronic sun exposure. The pattern of development includes the usual appearance in sun-

damaged skin—especially in individuals with a fair complexion. This skin is frequently erythematous, with a tendency to form keratotic scales and crusts (Fig. 16-2). In these skin disorders the surface squamous epithelium all too often shows microscopic maturational abnormalities representing epithelial

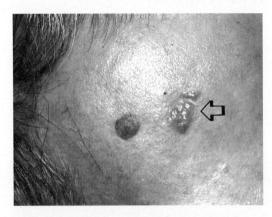

Fig. 16-1   Basal cell carcinoma and seborrheic keratosis. Raised, pearly, nodular basal cell carcinoma (*arrow*) has developed next to a long-standing, waxy, pebbled seborrheic keratosis on this patient's forehead.

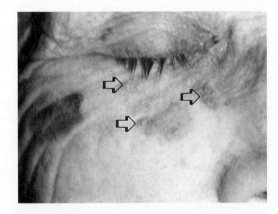

Fig. 16-2   Squamous cell carcinomas of skin. Numerous red, scaly carcinomas (*arrows*) on face of light-complexioned individual. Note the large seborrheic keratosis of the right cheek.

dysplasia. As discussed in Chapter 8, epithelial dysplasia is considered a frequent forerunner of SCC.

Squamous cell carcinoma of skin typically manifests itself as a somewhat irregular, destructive ulcer. In some cases this cancer may form a highly thickened hornlike keratin plug. With time, SCC will enlarge, producing prominent induration, extensive local destruction, and invasion into surrounding structures. As mentioned in Chapter 9, SCC sharply differs from basal cell carcinoma because of its significantly greater tendency to metastasize to regional lymph nodes. It is exceedingly important for the dental team to view with great suspicion any crusting or ulcerated lesion of skin that fails to heal within a 2-week period. Patients with suspicious crusted, erythematous, destructive, or ulcerative lesions should be referred for medical treatment.

Seborrheic Keratosis

Seborrheic keratosis is a benign neoplasm that originates from stratified squamous epithelium. This lesion is largely limited to sun-exposed skin, first appearing in middle age and becoming prevalent in the geriatric population. Although exceedingly common on the skin of individuals with fair complexions, it does not occur on oral mucosa. Multiple lesions of the skin are common.

The characteristic clinical appearance consists of a light to dark brown, finely pebbled plaque that often appears as if it is attached to the skin in a manner that would allow one to easily peel it off. The plaques appear sharply demarcated with a velvet texture and soft or waxy consistency (Figs. 16-1, 16-2). Size is quite variable, ranging from a few millimeters to over a centimeter in diameter. Common sites of occurrence include the skin of the face, back, extensor surfaces of the arms, and the scalp. A hallmark of this condition is slow, gradual enlargement over many years without any ominous signs

such as induration, crusting, and ulceration. The lesions are usually painless unless irritated. Cosmetic concerns constitute the usual rationale for excision.

By virtue of its pigmented appearance, seborrheic keratosis may bear some similarity to benign pigmented nevi (discussed next) and malignant melanoma (see Chapter 9). With experience and the taking of an accurate history, the dental hygienist can usually identify seborrheic keratosis reliably based on its clinical features. However, some cases may not be clear-cut, and one should promptly refer the patient in whom malignant melanoma is even remotely suspected.

Nevus

Benign pigmented nevi (moles) are commonly found on paraoral skin. They may appear either as flat (macular), light to dark brown lesions, or as nodular elevated growths. Extension of hair through benign nevi is a common finding and is generally considered indicative of their benign character. The types of pigmented nevi that may be seen include all of those described in Chapter 8. The clinical hallmarks of the benign pigmented nevus are its relatively static, or unchanging, appearance, largely uniform coloration, and lack of symptoms. Thus, pigmented lesions that change shape; become larger or smaller; display variation of color, including multiple shades of brown, blue, black, and pink; show crusting or ulceration; or produce symptoms such as itching or pain may be melanomas and must receive careful scrutiny. Prompt referral for biopsy is generally indicated in these situations.

INTRAORAL SKIN DISEASE
Lichen Planus

Lichen planus is widely considered to represent the most common dermatologic condition to occur in the mouth. It is a disease produced by a disturbance in chronic inflammation and the immune system, leading to local skin or mucosal damage with keratosis and irritation. Although the cause of this disease is unknown, we will see that in many instances this disorder may be produced or unmasked by a wide range of environmental factors.

An interesting characteristic of lichen planus is the remarkable range of clinical patterns it can demonstrate. The most common oral pattern of presentation is termed *reticular* lichen planus. It is so named because of the presence of a lacelike pattern of intersecting, somewhat angular to curved white striations—so-called Wickham's striae (Fig. 16-3). These striae are present to some extent in all forms of lichen planus. *Erosive* lichen planus shows striations, as well as irregular, painful ulcers (Fig. 16-4). In some cases of lichen planus, prominent striae are found superimposed on a red, atrophic background; this is termed *atrophic* lichen planus. While striae in lichen planus are generally separate and distinct, on occasion they appear closely situated, forming confluent white plaques. This describes *hypertrophic* lichen planus (Fig. 16-5). Finally, in rare cases, blister formation occurs on a background of characteristic Wickham's striae, yielding *bullous* lichen planus. It should be emphasized that individual cases of this disorder may combine characteristics of two or more forms. Thus a patient may exhibit striations, erythematous zones, and confluent white plaques. Although lichen planus is a chronic and generally static disorder, some cases may appear as reticular disease, and later progress unpredictably into an erosive pattern.

Lichen planus shows a predilection to occur in women, and is distinctly more common over the age of 40. Among the more common forms of lichen planus, the reticular and hypertrophic types are largely asymptomatic, whereas the atrophic and, in particular, the erosive forms can be very painful. Oral lichen planus has a striking predilection for

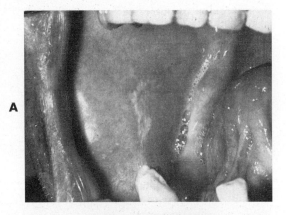

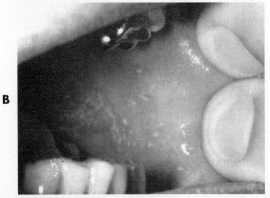

Fig. 16-3 Lichen planus (**A**). The white Wickham's striae (**B**) are present on the buccal mucosa.

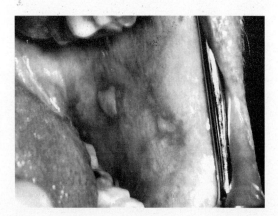

Fig. 16-4 Erosive lichen planus. Ragged ulcers with radiating striae.

the buccal mucosa, typically producing lesions bilaterally. However, virtually any oral mucosal site may be involved. It should be emphasized that the vast majority of cases show buccal mucosal involvement regardless of the degree and extent of oral involvement at other sites. These features, coupled with the distinctive striations, represent important factors in clinical diagnosis.

As mentioned earlier, the etiology of lichen planus is not understood. However, considerable attention has been directed toward the identification of predisposing factors. Drawing a firm distinction between predisposing and etiologic factors can at times be most difficult. Predisposing factors in lichen planus fall into two major categories, namely, metallic restorations and drugs. While it should be emphasized that metallic restorations only rarely induce lichen planus, two mechanisms are known. It is recognized that certain amalgam alloys in rare cases will induce development of lichen planus in the adjacent buccal or lingual mucosa. Even less common is lichen planus arising under the influence of galvanic (electrical) currents flowing between metallic restorations composed of dissimilar metals (Fig. 16-6). Typically, oral mucosa adjacent to the involved restorations will exhibit lichenoid

lesions, with all other mucosa spared, suggesting a likely relationship. Elimination of all contributory alloys, if followed by disappearance of adjacent mucosal disease, serves to confirm the role of these alloys in the disease. This, however, can be both expensive and ineffective, since the great majority of cases do not respond; therefore, such an approach is often unrealistic.

A far more common and important predisposing factor in lichen planus is drug ingestion. The list of drugs reported to induce oral and/or cutaneous lichen planus is quite extensive. Among the frequently used drugs that on occasion contribute to development of lichen planus are metal-containing drugs (gold sodium thiomalate, Pepto Bismol), antimalarial drugs used to treat systemic inflammatory disorders (quinacrine, chloroquine), antituberculosis drugs (para-aminosalicylic acid, streptomycin), thiazide diuretics, beta-blockers used in treatment of hypertension and cardiac arrhythmia (methyldopa, Inderal), angiotensin-converting enzyme inhibitors (Captopril, Vasotec), and a variety of frequently encountered drugs such as Lasix (diuretic), Diabinese (for diabetes mellitus), and penicillamine

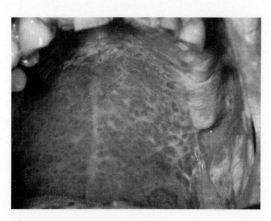

Fig. 16-5 Hypertrophic lichen planus. White plaques with associated striations.

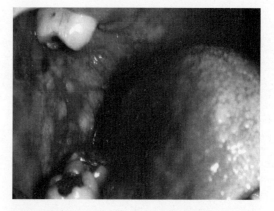

Fig. 16-6 Lichen planus—galvanism. Biopsy confirmed lichen planus. Lesions occurred when dissimilar metal (gold) crowns were placed, and diminished when alloy fillings were removed.

(for treatment of systemic inflammatory diseases). For all patients with lichen planus, there should be careful review of the health and drug histories in order to determine the possible contribution of patient drug ingestion to the disease. Elimination of the offending agent offers the strong possibility of significant clinical improvement in some cases. Of course, physician consultation is mandatory.

Clinical examination of a patient with suspected oral lichen planus should include examination of the patient's skin, and appropriate questioning. The most common location for lichen planus is the flexor surfaces of the extremities. In these locations lichen planus produces distinctive purple (so-called violaceous) rhomboid plaques covered by thin keratotic scales (Fig. 16-7). These lesions are noteworthy for their extreme itchy (pruritic) nature, often leading to patient scratching and self-inflicted trauma (excoriation). Thus the patient should be questioned regarding itching skin rashes.

Patient stress seems to play an important predisposing role in the development and exaggeration of lichen planus. Patients with lichen planus will frequently volunteer that they are under increased stress and correlate the stress to the severity and development of oral lesions. Commonly, patients also demonstrate

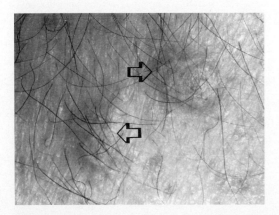

Fig. 16-7 Lichen planus. Scaly violaceous plaques of the wrist.

fear of developing cancer (cancerophobia) and worry that the oral lesions either are cancer or will develop into cancer. In only rare instances does the atrophic form become premalignant or malignant. If patients demonstrate the other forms of lichen planus, assurance can be given that the lesion is not cancerous or precancerous.

Because it is the oral expression of an important dermatologic condition, it would be reasonable to anticipate that oral lichen planus would usually occur with concurrent skin disease. In like manner, lichen planus of the skin would be expected to typically include oral disease. Interestingly, neither pattern is frequently observed. Paradoxically, oral lichen planus usually occurs in patients without cutaneous disease, and the majority of patients with lichen planus of the skin are free of oral disease. However, concurrent oral and cutaneous lichen planus do occur with some frequency. The finding of typical cutaneous lichen planus in a patient with suspected oral lichen planus provides additional support for the oral diagnosis.

The differential diagnosis of lichen planus is extensive, in large measure due to the many clinical patterns of presentation. Lichen planus in its more common forms may appear as a white lesion, a red and white lesion, or a combination of white and red lesions with ulceration. Important conditions that must be considered in the differential diagnosis include oral cancer, epithelial dysplasia, carcinoma in situ, candidiasis, contact allergy, and lupus erythematosus. When uncertainty exists, biopsy is necessary. Several differential diagnoses that include oral lichen planus are found later in this chapter. Treatment of oral lichen planus includes use of topical steroid creams, ointments, and rinses. Severe erosive cases are managed with systemically acting corticosteroids. Some management has also been accomplished with vitamin A precursors. Assurance of the patient that these lesions are benign is often necessary.

Pemphigus

Pemphigus is a disease of autoimmunity in which confused antibodies are produced that react with the cementing materials linking adjacent squamous cells of the skin and oral mucosa. These antibodies are readily detected in the blood of patients with pemphigus. They bind to cementing materials (also known as desmosomes), and lead to the destruction of cell-to-cell linkages. With the loss of intercellular linkages the surface epithelium becomes weakened and the cells separate, leading to blister formation and epithelial desquamation.

It should be emphasized that pemphigus often tends to affect the mouth long before skin disease appears. Over two thirds of all cases of pemphigus begin in the mouth, and involvement of skin may not occur until as much as 1 year later. Oral lesions consist of large superficial blisters and ulcers. The blisters are weak and quickly tear away under the normal mechanical forces of the mouth, leaving large, superficial, ragged, painful ulcers (Fig. 16-8). Commonly affected areas of the mouth include the soft palate, buccal mucosa, and lower lip. Application of mild lateral pressure on clinically normal mucosa in patients with pemphigus often produces some blister-ing and sloughing of the mucosa, leaving a raw, painful surface. This finding is referred to as *Nikolsky's sign.*

Oral symptoms include extreme pain and sore throat. An early symptomatic complaint is frequently related to gingival involvement. Patients often complain of painful, burning gums, and clinically the gingiva appears to be peeling, with ulcerations localized above the cervical aspects of multiple teeth (desquamative gingivitis). Although skin lesions occur in slightly more than half of all cases, it is typically a later manifestation indicating relatively advanced disease. Skin lesions consist of widely distributed vesicles (blistering) and bullae, leading to sloughing. In severe cases, nearly the entire skin surface may become ulcerated, mimicking the clinical appearance of the severe burn patient.

Diagnostic evaluation begins with a thorough clinical examination. Oral biopsy discloses characteristic histologic changes. Sophisticated tests may be performed to detect the presence of the abnormal epithelial antibody in the patient's tissues (direct immunofluorescence), as well as in the patient's serum (indirect immunofluorescence). In addition, the contents of intact vesicles can be examined microscopically for the presence of damaged, separated epithelial cells (the so-called Tzanck test).

Treatment for pemphigus is directed at suppressing the immune system. This therapy is usually delivered in the hospital setting, and can include high doses of corticosteroids and other immune suppressive drugs. These treatments are generally effective in suppressing the disease. However, the intensity and duration of therapy may produce significant and, all too often, life-threatening side effects. Treatment is usually coordinated by the physician.

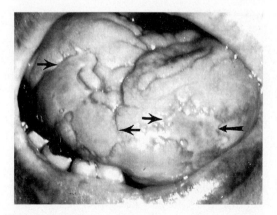

Fig. 16-8 Pemphigus. Large, ragged, superficial ulcers of the tongue (*arrows*). The patient has other oral and skin ulcers and vesicles.

Pemphigoid

Pemphigoid is also an autoimmune disease that effects the mouth, mucous membranes, and skin. Antibodies are directed against the constituents found in the basement membrane zone between epithelium and connective tissue. These autoantibodies lead to the destruction of the linkage between these tissues, leading to blister formation and epithelial desquamation.

Numerous patterns of pemphigoid are recognized. *Bullous pemphigoid* chiefly affects the skin, with concurrent oral involvement in approximately one third of cases. Skin lesions consist of vesicles and large blisters (bullae), and are often characterized by itching. *Cicatricial* (scarring) *pemphigoid* chiefly affects mucosa, including the oral cavity, upper aerodigestive tract, eye, and genital regions. Multiple regions of mucosa may be simultaneously involved. The mouth is frequently the first site to be affected. Oral lesions consist of vesicles, bullae, and ulcers (Fig. 16-9). Common sites of oral involvement include the gingiva, buccal mucosa, and palate. Gingival lesions produce a rather distinctive appearance, that of diffuse gingival erythema (see Chapter 17). Patients will generally complain of painful raw gums, although the pain is often described as quite mild. Clinically the gingiva is often ulcerated and blistered, and patients with cicatricial

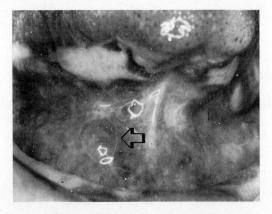

Fig. 16-9 Cicatricial pemphigoid. Ulcers of the ventral surface of the tongue and a vesicle of the floor of the mouth (*arrow*).

pemphigoid typically demonstrate Nikolsky's sign. In evaluating patients suspected of having oral cicatricial pemphigoid, appropriate questioning to elicit indication of involvement of other mucosal sites is necessary. Ocular disease often produces a "sandy" or "burning" sensation in the eyes, whereas involvement of the oropharynx may produce a sore throat, and genital mucosal disease may produce pain on urination.

The lesions of cicatricial pemphigoid heal with scar formation (cicatrix: scar). Such scarring may produce significant pathologic effects, including loss of oral function (such as reduced tongue mobility), dysphagia, and, in cases of ocular involvement, blindness. Treatment involves immune suppressive agents such as corticosteroids delivered locally (in mouthwash, adhesives) or systemically. When the gingiva is involved, meticulous oral hygiene is necessary to reduce plaque. However, hygiene procedures (brushing, flossing, scaling) can also damage the tissues; therefore, they must be accomplished judiciously. Chlorhexidine adjunctive therapy is helpful.

Lupus Erythematosus

Lupus erythematosus also represents an autoimmune disease with frequent oral lesions. Disease manifestations often arise as a result of the formation of antigen-antibody complexes (as in type 3 hypersensitivity), that through complement activation stimulate a destructive, chronic inflammation in many organs and tissues. (See Chapter 4.)

Lupus erythematosus manifests itself in several clinical patterns. The mildest form affects only the skin and mucous membranes, and is termed *discoid lupus erythematosus* (DLE). The name is derived from its characteristic disk-shaped, depressed, atrophic skin lesions. Skin involvement may also produce abnormal hair loss (alopecia) and local alterations in pigmentation. Lesions of the vermilion border are common, showing zones of atrophy surrounded by a raised, striated, keratotic border. Oral lesions are present in 25% to 50% of patients with chronic discoid lupus. The lesions are characterized by combinations of fine white striations radiating from an atrophic and often ulcerated central region (Fig. 16-10). The disease frequently affects the buccal mucosa, as well as the gingiva. Discoid lupus erythematosus has a predilection for onset in middle-aged women.

The most severe form of lupus erythematosus produces extensive disease involvement of both external body surfaces and internal organs. Known as *systemic lupus erythematosus* (SLE), it has a marked predilection for occurring in women, with the peak age of occurrence around 30. This disease characteristically produces extensive skin and oral disease, typically without scar formation. Skin lesions are erythematous and rashlike (Fig. 16-11). Oral lesions are present in between 50% and 70% of individuals affected, and are often described as red and ulcerative. Numerous oral sites may be involved, including the palate, buccal mucosa, and gingiva. Particularly significant are the effects of SLE on internal organs. Involvement of the heart valves often leads to thrombus formation and significant predisposition to subacute bacterial endocarditis (see Chapter 10). Marrow involvement leads to suppression of platelet and red blood cell formation, resulting in bleeding tendency (thrombocytopenia) and anemia. Disease of the kidney targets glomeruli, leading to renal failure. Joints often show arthralgia (pain) without permanent scarring or deformation. Numerous systemic manifestations, including fever and malaise, are also common.

Both DLE and SLE are characterized by photosensitivity: that is, development or worsening of skin rash when in sunlight. In addition, the malar region of the face including the bridge of the nose is a common location for this skin eruption, producing the very characteristic *butterfly rash* (Fig. 16-11).

The oral lesions of lupus erythematosus may bear a striking resemblance to those of erosive lichen planus. Both the location and the presence of white striations are characteristics shared by these disorders. Other white, and red and white conditions to consider include epithelial dysplasia, oral cancer, keratosis, cheek chewing, hypertrophic candidiasis, and local mucosal reaction to cinnamon flavoring agents (such as in chewing gum). In cases where the ulcerative nature of the disease predominates, conditions such as minor and major aphthous ulceration, pemphigus, pemphigoid, erythema multiforme, and allergic stomatitis must be considered. Clearly, attention to the presence of skin lesions, as well as signs or history of organ

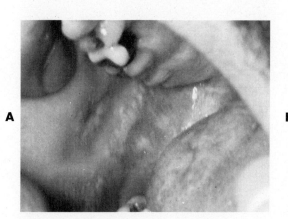

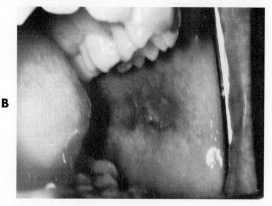

Fig. 16-10 A, Discoid lupus erythematosus. Lesions of the buccal mucosa in two patients who test positive for lupus. **B,** This ulcer is painful.

disease, aids in choosing between many of the diseases in these differential diagnoses.

Erythema Multiforme

Erythema multiforme may be defined as an acute mucocutaneous eruption of unknown cause. A number of precipitating factors associated with onset of this mysterious disease have been defined. Probably the most important are a recent history of upper respiratory tract infection or a recent eruption of herpetic infection. Other significant associations are seen with numerous drug therapies, vaccination, radiation therapy, and inflammatory bowel disease. It is important to emphasize that one third of all cases appear to be unrelated to any definable precipitating event.

Erythema multiforme typically has an abrupt onset, producing simultaneous eruptions of the skin and multiple mucosal sites. The disease shows a strong male predilection, with the majority of cases occurring in young adults. Skin lesions, when present, show a classic "target" or "iris" appearance, consist-

ing of concentric rings of red and pale color, often surrounding a vesicular center. In addition, a multiplicity of macular erythematous rashes are often present, involving wide areas of skin (Fig. 16-12), but characteristically found on the palms of the hands and soles of the feet. The lips demonstrate extensive ulceration with a fibrinosanguineous exudate, producing the classic blood-crusted lips (Fig. 16-13). Intraoral lesions are typically extensive, consisting of widespread, painful ulceration characterized by a copious fibrinous exudate (Fig. 16-14). Conjunctival involvement consists of photophobia and marked erythema. Severe ocular disease can lead to corneal involvement and blindness. Severe cases of erythema multiforme often show vesiculoulcerative disease affecting the mouth, eyes, genitalia, and skin. Such disease is termed *Stevens-Johnson syndrome.*

Erythema multiforme is often accompanied by systemic manifestations, including fever, malaise, and lymphadenopathy. Although many individuals experience single bouts of this disorder, some go on to experience multiple recurrent episodes. Emergence of this disease in individuals over the age of 50 is a particular cause for concern and is considered a sign that the patient may have an internal malignancy. Systemically acting corticoster-

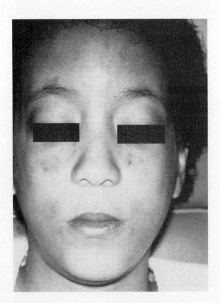

Fig. 16-11 Acute systemic lupus erythematosus. The patient developed simultaneous oral ulcers and malar rash.

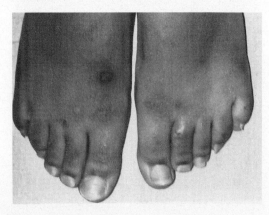

Fig. 16-12 Erythema multiforme. Rashlike and vesicular lesions of the feet.

oids usually provide adequate treatment for the skin and mouth lesions.

Contact Stomatitis, Medication Stomatitis, Allergy

In the foregoing portions of this chapter, mention has been made of oral inflammatory disease produced by either direct contact with or ingestion of medications. Thus direct contact of the mucous membranes with galvanic alloys or amalgam may on occasion produce lichen planus; cinnamon flavoring agents may produce a distinctive contact mu-

cositis (Fig. 16-15); and ingestion of various medications may alternatively mimic lichen planus, pemphigus, pemphigoid, lupus erythematosus, and erythema multiforme.

Contact stomatitis may result from a large number of agents in addition to those listed previously. These include toothpastes, mouthwashes, flavoring agents, topical medications, nickel-containing alloys, and dental impression materials (Fig. 16-16). An important paraoral form of contact dermatitis has recently been reported with increasing frequency, and has been related to latex glove allergy. Patients may actually demonstrate such an allergy to the gloves worn by the dental practitioner. Likewise, a significant number of dental personnel are allergic to latex gloves and must use glove liners or vinyl types of gloves to prevent such a reaction on their hands. Similar reactions have been seen following exposure to rubber dam and orthodontic rubber bands. Lesions of contact stomatitis may be red, white, red and white, ulcerated, or any combination at clinical presentation. Careful patient questioning—with emphasis on detecting substances that come in direct contact with the lesions on a recurrent basis—is necessary. Contact and medication stomatitis often arise through allergic mechanisms, although it is known that many skin and

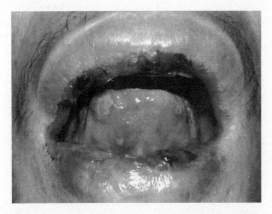

Fig. 16-13 Stevens-Johnson syndrome. Note the blood-crusted lips and ulcers of the ventral surface of the tongue.

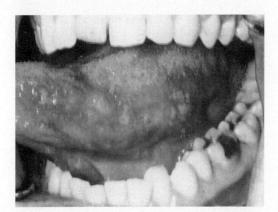

Fig. 16-14 Erythema multiforme. Multiple ulcers and vesicles of the tongue. The gingiva is not inflamed.

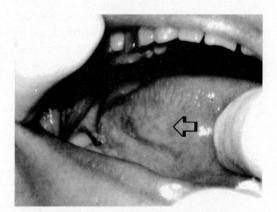

Fig. 16-15 Contact stomatitis. Lichen planus–like tongue lesions (*arrow*) secondary to habitual use of cinnamon candy.

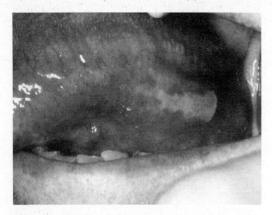

Fig. 16-16   Contact stomatitis.
Vesiculoulcerative lesion of the ventral surface of
the tongue developed as a reaction to dental
impression material.

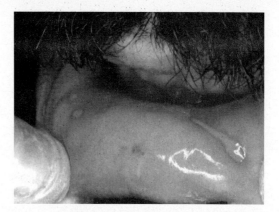

Fig. 16-17   Stomatitis medicamentosa.
Multiple ulcers of the oral mucosa developed after
an allergic reaction to an antibiotic.

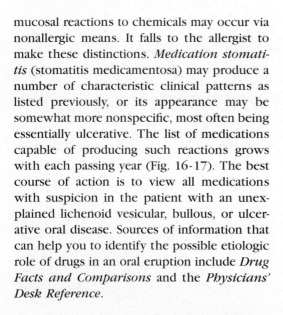

mucosal reactions to chemicals may occur via nonallergic means. It falls to the allergist to make these distinctions. *Medication stomatitis* (stomatitis medicamentosa) may produce a number of characteristic clinical patterns as listed previously, or its appearance may be somewhat more nonspecific, most often being essentially ulcerative. The list of medications capable of producing such reactions grows with each passing year (Fig. 16-17). The best course of action is to view all medications with suspicion in the patient with an unexplained lichenoid vesicular, bullous, or ulcerative oral disease. Sources of information that can help you to identify the possible etiologic role of drugs in an oral eruption include *Drug Facts and Comparisons* and the *Physicians' Desk Reference.*

Case Studies

Case 1
R.T. is a 49-year-old woman who went to her dentist for the first time in 5 years for tooth cleaning. At initial inspection, an indurated, crusting, 0.5-cm ulcer was noted on the cheek, adjacent to her nose. The area had been present for about 1 year and had grown slightly. R.T. admit-

ted rubbing and scratching the area from occasional itching. The dental team completed the cleaning without event and referred her to the dermatologist for evaluation. The lesion was diagnosed as squamous cell carcinoma. The physician noted that with careful surgery, the area was excised. There was no evidence of tumor in her lymph nodes or anywhere else.

Case 2
N.G. is a 66-year-old retired schoolteacher who complained of bilateral irritating ulcers of her buccal mucosa. She noted that the lesions worsened when she had a metallic partial denture constructed. Oral examination revealed ragged ulcers with radiating white striations on both sides of the buccal mucosa adjacent to crowned teeth and the partial denture clasps. Biopsy results were consistent with lichen planus. No skin lesions were apparent. N.G. confided that her sister had died of oral cancer and she was worried about the malignant potential of her lesion. She had never smoked tobacco. Neither removal of the denture for 3 weeks nor change in her hypertension medication gave any appreciable relief, and the lesions persisted for 10 years. Topical and occasional systemic corticosteroid therapy seemed to diminish lesion severity and duration. Extraction of the metal-crowned lower molar for periodontal reasons resulted in

marked regression of the lichen planus. She is presently on no medications and demonstrates mild reticular lesions.

Case 3

S.T. is a 31-year-old woman who had been diagnosed with systemic lupus erythematosus 6 years earlier. Her kidney and heart lesions were being controlled by her physician with quinine and corticosteroids. She went to her dentist with red and white striated lesions and ulcers of the lower lip of 3 months' duration and red persistent plaques of the hard palate. S.T. further noted an occasional rash across the bridge of her nose, especially after sun exposure. A clinical diagnosis of lupus versus drug-induced stomatitis was entertained. When the physician reduced her quinine medication, the oral lesions worsened rather than improved. Increased quinine decreased the incidence and duration of oral lesions. Biopsy of the oral lesions gave results consistent with lupus erythematosus.

Case 4

M.G. is a 60-year-old woman who complained of sudden bleeding gingiva of 6 months' duration. Her health history was negative and there was no history of skin lesions. Her gingiva was diffusely red and focally ulcerated, and superficially peeled with minor pressure. Biopsy revealed subepithelial vesicle formation, and immune staining gave results consistent with changes characteristic of pemphigus. M.G. was referred to a dermatologist, who discovered skin lesions of the elbow and skin consistent with early pemphigus. Both her skin lesions and gingival lesions are well controlled with systemically acting immune depressants.

Case 1

1. What is the usual etiologic agent for this type of skin cancer?
2. Who is at greatest risk for developing squamous cell carcinoma of the face?
3. Does this type of cancer ever metastasize? Should R.T. be further checked for metastasis?

4. Is it appropriate for dental personnel to initiate referral on paraoral skin lesions?

Case 2

1. Can lichen planus be ulcerated?
2. Give two reasons to justify removal of the denture for a period of time—even after diagnosis of lichen planus.
3. Why was N.G.'s hypertension medication changed?
4. Does the absence of skin lesions preclude the diagnosis of lichen planus?
5. How might the extraction of the molar tooth have reduced the severity of the lichen planus?
6. What is meant by a reticular lesion?

Case 3

1. Should lichen planus have been a consideration in this patient based on the clinical appearance of the oral lesions?
2. Do you think drug-induced stomatitis might resemble lupus or lichen planus?
3. What other symptoms might be associated with systemic lupus?
4. What is discoid lupus? Do discoid lupus patients develop oral lesions?

Case 4

1. What is Nikolsky's test?
2. Which oral lesions might show a positive Nikolsky's test?
3. Does the biopsy and immunological staining rule out most other bullous diseases including pemphigoid?
4. Are M.G.'s skin lesions expected?
5. Explain the rationale for treatment with corticosteroids.

SUMMARY

- Skin cancer incidence and duration are related to the location and amount of exposure to the sun. Individuals with a light complexion are most susceptible. The face is frequently involved.

- Basal cell carcinomas seldom metastasize but can be locally destructive.
- Seborrheic keratosis presents as common pigmented plaquelike growths of the skin of the face. They are benign in behavior but may be confused with some types of skin cancer.
- Pigmented nevi are common hamartomas or choristomas of the skin. Any change in color, surface characteristics, size, or shape of a nevus may indicate malignancy.
- Lichen planus most commonly is characterized by white lacy striations of the buccal mucosa and other mucosal locations. Other clinical subtypes including atrophic, erosive, and hyperplastic forms occur less commonly.
- Numerous medications, allergens, metals, and galvanic reactions can stimulate or cause oral lichen planus or lichenoid-appearing lesions.
- Cancerophobia is common in lichen planus patients.
- The clinical and microscopic changes of lichen planus are difficult to distinguish from those of certain other oral and systemic conditions.
- Pemphigus is an unusual autoimmune skin disease that may first present in the oral cavity. Large blisters of the oral mucosa and skin result in ulcerations and pathologic sequelae. Biopsy and immunofluorescent testing are usually necessary to establish a diagnosis.
- Pemphigoid usually affects mucous membranes and causes blisters and erosions. Scarring lesions of the conjunctiva produce blindness.
- Erythema multiforme is idiopathic but may be a reaction to herpes infection or certain medicines. Stevens-Johnson syndrome is severe oral erythema multiforme with ulcerations, hemorrhage, and crusting of oral

mucosa and lip lesions. This is a pathologic and sometimes fatal condition.

- Contact stomatitis may be caused by dental preparations, dental appliances, or even dental instruments.

Suggested readings

1. Laskaris. G, Sklavounou A, and Stratigus J: Bullous pemphigoid, cictricial pemphigoid and pemphigus vulgaris: a comparative clinical study of 278 cases, Oral Surg Oral Med Oral Pathol 54:656, 1983.
2. Lever WF and Schaumburg-Lever G: Histopathology of the skin, ed 6, Philadelphia, 1983, JB Lippincott, pp 476–481, 499–502.
3. Lozada-Nur F, Gorsky M, and Silverman S Jr: Oral erythema multiforme: clinical observations and treatment of 95 patients, Oral Surg Oral Med Oral Pathol 67:36, 1989.
4. Scully C and El-Kom M: Lichen planus: a review and update on pathogenesis, J Oral Pathol 14:431, 1985.
5. Vincent SD, Lilly GE, and Baker KA: Clinical, historic, and therapeutic features of cicatricial pemphigoid, Oral Surg Oral Med Oral Pathol 76:453, 1993.
6. Vincent SD and others: Oral lichen planus: the clinical, historical and therapeutic features of 100 cases, Oral Surg Oral Med Oral Pathol 70:165, 1990.
7. Walsh LJ and others: Immunopathogenesis of oral lichen planus, J Oral Pathol Med 19:389, 1990.
8. Zelickson BD and Rogers RS: Oral drug reactions, Dermatol Clin 5:695, 1987.
9. Drug facts and comparisons, St. Louis, 1994, Mosby.
10. Physicians' desk reference, ed 48, Montvale, N.J., 1994, Medical Economics Data.

17

Periodontal and Gingival Disease

IN THIS CHAPTER

1. Gingivitis
   - Gingivitis from local factors
   - Gingivitis from systemic disease
   - Acute necrotizing gingivitis
   - Desquamative gingivitis
2. Periodontitis
   - Chronic periodontitis
   - Acute and rapidly progressive periodontitis
3. Gingival tumors
   - Reactive gingival lesions
   - Parulis
4. Case studies

After studying this chapter, you should be able to meet the following objectives and define the key terms:

- List local factors that cause gingivitis.
- Explain the rationale for treating hormone-induced gingivitis.
- Explain the pathogenesis of leukemia-associated gingivitis.
- List the predisposing features for acute ulcerative gingivitis.
- Name the organisms responsible for acute ulcerative gingivitis.
- Treat acute ulcerative gingivitis based on understanding of its pathogenesis.
- Develop a differential diagnosis for acute ulcerative gingivitis and name other conditions that must be considered.
- List the different causes of desquamative gingivitis.
- Explain the rationale for treatment of desquamative gingivitis.

- Discuss chronic periodontitis.
- Relate acute periodontitis to systemic diseases.
- Differentiate pyogenic granuloma, peripheral giant cell granuloma, and ossifying fibroma by cause and clinical presentation.
- Discuss the treatment and prevention of gingival reactive lesions.

Gingival and periodontal diseases are very common conditions that frequently bring patients to the dental health team for treatment or are discovered by the dental health practitioner. These conditions may be confined to the gingival and periodontal structures, or may be a reflection of systemic disease (leukemia, diabetes, AIDS). In most instances, early diagnosis can lead to treatment and prevention protocols that markedly reduce the effects of disease.

GINGIVITIS

Gingivitis from Local Factors

Acute gingivitis simply represents an inflammatory reaction of the gingiva to a host of physical, chemical, and microbiologic agents. Patterns of involvement, exudation, appearance, and correlation with other signs and symptoms often give reliable clues to the cause. In general, acute gingivitis involves the free and, frequently, the attached gingiva. These areas appear red and swollen, with loss of stippling (Fig. 17-1). The gingiva may be painful or burning. The most common cause of gingivitis is accumulation of dental plaque on teeth. The bacteria of plaque and their

281

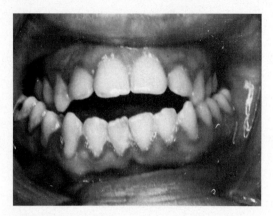

Fig. 17-1 Acute gingivitis. The red, swollen free gingiva is inflamed secondary to poor oral hygiene.

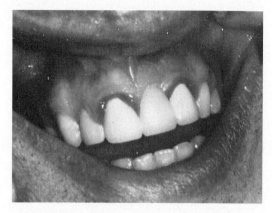

Fig. 17-2 Allergic gingivitis. The gingival reaction about teeth No. 8 and 10 is caused by allergy to the dental cement used beneath the crowns on these teeth.

byproducts initiate necrosis and inflammation of the free gingiva, which then rapidly spread to the attached gingiva. In severe cases ulceration and purulent exudation may occur. Poor oral hygiene and lack of gingival stimulation resulting from misalignment of teeth usually are the cause of the plaque accumulation and gingival inflammation. Control of this *acute nonspecific gingivitis* is based on plaque removal, antibacterial therapeutic agents (mouthwash, chlorhexidine), improved dental hygiene, and correction of stimulation problems such as misalignment, improper contour of dental hard tissues, and cavities.

Allergic gingivitis is another rather common acute inflammatory response of the gingiva. This type I hypersensitivity is most commonly caused by ingredients in dental preparations such as toothpaste (such as flavoring, antiplaque agents, preservatives) by mouthwash, candies (such as cinnamon), chewing gums, and other allergens. Usually the free and attached gingiva and alveolar mucosa are involved, and not uncommonly other contiguous areas of contact such as the tongue or buccal mucosa may also demonstrate lesions. The gingiva often appears intensely red to red-orange (Fig. 17-2). Blisters, desquamation, and burning pain are often accompanying

features. Diagnosis involves careful patient questioning concerning use of possible causative factors and concurrent development of symptoms. Sometimes this correlation is easy—especially in instances where symptoms result from use of a new product or overuse of a product. Occasionally, the diagnosis is difficult because the patient is reacting to a previously used product that has been reconstituted by the manufacturer. Diagnosis usually is based on a patient food-product diary with correlation to lesion development or disappearance. Allergy testing is sometimes useful; however, all "contact allergies" are not necessarily true type I hypersensitivities. Therefore, false negative results may occur. Treatment and prevention consist of discontinuance of use of the allergen, and antihistamine therapy.

Gingivitis caused by mouth breathing is not uncommon. This may occur in association with developmental deformities of the jaws or nasal areas, in individuals with large adenoid tonsils that restrict nasal air exchange, and in individuals who mouth breathe at night. In some instances, respiratory allergies or a severe upper respiratory tract infection (head cold) will contribute to mouth breathing and gingivitis. The free gingiva, attached gingiva,

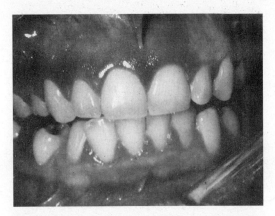

Fig. 17-3 Gingivitis from mouth breathing. The labial gingiva of the anterior teeth is red and swollen.

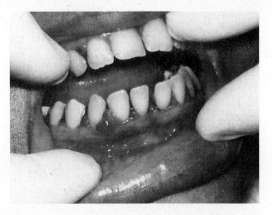

Fig. 17-4 Hormonal gingivitis. This patient is 7 months pregnant. Note the small pregnancy tumor between teeth No. 26 and 27.

and alveolar mucosa of the labial portion of the anterior maxilla are most commonly and severely involved, and are often intensely red-orange and swollen (Fig. 17-3). Pain is usually not very intense and frequently is absent. The mouth breathing habit may not be obvious to you or apparent to the patient; therefore, questioning and discovery based on the clinical signs and symptoms is important. Treatment involves use of salves and fluids for gingival lubrication and protection, and removal of the cause of mouth breathing.

Gingivitis from Systemic Disease

Several systemic conditions commonly contribute to bacterial gingivitis. These include the hormonal imbalances associated with pregnancy, puberty, and menopause. These conditions usually occur in women and result in red to red-blue edematous inflammation of the free gingiva and attached gingiva. Some pain and bleeding of the gingiva with toothbrushing or other stimulation is not uncommon (Fig. 17-4). The hormones do not cause the gingivitis, but rather seem to increase the intensity of inflammation associated with bacterial gingival infection. Therefore, plaque hygiene is important in controlling and preventing hormonal gingivitis. Estrogen therapy has

not been of proven therapeutic value in preventing these conditions. Tumorous pyogenic granulomas (pregnancy tumors) may accompany the hormonal gingivitis of pregnancy. We discussed pregnancy tumors in Chapter 13.

Gingivitis may be associated with leukemia in general and monocytic leukemia in particular. In leukemia, the gingiva becomes very swollen and hemorrhagic—often spontaneously. The free gingiva, attached gingiva, and alveolar mucosa appear red to red-purple, and there is loss of stippling. Ulcerations of the interdental papillae, purulent exudation, and tumorlike hyperplasia of the gingiva may occur (Fig. 17-5). These lesions are the result of (1) an accumulation of circulating leukemia cells in the gingival tissues, (2) infections secondary to bone marrow suppression, (3) immune deficiency, and (4) hemorrhage as a result of low platelet counts. In leukemia, although there may be 10 to 20 times as many white blood cells as normal, these cancer cells are not functional, and the formation of leukemic cells in the marrow reduces the number of other WBCs and platelets. Therefore, these patients have reduced WBC response and spontaneous bleeding problems (review inflammation, immunity,

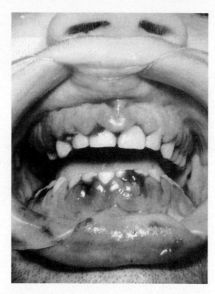

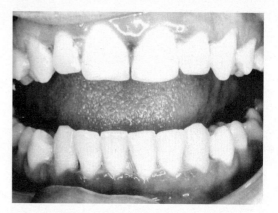

Fig. 17-6 Acute necrotizing ulcerative gingivitis. Note the ulcerations of the interdental papillae.

Fig. 17-5 Hemorrhagic hyperplastic gingivitis. These lesions are consistent with those of leukemia.

hemostasis, and hemorrhage). Occasionally, the leukemic gingivitis provides a clue to the dental practitioner of a previously undiagnosed disease. Treatment involves anticancer therapy and antibiotic and dental hygienic support.

We have previously discussed other forms of gingivitis, including those associated with immune suppression and HIV-G. Numerous other injurious agents (such as vitamin deficiency, leukopenia) can lead to gingivitis and subsequent periodontal destruction. We must make special effort to correctly diagnose and treat acute gingivitis so that we can avoid further morbid consequences.

Acute Necrotizing Gingivitis

Acute necrotizing ulcerative gingivitis (ANUG, trench mouth) is an extremely painful form of acute gingivitis that most frequently occurs in young adults. Clinically, this unpleasant condition is manifest as painful swelling of the free gingiva with classic ulcerations of the interdental

papillae—to the point of amputation of the papillae (Fig. 17-6). Both buccal and lingual maxillary and mandibular regions of the gingiva are usually involved. Extension of the inflammation to the alveolar mucosa and palate and into bone may occur (Fig. 17-7). Purulent exudation is common. In addition to pain, patients complain of metallic taste, increased saliva, and halitosis—which is readily clinically apparent. Some dental practitioners claim that they can smell ANUG and diagnose accordingly. Fever, malaise, and cervical lymphadenitis are common systemic symptoms. This gingivitis is caused by endemic fusospirochetal microorganisms that are normally found in the crevicular plaque environment of the teeth. These organisms overgrow and infect further when stimulated by several predisposing factors. These factors include poor nutrition to the point of malnutrition, extremely poor oral hygiene and plaque control, psychological stress, and immune suppression. Frequently, the patient exhibits all the predisposing factors in combination. We have previously discussed an association of ANUG with HIV-G and AIDS. Treatment consists of correction of the malnutrition, plaque removal (through scaling, polishing, home care), use of topical anesthetics, and

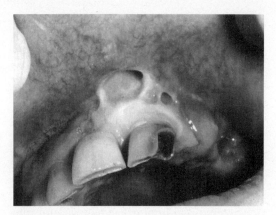

Fig. 17-7 Acute necrotizing ulcer of the gingiva. This patient is being treated with chemotherapy for leukemia.

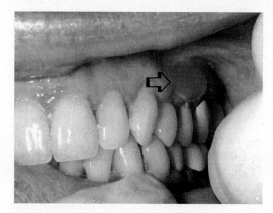

Fig. 17-8 Desquamative gingivitis. Note the swelling and vesicle *(arrow)* of the gingiva. This was proved to be cicatricial pemphigoid by biopsy.

use of topical and systemically acting antibiotics to reduce bacterial growth. Immune enhancement is beneficial in disease control. Dental hygiene procedures are very painful but necessary, and may have to be performed with adjunctive anesthesia.

Desquamative Gingivitis

The term *desquamative gingivitis* refers to a clinical type of diffuse gingivitis that is characterized by peeling of the gingival mucous membranes spontaneously or after slight pressure. The free and attached gingiva usually appear red and swollen, with red, bleeding, ragged ulcerations prominent. Vesicles are common and can frequently be created with slight pressure (Nikolsky's sign) (Fig. 17-8). Often the mucosa will peel off with minor dental manipulation such as pressured air blown into the gingiva from the air syringe. Lesion distribution involves both arches bilaterally, including lingual and buccal surfaces. Interestingly, patients usually are concerned about the appearance and bleeding associated with this condition, but seldom complain of extreme pain.

Desquamative gingivitis can be the clinical manifestation of at least five separate disease entities (Table 17-1). These are lichen planus, cicatricial pemphigoid, pemphigus, hormonal (menopausal) gingivitis, and idiopathic desquamative gingivitis. We have previously discussed lichen planus. This disease may appear as pure desquamative gingivitis or as gingivitis associated with the other common forms of lichen planus on other mucosal surfaces. Many times, the gingival lesions demonstrate the white reticular striations of lichen planus and this observation gives us information for diagnosis. When a patient has desquamative gingivitis—with or without striations—we must check other mucosal and skin surfaces for lichen planus.

It is not unusual for cicatricial pemphigoid to be manifest as pure desquamative gingivitis without accompanying lesions of other mucous membranes. Clinical signs and symptoms are generally those already described. The correct diagnosis is based on biopsy and immunologic testing. Patients with cicatricial pemphigoid should be referred for examination for the serious lesions of the other mucous membranes (such as those of the eyes) that may coexist. However, most frequently the lesions are confined to the gingiva.

TABLE 17-1

Desquamative Gingivitis

Cause (type)	Special features
Cicatricial pemphigoid	Results of antibody tests and biopsy
Lichen planus	Striated white areas
Hormonal	Association with menopause, hysterectomy
Idiopathic	None
Pemphigus	Skin blisters, results of antibody tests and specific biopsy

Pemphigus, the more serious autoimmune skin and mucous membrane disease, rarely appears as desquamative gingivitis. Again, general signs and symptoms occur that cannot be distinguished clinically from other forms of the condition. Gingival lesions frequently precede other mucosal and skin lesions and therefore the patient can be expected to develop other disease locations. Early diagnosis is based on biopsy and immunologic testing.

Many times, desquamative gingivitis occurs in postmenopausal women. This condition, termed hormonal desquamative gingivitis, is quite common. The signs and symptoms resemble those of the other types of the disease. Tests for lichen planus, pemphigoid, and pemphigus give negative results, and no specific testing mechanism is known to diagnose this entity. Hormonal therapy is not helpful. Psychological stress seems to play a role in increasing the severity of the disease.

Idiopathic desquamative gingivitis is a diagnosis by exclusion that is rendered when all of the preceding considerations have been ruled out. Again, signs and symptoms are similar to those of the previously listed entities. Rarely, contact allergy, systemic allergy, and physical irritation and habits (excessive gingival brushing) mimic this condition and must also be ruled out for this exclusive diagnosis.

All forms of desquamative gingivitis are basically controlled (not cured) in somewhat similar fashion. Therapy includes topical and/or systemic corticosteroid therapy to reduce the immune response, antibiotics and antiseptics to control secondary infection, and meticulous hygienic procedures to reduce plaque. Distinction of forms is nevertheless important because of variation in treatment and the more morbid prognosis of pemphigus and pemphigoid. Pemphigus and pemphigoid respond best to moderate to heavy doses of systemically acting corticosteroids—usually prescribed and monitored by the physician. Lichen planus, hormonal gingivitis, and idiopathic disease frequently can be controlled by low-dose systemically acting corticosteroids and/or topical steroids. Pastes, salves, and creams of these steroids can be useful. The dental team may need to construct custom trays to aid in application and adherence of these corticosteroids to the gingiva. Dental hygiene and plaque control is most difficult in these patients because both brushing and office cleaning procedures aggravate the condition. Bacterial plaque seems to increase the inflammation and the desquamation; therefore, plaque control is essential. This fact must be emphasized to patients, who must be meticulous in plaque removal without damaging the gingiva. Soft toothbrushes and topical antibacterials (chlorhexidine, sanguinaria) can aid this therapy. The idiopathic and hormonal types of desquamative gingivitis frequently fluctuate in intensity and may spontaneously resolve—usually after years of occurrence. Extraction of the teeth often leads to reduction or resolution of most types of the disease.

PERIODONTITIS

Chronic Periodontitis

We have described this condition previously as an infectious disease that is markedly affected by genetic and environmental factors. Plaque and calculus, smoking, irritation, salivary factors, and systemic disease all play important roles in cause and management of this condi-

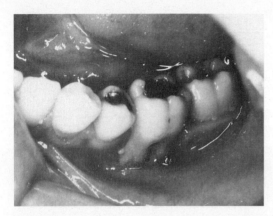 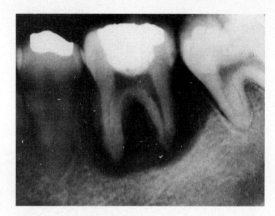

Fig. 17-9 Juvenile focal periodontitis. This 18-year-old patient has already had her maxillary central incisors extracted for periodontitis.

tion. Remember, occasionally such serious systemic conditions as diabetes mellitus, leukopenia, certain syndromes, and immune suppression can accelerate and exaggerate chronic periodontitis. These conditions must be considered when the disease advances beyond normal expectations or when periodontitis is resistant to therapy.

Acute and Rapidly Progressive Periodontitis

In some individuals periodontitis occurs as a more rapidly progressive disease or infection. Certain resident crevicular organisms—especially Gram-negative anaerobes—seem to play an important etiologic role. The overgrowth of these organisms may be the result of genetic influences and immune suppression. Acute and rapidly progressive periodontitis is probably not contagious. We have already noted the association of these conditions with AIDS and other immune deficiency diseases.

The so-called juvenile focal periodontitis falls within this category of disease. This uncommon condition usually arises in children or young adults. Rapid periodontal destruction, especially in the areas of maxillary incisors and mandibular molars, is often accompanied by bleeding, gingivitis, pain, and abscess formation (Fig. 17-9). The pattern and morphology of bone destruction is quite characteristic. Unless the disease is diagnosed and treated early in its course, tooth mobility and tooth loss is common. The condition tends to occur in families and in some racial populations. Often these individuals have clean mouths and good hygiene habits. Treatment includes antibiotic therapy, pocket reduction, and meticulous hygiene procedures. Even with therapy, the prognosis is not good. Some rare forms of juvenile periodontitis are more diffuse, and others occur in very young children and infants. Systemic conditions (diabetes, HIV, leukopenia) must be considered in all cases.

GINGIVAL TUMORS

Reactive Gingival Lesions

Some of the inflammatory and reactive lesions we studied in Chapters 12 and 13 frequently or exclusively occur on the gingiva. These lumps or tumors must be distinguished from other gingival lesions. Usually they must simply be treated or removed, but they sometimes may signal more severe oral and systemic conditions.

Pyogenic granulomas, peripheral giant cell reparative granulomas (PGCGs), and peripheral

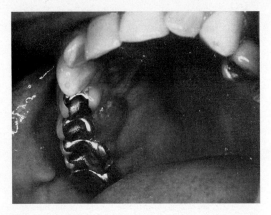

Fig. 17-10 Pyogenic granuloma. This lesion formed during pregnancy.

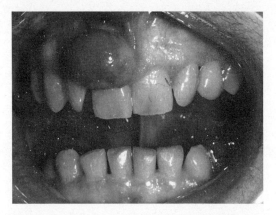

Fig. 17-11 Peripheral giant cell granuloma. The tumor is red and firm but not painful.

ossifying fibromas (POFs) are common reactive growths that most commonly occur on the gingiva and originate in the gingival sulcus area. These lesions appear quite similar to each other. They tend to be soft to firm, red or pink swellings with a somewhat granular, often ulcerated surface (Fig. 17-10). Although pyogenic granulomas occur elsewhere, PGCGs and POFs are found almost exclusively on the gingiva. This author believes that these three lesions represent stages of the same reactive condition, with the immature pyogenic granuloma representing the granulation tissue stage, the PGCG representing a slightly mature granulation tissue and osteoclast (periodontal cells) stage (Fig. 17-11), and the POF representing the more mature fibrotic and bony stage (Fig. 17-12). Indeed, microscopically, tissues representing two or even all three of these conditions are noted in some lesions. As with most hyperplastic lesions, a stimulus or irritant should be present. Once the irritant is removed, the reactive growth will stop growing or may begin to recede; however, surgical excision is frequently necessary to assure diagnosis and completely remove the lesion. If the stimulus is not located or removed, recurrence is likely. Pregnancy hormones stimulate reactive gingival lesions; therefore, such lesions—

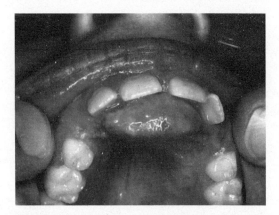

Fig. 17-12 Peripheral ossifying fibroma. The diagnosis was confirmed by biopsy.

especially pyogenic granulomas—frequently accompany pregnancy and pregnancy gingivitis. Certain drugs and medications like phenytoin (Dilantin) and cyclosporine can also stimulate reactive gingival lesions such as these. In both pregnancy- and drug-induced situations, the lesions can be controlled or prevented with careful oral hygiene. It is therefore speculated that bacterial factors (plaque, calculus) serve as the irritant and that systemic factors (hormones, drugs) stimulate connective tissue hyperplasia and metaplasia.

Parulis

The parulis represents the opening of an infected sinus tract to the surface of the attached gingiva or alveolar mucosa. The lesion appears as a painless red to yellow growth that may exude pus with pressure. As described previously, the parulis represents the distal portion of a draining sinus tract and abscess from the root area of an infected tooth. Often the apical infection is not readily apparent since it may not have attending symptoms. Parulides are usually quite recognizable clinically and should alert the health care practitioner to the possibility of dental infection.

We have previously discussed other reactive lesions such as fibromas, fibrous hyperplasia, and phenytoin hyperplasia. Please review these entities and remember, they occur commonly on the gingival tissues.

Case Studies

Case 1
M.J. is a 53-year-old woman who complained of red, raw, bleeding gingivae of 1 year's duration. Her health history was negative. Examination by the dentist revealed red, sloughing gingiva of all dental quadrants with ulceration of the lower lingual anterior and upper palatal gingiva. Biopsy ruled out pemphigus, pemphigoid, and lichen planus, and the condition was diagnosed as the chronic plasma cell type of gingivitis. No other oral or dermatologic lesions were detected. She had begun estrogen supplementation 2 years earlier. There was no history of allergy, and no mouthwash, toothpaste, gum, or candy use could be correlated with the chronology or severity of lesions. A diagnosis of hormonal gingivitis was rendered. Hormonal adjustment by her physician gave no relief. A therapeutic regimen of topical antibiotic rinse, topical steroid cream, and meticulous hygiene resulted in considerable reduction in the extent and severity of lesions.

Case 2
B.K. is a 21-year-old male student who developed pain, gingival ulcerations, and halitosis within a 3-day period. He had been studying for final exams and attempting to produce two 10-page papers during a 2-week period and had therefore neglected his diet and suffered from sleep deprivation. Oral exam by his dentist revealed large interpapillary ulcers, acute purulent gingivitis, increased salivation, and halitosis. Calculus, plaque, and materia alba were readily apparent on the dentition. His body temperature was 101° F, and there were bilateral swollen cervical lymph nodes. A diagnosis of acute necrotizing gingivitis was rendered. Scaling and cleaning using topical anesthetics was followed by topical antibiotic therapy for 10 days. Multivitamin therapy was prescribed and he was advised to get some rest. At 10 days' follow-up, healing of the gingiva was almost complete. However, B.K. did not finish his term papers by the deadline. At 2 months' follow-up, there was no sign of gingival disease.

Case 1
1. Does M.J. have desquamative gingivitis?
2. Why did the dentist ask about mouthwash, toothpaste, gum, etc?
3. Why was a biopsy performed?
4. What is the working diagnosis? Could there still be more than one condition?

Case 2.
1. What conditions frequently predispose the patient to acute necrotizing gingivitis?
2. What organisms are usually responsible for ANUG? Where do they come from?
3. What systemic disease should be suspected in patients who do not respond to treatment, have no other predisposing factors, or develop recurrent bouts of ANUG?

SUMMARY
- Acute gingivitis can result from local or systemic factors. Common local factors include dental plaque, allergies to foods and dental preparations, and mouth breathing.

- Systemic conditions such as puberty, pregnancy, leukemia, vitamin deficiency, and HIV infections can cause or aggravate acute gingivitis.
- Desquamative gingivitis is characterized by red, boggy sloughing of the gingiva and can be caused by several local and systemic factors including pemphigoid, pemphigus, lichen planus, hormonal changes, and idiopathic causes.
- Chronic periodontitis is caused by an interaction of dental plaque and the inflammatory and immune responses.
- Rapidly progressive periodontitis is related to the overgrowth of specific microorganisms in susceptible individuals.
- Reactive gingival lesions are common and usually result from connective tissue hyperplasia in response to local irritative factors. Phenytoin, cyclosporine, and other specific medications stimulate reactive gingival growth.
- Draining sinus tracts from periapical dental infections can result in parulis formation.

Suggested readings

1. Carranza FA: Glickman's clinical periodontology, ed 7, Philadelphia, 1992, WB Saunders, pp 149-159, 173-178.

2. Kerr DA, McClatchey KD, and Regezi JA: Allergic gingivostomatitis, J Periodontol 42:709, 1971.

3. Loesche WJ and others: The bacteriology of acute necrotizing ulcerative gingivitis, J Periodontol 53:223, 1982.

4. Rogers RS, Sheridan PJ, and Nightingale SH: Desquamative gingivitis: clinical, histopathologic, immunopathologic and therapeutic observations, J Am Acad Dermatol 7:729, 1982.

5. Ronbeck BA, Lind PO, and Thrane PS: Desquamative gingivitis: preliminary observations with tetracycline treatment, Oral Surg Oral Med Oral Pathol 69:694, 1990.

6. Stevens AW and others: Demographic and clinical data associated with acute necrotizing ulcerative gingivitis in a dental school population, J Clin Periodontol 11:487, 1984.

7. Winkler JR and Murray PA: Periodontal disease: a potential intraoral expression of AIDS may be rapidly progressive periodontitis, J Calif Dent Assoc J 15:20, 1987.

18   Nutritional Disease

IN THIS CHAPTER

1. Nutritional excess
2. Vitamin B complex
   - Vitamin B_1 (thiamine)
   - Vitamin B_2 (riboflavin)
   - Niacin (nicotinic acid)
   - Vitamin B_6 (pyridoxine)
   - Vitamin B_{12} and folic acid
3. Vitamin C (ascorbic acid)
   - Vitamin C deficiency—scurvy
   - Hypervitaminosis C
   - Vitamin C and disease
4. Vitamin K
5. Vitamin A
6. Vitamin D
7. Minerals
   - Iron deficiency
   - Calcium
   - Hypercalcemia
   - Hypocalcemia
   - Potassium deficiency
   - Zinc deficiency
8. Anorexia nervosa and bulimia
9. Nutrition: periodontal disease and caries
10. Case studies

After studying this chapter, you should be able to meet the following objectives and define the key terms:

- Discuss the role of diet and genetics in the development of obesity.
- List the significant sequelae of obesity.
- Define beriberi.
- Recognize oral and systemic signs and symptoms of vitamin B complex deficiency.

- Explain the pathogenesis of vitamin B_{12} deficiency.
- Compare and contrast the clinical features of vitamin B_{12} deficiency and folic acid deficiency.
- Evaluate the relationship of vitamin C with the common cold and with cancer.
- Relate the metabolic role of vitamin C to the clinical manifestations of vitamin C deficiency.
- List the sequelae of hypervitaminosis C.
- Discuss the function of vitamin K.
- Relate vitamin K metabolism to specific blood thinners.
- List diseases that predispose one to hypoprothrombinemia and vitamin K deficiency.
- Discuss chronic vitamin A deficiency and its possible role in several oral lesions.
- Define iron deficiency anemia and discuss the etiology and clinical manifestations.
- Define Plummer-Vinson syndrome and discuss its relationship to oral cancer.
- Explain the basic features of calcium regulation.
- List the causes of hypercalcemia.
- Relate the role of nutrition in dental caries and in periodontal disease.
- List common mineral deficiencies and relate them to the clinical signs and symptoms of the deficiency.

It is often said that "you are what you eat." Though assertions such as this may be viewed as falling somewhere between oversimplification and philosophical absurdity, it is undeniably true that personal health and appearance are affected by diet. Total caloric intake, dietary protein, vitamins, and minerals all represent important components of a complete, health-sustaining diet. It has long been known that diets with specific vitamin and mineral deficiencies cause well-defined clinical deficiency disorders. More recent investigation has linked dietary imbalance with a wide range of major diseases, including atherosclerosis, heart disease, and cancer. Public concern over such diet-disease relationships has not been lost on the food industry. Corporate marketing strategies have increasingly come to focus on suggested health-promoting nutritional values of retail food products, at times producing exaggerated claims and necessitating governmental corrective measures.

As health care professionals concerned with overall patient health, dental hygienists must be knowledgeable concerning basic concepts of nutrition and nutritional disease. In this chapter we will explore several aspects of nutritional disorders, frequently examining both general systemic and oral manifestations of nutritional imbalances and deficiencies.

NUTRITIONAL EXCESS

Appropriate body weight and appearance are major concerns of many Americans. Living in a country blessed with readily available and affordable food, its citizens paradoxically face the continuing dilemma of nutritional excess and obesity. Entire sections of supermarkets are stocked with "dietetic" foods. Post-holiday newspaper advertising inserts describing weight reduction programs that feature entire lines of special calorie-controlled foods and food substitutes (such as "milk shakes") receive national distribution, and similar television advertising is nationally aired. It is clear that many Americans are concerned with dietary excess, weight gain, and obesity.

Appropriate body weight, as well as obe-

sity, is generally determined through use of specific standards of comparison. Prepared statistical tables of average ratios of height to weight are useful, with ratios above the 85th percentile considered indicative of obesity. The Metropolitan Life Insurance Tables of Heights and Weights are a frequently used standard. In this publication, desirable body weights are identified through correlation with the lowest rates of mortality. Other measures of body fat content include the body mass index, and measurement of skin fold thickness at the biceps, triceps, and subscapular and supriliac areas. Using these and other measures, it has been estimated that 34,000,000 adult Americans are obese, with a slightly higher rate of obesity among women than men.

Research into the causes of obesity has been intense, and to date surprisingly few clear-cut explanations have emerged. It is clear that there is a genetic basis for a significant proportion of the obesity in the American population. It has been observed that obesity appears to run in families, although it is likely that both genetic and environmental factors have contributing roles. The influence of genetics is reflected in child adoption studies, where children born to obese parents but adopted by normal-weight individuals are more likely to become obese than children born to and adopted by normal-weight individuals.

Food intake, representing the major environmental factor, is of course at the heart of the obesity question. Conventional wisdom generally holds that obesity occurs through habitual overeating, and in large measure is attributable to ingestion of a high-calorie diet. It is surprising, then, that in controlled investigations, consistently elevated levels of food consumption (hyperphagia) have not been documented in the obese. Much speculation and interest centers around the possibility of defective function of the *satiety center*, that portion of the hypothalamus that tells an individual that enough food has been consumed. It is also suggested that food intake represents to some degree a conditioned response, thus amenable to behavioral modification.

It is known that there is considerable variation in *basal metabolic rate* (BMR) among individuals, differing by as much as 30% when variables such as age, sex, and body surface area are taken into account. However, studies of BMR in relation to obesity have failed to identify a significant correlation between BMR and obesity. Similarly, investigations into energy expenditures during physical activity and energy use after eating have also failed to suggest a consistent role for these factors in affecting body weight.

On occasion obesity may occur as a result of an underlying primary disease. Thus destruction of the satiety control center in the hypothalamus as a result of local tumor growth or surgery can lead to severe obesity. Excess adrenocorticotropic hormone (ACTH) production arising from pituitary hyperplasia or a secreting pituitary adenoma can result in Cushing's syndrome (see Chapter 19) with its clinically distinct pattern of weight gain. Ectopic ACTH production by various malignancies including certain lung cancers often produces much the same effect (see Chapter 7).

Chronic obesity has been shown to lead to a wide range of significant diseases, contributing to increased early mortality rates. Diabetes mellitus occurs with 3 times the incidence in the obese. Obesity is a major contributing factor in the development of type II diabetes mellitus (see Chapter 19).

The effects of obesity on the vascular system are significant, but by no means readily predictable. The incidence of hypertension in the obese is increased threefold; however, obesity's direct contribution to development of atherosclerosis appears minimal. An increased incidence of congestive heart failure is observed in overweight individuals, yet the brunt of vessel disease attributable to obesity appears to occur in the venous system. Varicose veins are more common and often severe in the obese, with increased incidence of thrombosis, thrombophlebitis, and pulmonary embolism (see Chapter 10).

Obesity in women appears to contribute to increased rates of cancer of the breast, endometrium, biliary system (bile ducts), and gallbladder. Increased rates of gallstones and cholecystitis are seen in both sexes. Men showing excessive weight are at increased risk for cancer of the colon, rectum, and prostate. A number of additional diseases occur with increased frequency and often increased severity in the obese. These include osteoarthritis in the weight-bearing joints as well as gout.

VITAMIN B COMPLEX

Vitamins may be defined as organic substances occurring generally in small amounts in a variety of foods, or in some cases synthesized by the body, that are necessary for normal metabolic function (Table 18-1). The B vitamins are a heterogeneous group of water-soluble substances that are found to varying degrees in certain meats, milk, yeast, grains, and a number of vegetables. The B complex vitamins include B_1 (thiamine), B_2 (riboflavin), niacin, and B_6 (pyridoxine). These vitamins are used to form essential coenzymes, agents that act in concert with protein enzymes to catalyze biochemical reactions. In this way, B-complex vitamins have a substantial role in carbohydrate and fatty acid oxidation (thiamine and riboflavin, respectively), electron transport (niacin), and amino acid and purine metabolism (pyridoxine and riboflavin, respectively).

Common conditions which contribute to the development of B-complex deficiency include alcoholism, pregnancy, malnutrition, severe diarrhea, severe burns, and debilitating diseases. Pyridoxine deficiency in infants is specifically associated with use of poor-quality commercial baby formula, and it also

TABLE 18-1.

Common Vitamin Deficiencies

Vitamin	Deficiency disease	Common Contributory Conditions	Clinical Presentation
B-complex	Avitaminosis	Alcoholism	Angular cheilitis Atrophic glossitis Dermatitis Psychosis
Thiamine (B_1)	Beriberi	Alcoholism Malnutrition Vomiting	Polyneuritis Psychosis Paralysis Heart failure
Niacin	Pellagra	Alcoholism Diarrhea	Dermatitis Diarrhea Dementia Atrophic glossitis
Riboflavin	Ariboflavinosis	Alcoholism	Angular cheilitis Atrophic glossitis Dermatitis
Pyridoxine (B_6)	Hypovitaminosis B_6	Infant formula Drug antagonism	Dermatitis Glossitis
Vitamin B_{12}	Pernicious anemia	Autoimmune gastritis Malabsorption*	Anemia Weakness Beefy tongue Burning mouth Paresthesia
Folic Acid	Megaloblastic anemia	Alcoholism Malabsorption* Chemotherapy	Anemia Burning mouth
Vitamin C	Scurvy	Diet	Weak bones ↓Wound healing Bleeding Cancer (?) Common cold (?)
Vitamin D	Rickets Osteomalacia	Diet	Hypocalcemia Weak bones Pitted enamel
Vitamin A	Hypovitaminosis A	Diet	Night blindness Keratinization Cancer (?) Xerophthalmia
Vitamin K	Hypoprothrombinemia	Liver disease Malabsorption* Anticoagulant Tx.	Petechiae Hemorrhage

*Malabsorption includes surgical removal and chronic diseases of segments of the gastrointestinal tract.

appears in patients undergoing isoniazid therapy (as for tuberculosis). These situations are often associated with B-complex deficiency because they contribute to a poor diet, create increased biochemical requirements, interfere with intestinal absorption, or disrupt normal metabolic pathways.

While clinical deficiency in multiple B vitamins is relatively common, deficiency in single B vitamins are quite rare. This is in large measure due to the fact that the preponderance of dietary sources of B vitamins contain multiple B vitamins. Specific B vitamin deficiencies are described in the next sections. However, the student should recognize that the majority of patients with B vitamin deficiency will exhibit clinical signs and symptoms of multiple B vitamin deficiency states.

Vitamin B$_1$ (Thiamine)

Signs of thiamine deficiency can be expected to appear relatively early in B-complex deficiency, as the body has only minimal means of storing this nutrient. The deficiency state is termed *beriberi* and occurs in three clinical patterns. One, in which signs of cardiovascular failure and peripheral edema are predominant, is termed *wet beriberi. Dry beriberi* targets the peripheral nervous system, producing bilateral polyneuritis with muscle paralysis and atrophy. Common clinical signs include loss of muscle tone in the extremities, leading to so-called wrist-drop and foot-drop. The third pattern of vitamin B$_1$ deficiency is called *cerebral beriberi.* In this form, tissue degeneration in and near the hypothalamus is responsible for disorganized eye movement and loss of coordinated skeletal muscle activity (ataxia). In addition, these patients often develop a form of psychosis characterized by loss of both memory and spontaneity, with a tendency to confabulate (tell false stories). This combination of motor and mental deficits is termed the *Wernicke-Korsakoff syndrome.*

There are no specific oral manifestations ascribable to B$_1$ deficiency.

Vitamin B$_2$ (Riboflavin)

It has been documented that the body is capable of storing riboflavin in amounts adequate for many months. Clinical deficiency would not be expected to occur rapidly as the result of a riboflavin-deficient diet. Clinical deficiency (ariboflavinosis) has prominent oral and paraoral manifestations. The lips demonstrate a characteristic angular cheilitis (Fig. 18-1), with desquamation of the vermilion border, and the tongue exhibits a painful atrophic glossitis with filiform papillary atrophy and prominent fungiform papillae. The skin is affected by a greasy, scaly dermatitis that is typically prominent at the nasolabial folds, nasal bridge, zygomatic areas, and ears, as well as on the extremities, trunk, and genitalia. Ocular disease consists of an inflammation of the cornea (interstitial keratitis) that can lead to cataract formation. Anemia is frequently encountered.

Niacin (Nicotinic Acid)

Although niacin is an important component of the diet, humans are usually able to synthesize

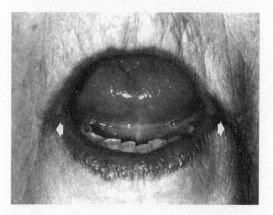

Fig. 18-1 Angular cheilitis—Ariboflavinosis. This woman admits to alcoholism. Note the mild atrophic glossitis and mucositis.

niacin from the amino acid tryptophan. This endogenous synthesis may be blocked if excess dietary leucine is present. The deficiency state produced by inadequate niacin is termed pellagra, and remembrance of its clinical characteristics is aided through use of the following mental prompt: the three D's—dermatitis, diarrhea, and dementia. The dermatitis shows marked scaly roughening with redness, can be widespread, and is typically more severe on sun-exposed areas. Alternating zones of depigmentation and hyperpigmentation may develop. Analogous disease of the oral mucous membranes is present, consisting of a red, swollen, "beefy" tongue that commonly shows ulceration and atrophy (Fig. 18-2). Similar changes occurring in the intestinal lining are responsible for the diarrhea. The dementia is related to degeneration of nerve cells in the brain and spinal tract.

Vitamin B_6 (Pyridoxine)

Deficiency of pyridoxine leads to seborrheic dermatitis, glossitis, cheilosis, diarrhea, pe-

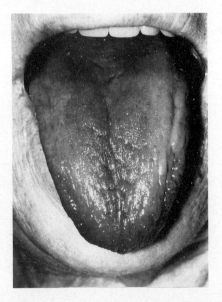

Fig. 18-2 Atrophic glossitis—pellagra. This chronic condition has occurred in an alcoholic. The patient also has dermatitis.

ripheral neuropathy, and hyperirritability that can lead to seizures. It should be noted that many of the features listed are similar to those attributed to deficiencies of other B-complex vitamins.

Vitamin B_{12} and Folic Acid

Vitamin B_{12} and folic acid, though chemically distinct, are closely related metabolically and, not surprisingly, in the clinical patterns of their deficiency states. Folic acid is readily available from such dietary sources as liver, kidney, fresh leafy vegetables, and asparagus. The body is capable of storing only a few months' supply. Folic acid fulfills a pivotal role in the synthesis of DNA and synthesis of the amino acid methionine. Many of folic acid's actions are dependent upon concurrent availability of vitamin B_{12}.

Deficiency of folic acid results in development of megaloblastic anemia, an anemia in which abnormally large circulating red blood cells are present. These red blood cells are decreased in number and have a decreased survival time in the bloodstream. Oral manifestations of anemia include such symptoms as soreness of the tongue and lips, and general complaints of so-called burning mouth.

Vitamin B_{12} has a molecular structure that is similar to that of the heme of hemoglobin. It includes multiple rings and a metal atom—though, in the case of B_{12}, it is cobalt rather than iron. This vitamin is synthesized by microorganisms in the environment, with particularly rich sources being sewage sludge and manure. The vitamin finds its way into the food chain, and is available to humans through a wide range of meats, as well as eggs. Vitamin B_{12} is closely involved with folic acid in the synthesis of nucleic acids, and is probably active in the synthesis of lipids incorporated into the nervous system.

With the exception of the strict vegetarian, humans rarely have a diet sufficiently low in vitamin B_{12} as to produce the deficiency state, known as pernicious anemia. It is recognized that the usual basis for vitamin B_{12} deficiency is a failure of the stomach to secrete a substance termed intrinsic factor (IF). IF normally binds dietary vitamin B_{12}, facilitating its absorption in the small intestine. Without IF, little vitamin B_{12} will enter the circulation to be available for biochemical activity. The reason that IF is not produced is that the stomach lining has been previously damaged by an abnormal chronic immunologic reaction that is entirely unrelated to vitamin B_{12} deficiency. The immune system destroys cells in the lining of the stomach and renders the stomach lining atrophic and inflamed (atrophic gastritis). The resultant lack of IF secretion prevents vitamin B_{12} absorption (Fig. 18-3). Thus vitamin B_{12} is not available to perform its important biochemical functions. Therefore, adverse effects on the blood and the nervous system occur and are recognized clinically as pernicious anemia. It must be emphasized that pernicious anemia is an autoimmune disorder affecting the stomach that secondarily prevents dietary B_{12} absorption, and not a dietary deficiency disease resulting from inadequate consumption of vitamin B_{12}.

The major clinical features of pernicious anemia are similar but not identical to those of folic acid deficiency. Patients demonstrate a megaloblastic anemia with sore mouth. The tongue is red, smooth, and beefy (Fig. 18-4). As mentioned previously, the stomach lining is atrophic, and these patients therefore have an increased risk of gastric cancer. Central nervous system damage focuses on the spinal cord, where myelin sheath degeneration leads to loss of axons. This produces clinical neurologic disturbances in motor and sensory function, with a major impact on the lower limbs. Specific manifestations include paresthesia ataxia and weakness.

Treatment of folic acid deficiency often consists merely of dietary supplementation. However, in some cases an underlying disorder in intestinal absorption blocks uptake of folic acid. In still other circumstances (such as infancy, pregnancy, disseminated cancer), increased folic acid requirements outstrip dietary supply. Clearly, management and treatment must include detection of any underlying basis for the deficiency.

As the vast majority of patients with vitamin B_{12} deficiency are unable to absorb this substance from the diet, alternative methods of administration must be used. Parenterally administered vitamin B_{12} is very effective in reversing the clinical effects of pernicious anemia if the vitamin can be administered before extensive central nervous system damage occurs. When central nervous system damage has occurred, such damage is generally irreversible.

VITAMIN C (ASCORBIC ACID)

Vitamin C Deficiency—Scurvy

The clinical deficiency state of vitamin C is scurvy. Although rare in the United States, it is seen with increased frequency among those with irregular and often poor eating habits, such as elderly and alcoholic persons. A child with a poor diet, or an infant maintained on a poor formula, is at significant risk for this disease.

Dietary sources of vitamin C include many fruits and vegetables, as well as fruit and vegetable juices. The vitamin is absorbed in the intestine, and a supply adequate for many months can be stored.

The clinical features of scurvy are extensive and reflect the many biochemical roles in which ascorbic acid is involved. These functions include significant contributions to the following: (1) collagen synthesis; (2) neutrophil and macrophage mobility and phagocytosis; (3) interferon synthesis; (4) electron transport (intracellular energy production); (5) folic acid metabolism and nucleotide synthesis; (6) iron absorption and transport; and (7) neurotransmitter synthesis. Deficits of these and other metabolic functions translate into the classic clinical manifestations of scurvy,

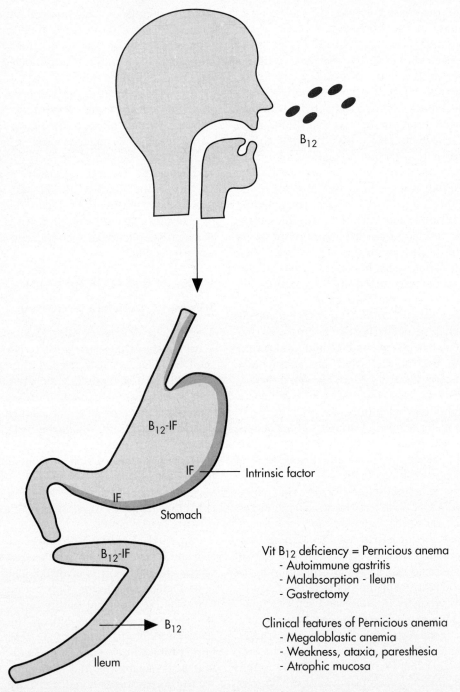

B$_{12}$

B$_{12}$-IF

IF —— Intrinsic factor

IF

Stomach

B$_{12}$-IF

B$_{12}$

Ileum

Vit B$_{12}$ deficiency = Pernicious anema
- Autoimmune gastritis
- Malabsorption - Ileum
- Gastrectomy

Clinical features of Pernicious anemia
- Megaloblastic anemia
- Weakness, ataxia, paresthesia
- Atrophic mucosa

Fig.   18-3   Vitamin B$_{12}$ in the diet is complexed with intrinsic factor IF in the stomach and absorbed in the ileum. The common causes of vitamin B$_{12}$ deficiency are presented, and the clinical signs and symptoms are listed.

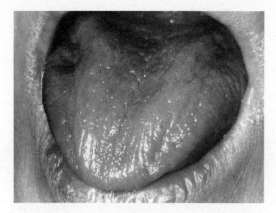

Fig. 18-4 Atrophic glossitis. This patient presented with burning mouth and atrophic mucositis. Blood testing confirmed a diagnosis of pernicious anemia.

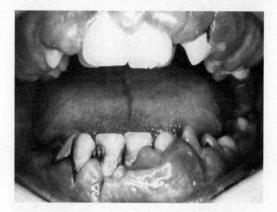

Fig. 18-5 Vitamin C deficiency gingivitis. This 12-year-old girl had swollen hemorrhagic gingivitis. Results of biopsy and specimen examination were considered consistent with changes associated with scurvy. The patient admitted to a "fast-food" diet.

including extensive hemorrhagic tendencies, weak bones, fractures and poor bone healing, poor wound healing and infection, anorexia, weight loss, and listlessness. Depression of the sternum coupled with weakened ribs produces a "scorbutic rosary"—two parallel rows of knobby hard elevations down the midline of the chest. A distinctive hemorrhagic, hyperkeratotic, papular rash is often visible on facial skin. The major oral features of scurvy are multiple loose teeth and swollen, painful, bacterially infected bleeding gingiva (Fig. 18-5). The effects on bone, healing, and teeth are closely related to defective collagen formation, whereas the vulnerability to infection is probably related to deficient neutrophil and macrophage function.

Hypervitaminosis C

Interestingly, excess consumption of vitamin C can also produce a disease state. Hypervitaminosis C brings with it a low but increased risk of renal stones, and can produce increased gastric sensitivity to aspirin. Among predisposed individuals, excess vitamin C can lead to build-up of increased amounts of iron, leading to the systemic disorder hemochromatosis with severe pancreatic and hepatitic damage. Clearly this is an example of "too much of a good thing."

Vitamin C and Disease

The history of vitamin C has been filled with dramatic claims and controversy. There is no question as to the beneficial effects of dietary and supplemental vitamin C in proper doses. However, recent claims of dramatic health benefits of "megadose" vitamin C "therapy" have created much confusion, not to mention much sales volume. Nobel laureate Dr. Linus Pauling made headlines with claims of the prophylactic properties of vitamin C as it concerned the common cold. More recently it has been claimed that high-dose vitamin C prevents certain forms of cancer. Neither of these claims for vitamin C has been corroborated through controlled scientific investigation. However, the dangers of excessive vitamin C consumption have been confirmed (as we have just discussed).

VITAMIN K

Vitamin K is a fat-soluble vitamin that is present in a variety of vegetable sources including vegetable oils. In children and adults this vitamin is produced by symbiotic intestinal bacteria; however, quantities produced are sometimes insufficient, making dietary consumption necessary. Newborn infants typically lack the intestinal bacteria to produce vitamin K and require dietary supplementation to avoid development of the deficiency state. In the adult, vitamin K stores are sufficient for several weeks in the absence of adequate dietary vitamin K. Endogenous (intestinal bacterial) synthesis of vitamin K significantly delays the onset of the clinical deficiency state, *hypoprothrombinemia*. Vitamin K biochemically serves as a cofactor in the synthesis of biologically active clotting factors II (prothrombin), VII, IX, and X, as well as several additional plasma proteins that have an impact on the coagulation system. As vitamin K participates in the synthesis of these proteins, it becomes inactivated and then recycled through an enzymatic reactivation process. This vitamin K reactivation step can be efficiently suppressed by "blood thinners" such as warfarin (coumarin).

Hypoprothrombinemia is more likely to occur in (1) patients with extensive liver disease, (2) patients with intestinal malabsorption, (3) patients taking anticoagulants (such as warfarin), and (4) neonates. As the liver is a major site for coagulation factor synthesis and for vitamin K utilization, extensive liver disease can limit synthesis of coagulation factors including prothrombin. Intestinal malabsorption often interferes with absorption of dietary fat, including fat-soluble vitamins such as vitamin K. The action of coumarin on recycling of vitamin K has been discussed, as has the relative lack of vitamin K–producing intestinal bacteria in newborns. All of these circumstances tend to reduce the availability of active vitamin K for coagulation factor synthesis.

An important clinical feature of vitamin K deficiency is an increased tendency toward hemorrhage. In the adult this chiefly affects the skin and mucous membranes, resulting in easy bruising (ecchymosis), pinpoint hemorrhages (petechiae) (Fig. 18-6), and hematomas. Spontaneous gingival bleeding may occur, and blood may be present in urine (hematuria) and stool (melena). There is also increased risk of life-threatening hemorrhage into major organs, with neonates at particular risk for intracranial bleeding.

Adequate administration of vitamin K (dietary or parenteral) can readily reverse many cases of hypoprothrombinemia. However, underlying diseases contributing to the disorder (such as liver disease, malabsorption) and any concurrent anticoagulant therapy will obviously influence the effectiveness of vitamin K.

VITAMIN A

Vitamin A is a fat-soluble vitamin that plays a major role in epithelial cell differentiation. Dietary sources include eggs and whole milk. Carotenoids also represent a major dietary source of vitamin A and are found in carrots, squash, and pumpkins. The most com-

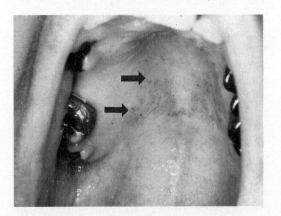

Fig. 18-6 Petechial hemorrhage. These spontaneous lesions are present in a patient taking vitamin K antagonist medication.

mon and biologically active form of vitamin A is termed retinol. Adequate absorption of dietary vitamin A is dependent on good hepatic, pancreatic, and intestinal function. The typical adult is able to store up to a 6-month supply of vitamin A in the liver.

Deficiency of vitamin A has dramatic effects on the eyes, exocrine glands, and skin. Chemical derivatives of the vitamin are required to maintain vision in reduced lighting (so-called night vision), and to maintain lacrimal (tear) gland function, and healthy conjunctiva and cornea. With vitamin A deficiency, patients develop night blindness, dry eyes with conjunctival keratinization (xerophthalmia), and corneal softening and ulceration (keratomalacia). Vitamin A deficiency is a leading worldwide cause of permanent blindness, although blindness resulting from vitamin A deficiency is uncommon in the United States.

Vitamin A is also necessary for the secretory function of exocrine glands. With vitamin A deficiency, exocrine cells (such as mucous cells) lose their secretory ability, leading to inadequate glandular secretions. In addition to dry eyes, the deficiency reduces salivary gland function, producing xerostomia and parotid swellings. Similar adverse effects occur along the gastrointestinal and respiratory tracts. Ciliary function is often lost in the trachea and bronchi, impairing local defense mechanisms and increasing the risk for upper respiratory tract and lung infections.

The oral mucosa is affected by vitamin A deficiency. Oral white lesions can result and are probably related to increased mucosal epithelial keratinization. There is also some evidence to suggest that chronic vitamin A deficiency increases the risk of a number of cancers, including oral squamous cell carcinoma and some salivary gland carcinomas. Vitamin A is also necessary for ameloblast specialization. A deficiency of this vitamin during tooth formation is a recognized cause of enamel hypoplasia.

VITAMIN D

Individuals are generally able to obtain vitamin D through two sources. Up to 80% of the body's requirement may be synthesized in the skin, requiring the action of the sun's ultraviolet light. Dietary sources of vitamin D include various ocean fish and grains. In order for vitamin D to be chemically active, it must be acted upon sequentially by the liver and kidney, converting vitamin D to calcitriol, the active form of the vitamin.

The primary effect of the presence of calcitriol is maintenance of normal serum concentrations of calcium ion. The serum concentration of calcitriol is closely regulated to prevent abnormal elevation of serum calcium levels. Calcitriol aids in controlling serum calcium concentration through direct actions on several organs. Calcitriol stimulates the intestine, increasing absorption of dietary calcium and phosphate. Calcitriol also acts together with parathyroid hormone to release calcium from bone, and to increase kidney reabsorption of calcium. In aggregate, calcitriol serves to regulate blood calcium concentration, making this ion available for action in a variety of important metabolic pathways (Fig. 18-7).

Dietary deficiency in vitamin D leads to hypocalcemia—reduced calcium ion concentration in the blood—creating important adverse effects on bone formation and maintenance. In the growing child, calcium is needed to achieve proper cartilage and skeletal bone growth with mineralization. The distinctive combination of clinical features resulting from vitamin D deficiency in these patients is termed rickets, and this condition shows a number of skeletal abnormalities. The chest often exhibits a ringlike distribution of firm, knobby overgrowths of cartilage occurring at the rib costochondral junctions—the so-called rachitic rosary. Weakened ribs are deformed by the normal stresses of respiratory muscle action, producing a protuberant sternum (pigeon breast deformity) and a roughly horizontal circumferential depression at the base of the rib cage (Harrison's groove). As all of the weight-bearing bones are softened, the effects of gravity during walking lead to bowing of long bones, reduced body height, and distortion of the spine and pelvis. The bones of the calvaria of the skull are also softened and flexible, buckling under externally applied pressure and then snapping back into position (craniotabes). Frontal bossing and a squared shape of the head are also common.

Whereas the major impact of rickets on the head and neck is seen in its effects on the skull, the enamel of teeth often shows generalized enamel hypoplasia. Only enamel formed during the period(s) of vitamin D deficiency, with its associated reduced blood calcium concentration (hypocalcemia), is affected. The enamel is typically pitted and cannot be clinically distinguished from environmental enamel hypoplasia caused by other etiological influences (see Chapter 11).

Vitamin D deficiency in the fully grown adult leads ultimately to softened bones, producing osteomalacia. Clinical signs in advanced cases consist primarily of bone fractures in weight-bearing and high-stress areas (spine, rib, wrist, and femoral neck). Deformity of the vertebral column is also common. As the dental enamel is fully formed in adults, there are no significant clinical dental abnormalities in osteomalacia.

MINERALS

Iron Deficiency

Iron is a critical mineral nutrient required for a variety of metabolic processes, including blood oxygen transport and normal muscle function. Dietary sources include various animal meats, vegetables, and grains. Animal sources of iron are absorbed in the small intestine with significantly greater efficiency than plant sources.

Systemic iron deficiency may occur as a result of inadequate diet, poor intestinal absorption, increased need for iron, or chronic bleeding. Iron deficiency due to poor diet is distinctly less common in the United States than in other parts of the world. However, specific populations in this country are at increased risk for iron deficiency, including elderly persons, infants, and the poor. These individuals may be restricted to iron-poor diets by economic factors, or merely by oversight (as in the use of iron-poor baby formula).

Iron absorption in the intestine under normal circumstances is only moderately efficient, with no better than 20% to 25% of dietary iron absorbed. Thus any disease that interferes with normal intestinal function (such as a disease producing chronic diarrhea) has the potential to diminish iron absorption to a significantly low level. Individuals with increased demand for iron include pregnant women, infants, and children. Dietary intake and absorption must keep pace to prevent systemic deficiency.

Chronic bleeding is an important cause of iron deficiency. Menstruating females frequently become iron deficient secondary to bleeding. With slow and continuous loss of blood, iron stores can become dramatically reduced. Other common causes of chronic bleeding include a number of malignant tumors, in particular those of the gastrointestinal tract. It is generally recommended that such tumors and other bleeding gastrointestinal diseases (e.g., peptic ulcer) be strongly suspected in men or postmenopausal women with iron deficiency.

Clinical manifestations of iron deficiency include anemia, as well as impaired immunologic and inflammatory responses, abnormalities in thermoregulation, and altered mental efficiency in children. Iron is a required constituent of heme. If supplies are inadequate, hemoglobin cannot be synthesized, leading to anemia. Generally signs of anemia include paleness, weakness, and failure to thrive. With iron-deficiency anemia, a distinctive combination of effects may be seen, referred to as Plummer-Vinson syndrome (see Chapter 9). As noted previously, this syndrome includes anemia, atrophic glossitis, and esophageal webs, with a predisposition to cancer of the upper digestive tract, including the oral cavity. Atrophic glossitis appears red and smooth, owing to atrophy of filiform papilla. Patients often complain of oral soreness, either restricted to the tongue or in connection with oral mucosal sites also affected by atrophy. The esophageal webs are scarlike strictures that reduce the internal diameter and flexibility of the esophagus, interfering with swallowing. Other characteristic clinical changes seen in iron deficiency include spoon-shaped fingernails, brittle fingernails, and atrophic gastritis.

Calcium

Calcium, like iron, is a critically important mineral nutrient active in a variety of metabolic pathways. The role of calcium as a major component of mineralized tissues renders it of immediate and central importance in oral health and disease. The concentration of calcium in the serum is very closely regulated through the action of a large number of organs and hormones. Comment has already been made concerning vitamin D, a substance whose actions as calcitriol are intimately involved in maintaining appropriate serum calcium concentrations, and parathyroid hormone (PTH), a hormone released by the parathyroid gland that acts with calcitriol when serum calcium concentration drops below optimal levels. In aggregate, calcitriol and parathyroid hormone tend to raise serum calcium levels through individual or joint actions on the intestine, bone, and kidney. Balancing these effects is calcitonin, a hormone synthesized by cells in the thyroid gland and released in response to raised serum calcium concentration (Fig. 18-7). Through inhibitory effects on both vitamin D transformation to calcitriol and release of calcium from bone, calcitonin acts to reduce serum calcium concentration.

Hypercalcemia. A wide range of diseases may produce abnormalities in serum calcium concentration. Elevated serum calcium concentration (hypercalcemia) is typical of primary hyperparathyroidism (including that caused by parathyroid hormone–producing tumors), hyperthyroidism, hyperpituitarism, Addison's disease, excess consumption of vitamin D, presence of disseminated bone-destroying (such as metastatic) tumors, sarcoidosis, milk-alkali syndrome (caused by excess consumption of milk and antacids), and prolonged body immobilization (as in space flight or bed rest following hip fracture) (Table 18-2). It is emphasized that excess consumption of dietary calcium is not a clinically significant cause of hypercalcemia. The most significant effect of hypercalcemia is diffuse calcification occurring in many tissues throughout the body. Termed *metastatic calcification,* this process produces its most dramatic effects on the kidney, and can lead to renal failure.

Hypocalcemia. Hypocalcemia (reduced serum calcium concentration) also may arise from many causes, including hypoparathyroidism, fluoride poisoning, inadequate dietary vitamin D, and failure to metabolically convert vitamin D to calcitriol (for example, as a result of diffuse chronic liver or renal disease). In some patients there may be a failure to absorb dietary vitamin D and calcium, such as is seen with chronic intestinal diseases causing diarrhea and poor absorption of dietary fats. These patients are also at increased risk for hypocalcemia.

The most dramatic clinical manifestation of hypocalcemia is tetany, characterized by severe (involuntary) muscle spasm, with spasms of the feet and hands. It is produced by cuff pressure on the ulnar and radial nerves. It is emphasized that hypocalcemic tetany is etiologically unrelated to the clinical tetany observed in patients with *Clostridium tetani* infection. Tetanus immunization is directed against the toxin produced by this bacterium

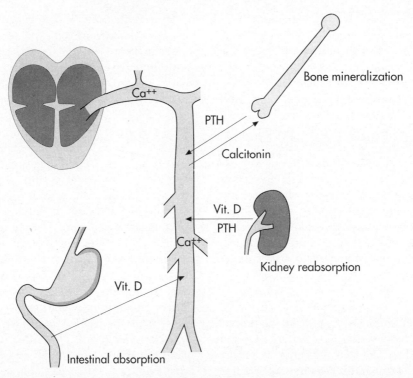

Fig. 18-7 Vitamin D helps intestinal absorption of calcium and with parathyroid hormone (PTH) helps save calcium at the level of the kidney. In Vitamin D deficiency, hypocalcemia results in poor bone mineralization (rickets, osteomalacia).

and is unrelated to hypocalcemic tetany. Chronic hypocalcemia often leads to poor bone and tooth mineralization. In growing children this effect can be dramatic, resulting in soft bones with increased risk of fracture, as well as enamel hypoplasia. As most causes of hypocalcemia are closely related to inadequate vitamin D, the reader is referred to that section of this chapter for further clinical description.

Potassium Deficiency

Potassium is a necessary mineral that plays an important role in nerve synaptic function, muscle contractibility, and renal tubular function. Potassium is common in many foods, and thus dietary deficiency is extremely rare. Potassium levels in the blood are regulated by adrenal mineralocorticoids acting on the kidney, affecting potassium reabsorption at the level of the kidney tubules. Hypokalemia usually results from such secondary causes as (1) certain antihypertensive diuretics (see Chapter 10) that interfere with tubular reabsorption of potassium and water, (2) intestinal fluid loss from vomiting and diarrhea (as in bulimia), and (3) adrenal hypercorticolism (Conn's syndrome, Cushing's Syndrome), which promotes renal tubular loss of potassium. The first two conditions are rather common. Hypokalemia can result in muscle weakness and paralysis, arrhythmia and cardiac arrest, and renal impairment; therefore, morbidity may be significant. In order to prevent hypokalemia during diuretic therapy, many of these diuretic preparations now contain potassium-sparing ingredients. Alternatively, patients may be given potassium supplementation during

TABLE 18-2

Hypercalcemia

Causes
Hyperparathyroidism
Secondary hyperplasia
Adenoma
PTH-producing cancers
Other endocrine imbalances
hyperthyroidism
hyperpituitaryism
Addison's disease
Immobilization
Fractures, cast, bed rest
Space flight
Dietary imbalances
Hypervitaminosis D
Milk-alkali syndrome
Sarcoidosis

Sequelae
Metastatic calcifications

diuretic therapy to prevent the complications of hypokalemia. Dental patients considered to be at risk of developing hypokalemia should be questioned and evaluated as part of the dental treatment planning.

Zinc Deficiency

Zinc deficiency is exceedingly uncommon in the United States but has been seen in populations in certain geographic regions with highly restricted diets. The element is required in trace amounts and is present in a wide variety of foods, including meats, fish, and legumes. Zinc is a mandatory component of a large number of enzymes involving virtually every aspect of human biochemical activity. Accordingly, it would be expected that a deficiency in this trace element would have wide-ranging effects.

Oral manifestations of zinc deficiency include altered taste sensation, possible burning mouth syndrome, delayed healing of oral wounds, and clinical features similar to those of vitamin A deficiency.

ANOREXIA NERVOSA AND BULIMIA

Anorexia nervosa and bulimia are related and represent psychological disturbances that frequently can result in numerous nutritional deficiencies and other resultant disease. Both conditions tend to occur in young female patients, and occasionally the two conditions coexist. Persons with anorexia nervosa are overly concerned with weight gain and therefore become consumed with total diet restriction. Both protein and total caloric malnutrition can result. The patients often appear emaciated and pale and frequently exhibit menstrual and other endocrine irregularities.

Persons with bulimia tend to eat increased amounts of food (binge eating) and subsequently induce vomiting or bowel irritation in order to purge the increased calories. Such binging and purging often occur on a daily basis and continue for long periods of time. In addition, these individuals often abuse both weight-loss medications and laxatives. Bulimic patients usually appear to be of normal weight and size.

Boths groups of patients exhibit multiple morbid systemic and oral sequelae. These include multiple endocrine disturbances (hypothyroidism, amenorrhea), vitamin deficiencies (B-complex deficiency, hypovitaminosis A), and potassium deficiency from chronic vomiting or diarrhea. The resultant hypokalemia may produce a fatal cardiac arrhythmia. Signs of anorexia nervosa and bulimia may be detected orally and during health history evaluation. In addition, these patients may also have relatively specific oral lesions such as chemical erosion of the teeth (see Chapter 13) and nonspecific parotid swelling (Chapter 15). Unfortunately, when questioned or confronted with these disorders, patients often deny the existence of such dietary habits. When indications of these diseases are detected by the dental team, the patient should be counseled and referred to a physician for evaluation.

NUTRITION: PERIODONTAL DISEASE AND CARIES

With our survey of nutritional diseases largely completed, we can now examine the effects of nutrition on periodontal disease and caries. It is currently accepted that bacterial colonization and infection play a central role in periodontal disease. Through the accumulation of bacteria-harboring and bacteria-rich plaque and calculus on teeth, conditions for development of periodontal disease with soft tissue and bone loss are created. Whether periodontal disease will indeed follow is to a major degree dependent on the periodontal tissue responses to these oral environmental conditions.

Nutritional status has a major impact on both tissue inflammation and repair. Diets with significant protein deficiency have an adverse effect on healing. Without the amino acid building blocks for collagen, granulation tissue and mature fibrous connective tissue cannot form (see Chapter 3). Vitamin C deficiency (scurvy) has a direct impact on collagen formation. Not surprisingly, a prominent clinical manifestation of scurvy is multiple early tooth loss. Effective inflammatory and immune responses are also needed in the maintenance of the gingiva. These responses are adversely affected in scurvy, iron deficiency, and zinc deficiency. The integrity of gingival epithelium is affected by dietary intake of vitamin A, vitamin B complex, and zinc, as well as folate, B_{12}, and by iron-related anemias. Although it is not possible to state categorically that one or more specific nutritional diseases cause periodontal disease, it is clear that the inflammatory and reparative mechanisms of the periodontal soft and hard tissues are closely tied to nutritional status. Clearly, good patient nutrition is an appropriate component in any program of periodontal care.

The role of nutrition in caries is somewhat more restricted. We have observed specific nutritional disorders in which there is an association with generalized enamel hypoplasia.

Examples include hypocalcemia, rickets, and vitamin A deficiency. Common sense would suggest that individuals with generalized enamel hypoplasia arising from these nutritional deficiencies would have an increased risk of caries. However, clinical experience fails to support an association.

The powerful effect of fluoride on reducing caries incidence is well known (see Chapter 12). Inclusion of dietary fluoride during tooth formation has dramatically reduced caries rates in many segments of the U.S. population. It is also recognized that diets high in simple carbohydrates help create an oral environment that favors the growth and proliferation of caries-producing bacteria. The resulting bacterial population materially contributes to caries production. Nutritional deficiency in vitamin A often leads to xerostomia, a condition also known to contribute to caries. In closing, it would be exaggeration to speak of caries as a nutritional disease. The involvement of bacteria, tooth development, and a host of local oral factors would suggest a far greater complexity in causation of this disorder. However, it would be equally erroneous to overlook the substantial impact of nutrition on dental caries and the larger issue of oral health.

Case Studies

Case 1

R.K. is a 47-year-old woman who has been obese her entire life. She is 5 feet 2 inches tall and weighs 205 lbs. Her mother and maternal grandparents were also obese. Her health history reveals non-insulin-dependent diabetes mellitus of 4 years' duration treated with oral pancreatic stimulant. Her hypertension is partially controlled with antihypertensive medications. She had gallstone surgery and a cholecystectomy 5 years ago. She is presently on a 1000-calorie, restricted diet and has lost 10 lbs in the past 4 months. Four previous attempts at dieting have failed. At a recent dental appointment, her blood pressure averaged 160/120. She was referred to her physician for further evaluation of hypertension with a note from her dentist detailing the hypertensive findings. She returned to her dentist 2 months later with an additional antihypertensive prescription. Her blood pressure was now 130/90. Routine dental care proceeded without complication.

Case 2

G.P. is a 52-year-old woman who complained of a burning tongue of 12 weeks' duration. Her health history revealed that she had had a gastric staple procedure 3 years earlier to correct obesity and had lost 125 lbs in the subsequent 3 years. She has been taking multiple vitamins and iron since the gastric surgery. On questioning by her dentist, she also noted tingling of her fingers and progressive weakness and malaise. Oral examination revealed a red atrophic glossitis and mucositis of the labial and buccal mucosa. Her dentures fit poorly. Cytologic smear tests for candidiasis gave negative results. G.P. was referred to her physician for a workup for anemia, iron deficiency, vitamin deficiency, and possible pernicious anemia. She was found to have megaloblastic anemia and a serum deficiency of cobalamin (B_{12}). Monthly intramuscular injections of vitamin B_{12} resulted in normal-appearing, asymptomatic mucous membrane and reversal of the fatigue and malaise within 4 months of commencement of treatment.

Case 3

D.J. is a 43-year-old male alcoholic who went to a dental clinic for extraction of his periodontally involved remaining teeth. His health history revealed a 20-year history of alcoholism and recent hospitalization for hemorrhage and a clotting disorder. He had two previous hospitalizations for psychiatric illness. Oral examination revealed severe hemorrhagic chronic periodontitis with 90% bone loss about his 12 remaining teeth. His oral hygiene was extremely poor, and calculus was apparent on all remaining tooth roots. He further demonstrated patchy atrophic glossitis and angular cheilitis. His face appeared dry, and areas of reddened dermatitis were apparent. He appeared thin and wasted. Oral surgery was deferred and D.J. was referred to the hospital for physical evaluation. Hospital diagno-

sis confirmed vitamin B complex deficiency and folate deficiency secondary to alcoholism and alcoholic cirrhosis. He was placed in a detoxification program in a psychiatric hospital and medicated with multivitamins, zinc, and vitamin K supplements. Three months later his teeth were extracted without incident. The pathology report confirmed severe chronic periodontitis. Healing was not remarkable, and dentures were fabricated.

Case 1

1. Is there a relationship between non-insulin-dependent diabetes mellitus and obesity?
2. Is there a familial/hereditary pattern for obesity?
3. Is there a relationship between obesity and hypertension?

Case 2

1. Why did the dentist perform a smear test on G.P.'s mouth for candidiasis?
2. What are some oral and systemic signs of anemia?
3. Why do you think G.P. developed pernicious anemia?
4. What is the significance of megaloblastic anemia?
5. Why does vitamin B_{12} have to be injected?

Case 3

1. Do you think that the alcoholism contributes to his psychiatric disease?
2. How do you explain D. J.'s periodontitis?
3. Why was elective oral surgery deferred?
4. What tests might help determine if D. J. was a surgical risk after his detoxification? Are these tests necessary after detoxification?

SUMMARY

- Obesity is the most common known nutritional disease in the United States.

Chronic obesity contributes to the development of diabetes, hypertension, pulmonary disease, vascular disease, cancers, and other common systemic conditions.

- Patients with poor diets or with gastrointestinal disorders are most susceptible to vitamin deficiencies.
- Patients with vitamin B deficiencies usually manifest signs and symptoms of B-complex diseases.
- Signs and symptoms of pernicious anemia can result from vitamin B_{12} or folic acid deficiency.
- Most vitamin B_{12} deficiency is related to autoimmune gastritis with lack of intrinsic factor to facilitate dietary B_{12} absorption. Therefore, vitamin B_{12} injections are necessary to reverse the disorder.
- Vitamin C deficiency has been implicated (but not proven to be involved) in the pathogenesis of cancer and the common cold.
- Vitamin K is important in clotting factor synthesis and activation. Vitamin K deficiency is usually secondary to interference with intestinal flora or the interference by anticoagulant drugs with vitamin K reactivation. The sequela is prolonged and excessive bleeding.
- Vitamin A plays an important role in epithelial maturation. Deficiency has been implicated in an increased risk of squamous cell cancer formation and other forms of epithelial dysmaturation of metaplasia.

- Vitamin D helps regulate serum calcium levels in concert with other hormones. Vitamin D deficiency leads to soft bones.
- Anemia results from iron deficiency. The most common cause of iron deficiency is bleeding. Iron deficiency anemia is a component of Plummer-Vinson syndrome.
- Hypercalcemia will lead to metastatic calcification of some tissues. Hypocalcemia may lead to tetany and poor bone and tooth formation.

Suggested readings

1. Chanarin I: Megaloblastic anemia, cobalamin and folate, J Clin Pathol 40:978, 1987.
2. Falconer DT: Scurvy presenting with oral symptoms, Br Dent J 146:313, 1979.
3. Garewal HS: Potential role of beta-carotene in prevention of oral cancer, Am J Clin Nutr 53:2945, 1991.
4. Hjorting-Hansen E and Bertram U: Oral aspects of pernicious anemia, Br Dent J 125:266, 1968.
5. Kumar V, Cotran RS, and Robbins SL: Basic pathology, ed 5, Philadelphia, 1992, WB Saunders, pp. 244-256.
6. Rubin E and Farber JL: Pathology, Philadelphia, 1988, JB Lippincott, pp. 314-325.
7. Shaw JH: Nutrition. In Shaw JH and others, editors: Textbook of oral biology, Philadelphia, 1978, WB Saunders.

19   Endocrine Disease

IN THIS CHAPTER

1. Pituitary gland
   - Hypopituitarism
   - Hyperpituitarism
2. Thyroid gland
   - Hypothyroidism
   - Hyperthyroidism
   - Thyroglossal duct cyst
   - Lingual thyroid gland
   - Thyroid cancer
3. Adrenal glands
   - Adrenal cortical hyposecretion
   - Adrenal hypersecretion
4. Parathyroid glands
5. Pancreas
6. Case studies

After studying this chapter, you should be able to meet the following objectives and define the key terms:

- Compare and contrast the clinical aspects of hyper- and hypopituitarism.
- Define diabetes insipidus.
- Draw the route of development of the thyroid gland and explain the thyroglossal duct cyst and the lingual thyroid gland.
- List common causes of myxedema.
- Discuss the etiology of Hashimoto's disease.
- List the etiology and clinical symptoms of Graves' disease.
- Relate types of thyroid cancer to radiation or genetic etiology.
- Define goiter.
- Define and discuss the etiology of Friderichsen-Waterhouse syndrome.

- Name the common causes of Addison's disease.
- Recognize the clinical features of Addison's disease.
- Discuss the etiology, pathogenesis, and clinical features of Cushing's syndrome.
- Name diseases caused by hypersecretion of aldosterone and adrenal sex hormones, and explain the pathogenesis.
- List the clinical and radiographic changes indicative of hyperparathyroidism.
- Differentiate type I and type II diabetes by etiology, pathogenesis, and clinical course.
- Explain the major metabolic disturbances that result from diabetes mellitus.
- Explain the major pathogenic lesions that result from diabetes mellitus.
- List common dental problems associated with diabetes mellitus.

Organs that manufacture and secrete chemicals needed for body functions are called glands. Exocrine glands secrete their products into ducts that transport the secretion onto a body surface or into the lumen of a hollow organ where these chemicals have a direct local effect. Endocrine glands are ductless and secrete their products directly into the blood. These products called *hormones* are secreted in minute quantities and act as chemical messengers causing regulatory changes in distant target cells or tissues. The stimulus for hormone secretion is often a chemical signal in the blood that is turned off once the hormone is released. When hormone again becomes necessary, this chemical signal reappears to stimulate more hormone secretion. For example, high levels of glucose will stimulate insulin secretion by the endocrine pancreas. Insulin secretion reduces blood glucose levels, which in turn reduces the demand for insulin. When the blood sugar (glucose) again rises, more insulin will be stimulated. Such a system of "negative feedback" ensures that hormone is supplied in optimal amounts and only in response to a need.

The major endocrine glands include the pituitary gland, thyroid gland, adrenal gland, parathyroid glands, the islets of Langerhans of the pancreas, and the gonads (testes and ovaries). When diseases affect these glands, the hormones may be underproduced, overproduced, or inappropriately produced, causing profound physical and biochemical changes that have far-reaching effects on the body, including the oral cavity.

We will study each of the major endocrine glands with the exception of the gonads, briefly reviewing the anatomy, development, and normal functions before discussing the diseases and the effects of underproduction or overproduction of its hormones. Table 19-1 provides an overview.

PITUITARY GLAND

The pituitary gland or hypophysis anatomically sits at the base of the brain within a bony cup called the *sella turcica*. It consists of two portions—an anterior lobe originating from an outpocketing of the embryonic oronasal cavity called *Rathke's pouch,* and a posterior lobe derived from the base of the brain. Table 19-1 lists the major hormones of the anterior lobe and describes their functions. The pituitary gland is often called the master gland because

TABLE 19-1

Endocrine Function and Disease

Hormone	Organ	Function	Deficiency	Excess
Thyroxin (T_3, T_4)	Thyroid gland	Increases metabolism	Myxedema, cretinism	Graves' disease, hyperthyroidism
Aldosterone	Adrenal cortex	Saves sodium and water	Addison's disease	Conn's syndrome
Cortisol	Adrenal cortex	Protein to sugar, activates stress-response	Addison's disease	Cushing's syndrome
Growth hormone	Anterior pituitary gland	Enhances growth	Dwarfism, Simmonds' disease	Giantism, acromegaly
Adrenocorticotropic hormone (ACTH)	Anterior pituitary gland	Stimulates adrenal cortex	Addison's disease	Cushing's syndrome
Antidiuretic hormone (ADH)	Posterior pituitary gland	Saves water and sodium	Diabetes insipidus	?
Parathyroid hormone	Parathyroid glands	Calcium from bone, raises serum calcium	Hypoparathyroidism, tetany	Hyperparathyroidism, brown tumors
Insulin	β pancreas	Decreases blood sugar, increases glucose anabolism	Diabetes mellitus	Hypoglycemia

it produces trophic hormones that regulate other endocrine glands.

The posterior lobe secretes antidiuretic hormone (ADH) that causes the kidney to resorb and conserve water in response to dehydration.

The major pathologic conditions affecting the anterior pituitary gland include diseases that destroy the gland, causing undersecretion of hormones, and neoplastic tumors, which may secrete excessive quantities of hormones.

Hypopituitarism

Three major syndromes result from the destruction of the hypophysis. If the anterior gland is diminished in childhood, the loss of growth hormone results in *dwarfism*. The entire body is affected, and thus the reduction in size is proportionate; the individual shows small arms, legs, torso, head, and teeth. This is not to be confused with the more common achondroplastic dwarf whose head and torso are of normal size and whose extremities are disproportionately short. If the onset of pituitary failure occurs in adulthood, dwarfism does not occur since the individual has already achieved normal stature; instead, *Simmonds' disease* results. Affected people fail to produce trophic hormones, the lack of which causes inactivity and atrophy of the thyroid gland, adrenal cortex, gonads, and pigment-producing cells (melanocytes). This results in sluggish activity, sterility, amenorrhea (in women), loss of body hair, and light-colored skin. *Diabetes insipidus* is the condition resulting from hypofunction of the posterior pituitary gland wherein lack of ADH causes extreme water loss manifested as continual urination with compensatory thirst and fluid consumption. We have already seen diabetes insipidus resulting from the proliferation of histiocytes about the pituitary gland in chronic disseminated idiopathic histiocytosis (Chapter 14).

Hyperpituitarism

Certain tumors of the pituitary gland cause excessive hormone secretion. The resulting condition depends on the cells involved and the action of the specific hormone that is hypersecreted. When growth hormone is involved, massive growth of the individual results. Affected children develop *giantism,* becoming extremely tall and proportionately large. If the tumor occurs in an adult after long bones have already finished growing, there can be little further growth in height. However, some bones will thicken with concomitant enlargement of hands, feet, mandible, and tongue. This condition is called *acromegaly.* Unhappily, these large individuals are medically compromised by the fact that the growing tumor within the skull acts like a brain tumor, causing pressure, visual disturbance, headache, and possible death.

Some pituitary tumors produce adrenocorticotropic hormone. This trophic hormone stimulates the adrenal cortex to become overactive, resulting in excessive cortisone production and consequent *Cushing's syndrome* (see the discussion of adrenal glands).

THYROID GLAND

The thyroid gland is located in the neck along either side of the larynx. As noted previously, it develops from the midposterior region of the tongue from an embryonic invagination called the *foramen cecum* and it grows downward as the *thyroglossal duct.* When the duct reaches the level anterior to the larynx, it proliferates to form the thyroid gland. The major hormone produced and stored by the thyroid gland is *thyroxin,* which regulates the basal metabolic rate (the metabolic activity at rest, including heartbeat, respiration, and maintenance of normal body heat). Production of thyroxin requires dietary iodine, and its secretion is regulated by pituitary thyroid-stimulating hormone (TSH).

Hypothyroidism

Hypothyroidism occurring in an infant results in *cretinism*. Affected children are underdeveloped, showing short stature and a severe mental handicap that becomes permanent if the condition is not reversed promptly. The skin becomes puffy and the tongue becomes enlarged (*macroglossia*). Tooth development, exfoliation, and eruption are delayed. Cretinism can be caused by iodine deficiency or by birth defects whereby the infant is born without a thyroid gland or with a gland that produces defective thyroxin.

Hypothyroidism in adults is termed *myxedema*. There is usually lowered basal metabolic rate (resulting in decreased blood pressure, heart rate, and respiration, and intolerance to cold weather) and obesity. The skin is edematous, dry, and cool, and macroglossia is often present. Mental sluggishness occurs but is reversible if thyroxin levels are restored. Dietary iodine deficiency is an important cause of myxedema. Individuals who do not eat seafood and do not use salt with iodine supplementation are at greatest risk. Additionally, certain foods such as turnips, cabbage, and rutabaga impair the body's ability to use iodine and may contribute to myxedema. With iodine deficiency, the lowered thyroxin level stimulates the pituitary gland to secrete excessive TSH, causing thyroid gland enlargement (goiter). Another important cause of myxedema is *Hashimoto's disease*. This disease, most common in adult women, is an autoimmune condition in which the body makes antibodies against its own thyroid gland and thyroxin. White blood cells infiltrate and destroy the gland, causing it to become symmetrically enlarged. Pituitary failure (Simmonds' disease) is also a rare cause of hypothyroidism resulting from reduced TSH stimulation.

Hyperthyroidism

The effect of excessive thyroxin includes elevation of the basal metabolic rate (increased heart rate, blood pressure, respiration, and temperature). The individual loses weight in spite of increased appetite. The skin is warm and flushed, and patients complain of heat intolerance. Anxiety and nervousness may prevent these people from engaging in productive activity. Affected children may show accelerated tooth development and exfoliation. The condition requires treatment because sudden release of thyroxin induced by illness, neck trauma, or stress—as may be caused by dental treatment—can trigger fatality.

Graves' disease is the most important cause of hyperthyroidism. Like Hashimoto's disease, Graves' disease is autoimmune in origin; but rather than destroying the thyroid gland, the autoantibody stimulates the gland, mimicking the action of pituitary TSH. The stimulated gland becomes hyperplastic and produces excessive thyroxin. As a side effect unrelated to hyperthyroidism, Graves' disease also features *exophthalmos* or severe bulging of the eyes.

Some benign tumors of the thyroid gland may also produce hyperthyroidism by production of thyroxin.

Other Diseases

Not all thyroid diseases interfere with hormone levels. The following diseases do not produce hyperthyroidism or hypothyroidism.

Thyroglossal duct cyst. The thyroglossal duct cyst is an often large cyst that develops from embryonic remnants of the thyroglossal duct. Because of its anatomic origin, the cyst must be located in a midline location usually overlying the larynx (Fig. 19-1). It appears as a lump that elevates when the patient swallows or protrudes the tongue. We have studied this cyst previously in Chapter 11.

Lingual thyroid gland. Thyroid tissue may persist at its point of embryonic origin, forming a lump in the midline posterior region of the tongue. In some patients, the lingual thyroid gland may represent the only thyroid tissue that the patient has; therefore, testing

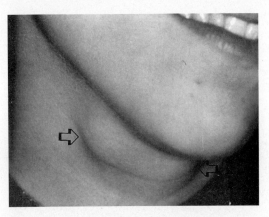

Fig. 19-1 Thyroglossal duct cyst. This neck cyst was soft and took a year to develop. The diagnosis was confirmed at excision by microscopic examination.

for presence of a normal thyroid gland is necessary before surgery is considered to remove the lingual glandular material.

Thyroid cancer. Thyroid cancers are important to the dental profession. One type (papillary adenocarcinoma) has been etiologically related to neck irradiation. Even though dental radiographs are insufficient to cause such cancers, lead thyroid shields should be used when taking dental radiographs to avoid unnecessary exposure of this area. Another variant of thyroid cancer has a tendency to metastasize through the blood and spread to the jaws. A third thyroid cancer (medullary carcinoma) is part of the genetic syndrome called multiple endocrine neoplasia (MEN III) in which patients develop multiple small nerve tumors throughout their mouth before the inevitable onset of thyroid cancer.

Before leaving the subject of thyroid disease, it is well to define the term *goiter*. This term simply refers to a thyroid gland enlargement. Since many diseases cause goiters (Graves' disease, Hashimoto's disease, iodine deficiency), the term does not imply a specific disease and does not denote whether the thyroid gland is producing too little or too much hormone.

ADRENAL GLANDS

The adrenal glands are paired organs that sit like caps on each kidney. Each gland actually contains cells of different embryonic origins. The outer *cortex* is derived from mesenchymal cells, whereas the inner *medulla* is of neuroendocrine origin. Hormones secreted by the cortex are listed and described in Table 19-1. The adrenal medulla produces catecholamines (epinephrine and norepinephrine).

Adrenal Cortical Hyposecretion

The *Friderichsen-Waterhouse syndrome* represents sudden adrenal failure usually on the basis of an overwhelming blood infection (septicemia) by gram-negative bacteria such as meningococci. There is sudden and profound functional collapse characterized by a precipitous fall in blood pressure and cardiac output followed by septic shock and death often within 24 hours of onset. The development of large skin hemorrhages (purpura) usually precedes death. The disease is so fulminant that death often intervenes before a diagnosis can be established. If the disease is detected, immediate institution of antibiotics, hormone replacement, and maintenance of vital signs may prevent a fatal outcome.

Addison's disease represents chronic adrenal cortical failure resulting from autoimmune mechanisms, chronic infections, metastatic tumors, or severe back trauma. Addison's disease can be caused by adrenal cortical depression secondary to long-term high-dose corticosteroid therapy—a common treatment for autoimmune diseases. Therefore, individuals on long-term cortisone therapy should be slowly "weaned" with decreasing doses of steroid taken over a long period of time. This allows the adrenal cortex to recover normal function and therefore avoids the risk of hyposecretion. In Addison's disease, the lack of aldosterone causes massive electrolyte imbalance with potassium retention and sodium loss, resulting in dehydration, hypotension, and reduced cardiac output. The lack of cortisone results in reduction of the stress response. The pituitary gland, responding to the diminished cortisone level, produces excessive ACTH, but to little avail, because the adrenal glands cannot respond. The excessive ACTH does, however, cause the skin and mouth to develop diffuse dark brown pigmentation resembling a suntan (Fig. 19-2). Sufferers of Addison's disease are emaciated and have low blood pressure with increased pigmentation of the skin and mucosa. They are dehydrated and crave salt. Death may result.

Adrenal Hypersecretion

Cushing's syndrome, resulting from cortisone overproduction, is the most common of the adrenal hypersecretion syndromes. It results from any of four causes: an adrenal cortical neoplasm spontaneously producing cortisone, an ACTH-producing adenoma of the pituitary gland causing bilateral stimulation and hyperplasia of both adrenal glands, a lung cancer producing ACTH, and chronic systemic long-term high-dose steroid therapy (prescribed for chronic inflammatory and autoimmune diseases). For whatever cause, the excessive steroids induce a protein deficiency and a carbo-

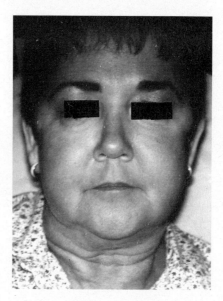

Fig. 19-3 Cushing's syndrome. The moon face is one of the characteristic signs. This patient has been taking corticosteroids for an immune disease.

hydrate excess because of the ability of cortisone to convert protein to carbohydrates. Protein deficiency encourages poor healing, immune deficiency, thin skin, and abdominal stretch marks, whereas excessive carbohydrates cause high blood sugar and obesity. Patients frequently notice a "moon face" and "buffalo hump" obesity of the face and back, respectively (Fig. 19-3). The antiinflammatory effect of cortisone reduces the body's ability to fight infection and therefore increases the susceptibility to infections including oral candidiasis. The anti–vitamin D effect and gastric acid–stimulating effect of steroids lead to weak, soft bones and gastrointestinal ulcers, respectively.

Oversecretion of aldosterone is often attributable to a tumor of the cortex and produces *Conn's syndrome.* Patients experience hypertension because of sodium retention, and periodic paralysis because of lowered serum potassium.

Oversecretion of steroid sex hormones (17-ketosteroids) results in a condition termed

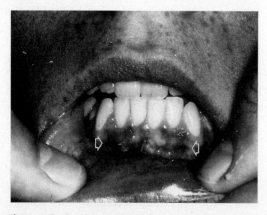

Fig. 19-2 Pigmentation of the gingiva can be an early sign of Addison's disease.

adrenogenital syndrome. Affected girls and women develop a male body form including hair, male muscular development, small breasts, and clitoral enlargement. These hormones can also cause hypertension, liver tumors, and heart disease. The profile of these complications should be considered by anyone contemplating the voluntary use of similar steroids for body building.

An excess of catecholamine is caused by an adrenal medullary tumor called a *pheochromocytoma.* It causes extremely high blood pressure. This tumor is noteworthy because it is associated with MEN III, which, as explained under thyroid disease, is frequently accompanied by oral neuromas and thyroid cancers.

PARATHYROID GLANDS

The parathyroids are four tiny glands embedded near the surface of the thyroid gland. They are embryologically and functionally unrelated to the thyroid gland, being derived from the branchial arches. The parathyroid glands produce parathyroid hormone (PTH), which raises the level of serum calcium. Calcium is needed for conduction of nerve impulses in muscle, for blood clotting, and for strong bones.

The oversecretion of PTH is usually attributable to a benign tumor. It results in mobilization of calcium out of the body. Blood calcium is elevated because calcium is depleted from bone into the blood and through the kidney, where it is lost. This leads to soft bones and predisposition to kidney stones. Affected individuals also report abdominal pains and psychological disturbances. Oral findings may include large jaw radiolucencies that are central giant cell granulomas or *brown tumors.* They are named after their brown color noted at biopsy. Another classic radiographic sign is the disappearance of the lamina dura around dental roots due to calcium loss. Early diagnosis based on these oral

findings allows for removal of the tumor, which restores normal calcium to the bone and protects the kidney from damage. Secondary hyperparathyroidism usually results from chronic renal diseases in which excess calcium is lost into the urine. The parathyroid glands become hyperplastic as a result of the loss of negative feedback resulting from reduced serum calcium. Clinical manifestations are similar to those of primary hyperparathyroidism.

PANCREAS

The islets of Langerhans are small clusters of endocrine cells distributed within the pancreas. The major hormone product is insulin, which lowers blood sugar (glucose). Maintenance of normal blood sugar level is important. If the level falls too low, the brain, which needs a constant supply of glucose, is denied this nutrient and will malfunction. If blood glucose level is too high (hyperglycemia), some will be lost through the kidneys. When a high-glucose meal is eaten, insulin is secreted to prevent blood sugar elevation. Insulin lowers blood sugar level by (1) allowing glucose into cells so that it can be used as energy, (2) allowing the conversion of glucose to glycogen so that it can be stored in liver and muscle, or (3) allowing its conversion to fat for storage in adipose tissue. The actions of insulin are counteracted by other hormones such as glucagon (also secreted by the pancreatic islet cells), epinephrine (which converts liver glycogen back to glucose), and cortisone (which converts proteins to glucose).

Diabetes mellitus (DM) is the condition resulting from failure of insulin production or utilization (Fig. 19-4). It should be considered in detail because it affects 1% to 2% of adults and up to 10% of all elderly individuals. Diabetes mellitus shortens life expectancy and is the seventh leading cause of death in the United States. Observant dental hygienists may detect early signs and symptoms of

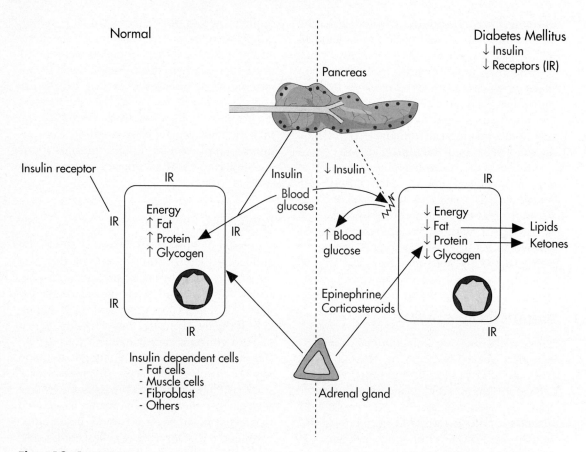

Fig. 19-4 The action of insulin in normal tissues is compared to the biochemical defect in diabetes mellitus in insulin-dependent cells. The result of decreased insulin formation or cell reception include increased blood lipids and ketones and decreased cell metabolism.

undiagnosed diabetes, hastening patient treatment for it. Conversely, invasive dental procedures on diabetic patients can have severe and life-threatening consequences.

There are two major types of diabetes mellitus. *Type I insulin-dependent diabetes mellitus (IDDM)* represents about 10% of all the cases of diabetes and occurs predominately in children and adolescents. It is most likely caused by several factors working in combination. In certain genetically predisposed individuals, a trivial viral infection stimulates the production of an immune

response against the pancreatic islet cells, resulting in destruction of many insulin cells. In order to develop this type of diabetes, the individual must have the susceptible genotype and contract the specific virus. *Type II non-insulin-dependent diabetes mellitus (NIDDM)* occurs in adults. There is a very strong genetic propensity, but viral infection and autoimmunity are not involved. In fact, the insulin cells are not necessarily destroyed. Instead, the problems result because the insulin that is produced does not function properly; either it is released in inadequate amounts to meet demand, or the body cells lose their sensitivity to the insulin. NIDDM develops slowly over a course of years but can be initiated, accelerated, or aggravated by stress, infection, pregnancy, and, most importantly, obesity (Table 19-2).

The biochemical alterations in diabetes mellitus make the pathology and symptoms easy to understand. Therefore, we can consider these first. When hyperglycemia is severe, glucose spills into urine, carrying excess water out with it. This causes excessive urination (polyuria) and compensatory thirst (polydipsia). Since in the absence of insulin, glucose cannot be used by many cells as a food source, the affected individual remains hungry even though he or she is eating normally (polyphagia). The person loses weight and becomes weak. The preceding symptoms typify type I diabetes, where the insulin deficiency is complete. Even when the insulin deficiency is less pronounced, as in type II diabetes, and the hyperglycemia is only moderate, over a period of years the constant high sugar levels can damage blood vessel linings, neural tissue, eyes, hemoglobin, and platelets. Excessive blood sugar also fosters bacterial and fungal infections, especially candidiasis.

Because many cells are unable to use glucose, the diabetic person's tissues turn to stored fat and protein as an energy source. Increased fat metabolism raises blood lipid and cholesterol levels promoting atherosclerosis. In addition, extremely high lipid breakdown in the glucose-starved cells causes the buildup of acid byproducts in the blood (ketoacidosis), which can be fatal. Protein, normally used for healing and building protoplasm, is also converted as an energy source in diabetic patients. This protein wasting compromises the diabetic patient's ability to manufacture white blood cells and antibodies, fight infections, and heal wounds.

As a dental patient, the diabetic patient should be considered a potential risk. The severe and accelerated arteriosclerosis predisposes these individuals not only to early heart attacks and strokes but to necrosis (gangrene) of the legs, kidney disease, blindness, and infections. The most important aspect in medically managing diabetic patients is control of blood sugar levels. Most diabetic complications can be reduced or delayed if the blood sugar can be stabilized at a normal level.

TABLE 19-2

Diabetes mellitus

Type	Cause	Age of onset	Pathogenesis	Treatment
IDDM (I)	Genetic (human lymphocyte antigens) factors Virus Autoimmune response	Child	Lack of insulin	Insulin
NIDDM (II)	Polygenic factors Environmental factors Obesity Stress Pregnancy Infection	Adult	Increased demand for insulin Fewer insulin receptors Decreased insulin function Decreased insulin	Diet β-stimulation

Mild type II diabetes can be controlled through diet by substituting starches for refined sugars. Other patients can take oral medications that stimulate insulin production. Type I diabetic patients and severe type II diabetic patients require insulin injections and are more prone to fluctuations of blood sugar level. These individuals, as well as those who refuse to practice diet control, are apt to develop early complications, including severe periodontitis and candidiasis. They also may respond poorly to dental treatment, showing accelerated bone resorption, infections, and impaired healing.

Case Studies

Case 1
M.B. is a 47-year-old woman who visited her dentist for routine examination. Oral examination revealed brown pigmentation of the mandibular and maxillary gingiva and alveolar mucosa that had not been noted 18 months previously. Her health history revealed that she was being treated for tuberculosis with medication and that she had been undergoing treatment for 1 year. She noted that her nail beds and portions of her skin appeared darkened. Her blood pressure was 90/60. She further complained of weight loss, thirst, and salt craving for the past 3 months. Biopsy of her gingival tissues revealed increased melanin pigmentation. M.B. was referred to her physician, who diagnosed Addison's disease. She was provided medication for Addison's disease and new medication for tuberculosis. She began to regain her weight, and her gingival pigmentation resolved 1 year after diagnosis.

Case 2
R.W. is a 65-year-old man who complained of a progressive swelling in his mandible of 2 years' duration. Health history was essentially negative. Oral and radiographic examination revealed a fairly well demarcated radiolucent area of the right side of his mandible in the area of teeth No. 18 to 20. The teeth were vital and there was no sign of infection; however, the buccal plate was expanded. The lamina dura about the mandibu-

lar teeth appeared less distinct than normally. Biopsy of the lesion resulted in a diagnosis of central giant cell granuloma. It was recommended that serum calcium and parathyroid hormone levels be determined. Both were elevated. Physical examination revealed a small parathyroid adenoma of the left side of the neck. After the adenoma was removed, the serum calcium level returned to normal. The mandible healed and remodeled to a normal form.

Case 3
C.C. is a 63-year-old man who is being treated for chronic severe periodontitis with bone loss and tooth loss. He is a type II (NIDDM) diabetic patient who has taken an oral islet cell stimulant for the past 8 years. C.C. exceeds standard weight by approximately 25% and has been retired for 8 years because of coronary atherosclerosis. He has been legally blind for the past year, is hypertensive, and complains to his physician of tingling and pain with ulcerations of his feet. He frequently detects glucose in his urine, and his fasting blood sugar level is elevated approximately 30%. Healing following periodontal scaling and minor surgery has previously been delayed, and he developed a gingival abscess after previous periodontal scaling. His present dental treatment plan includes antibiotic prophylaxis accompanying periodontal therapy and dental surgery. C.C. was recently placed on insulin therapy by his physician.

Case 1

1. What is the reason for pigmentation of the skin and gingiva?
2. What other systemic signs of Addison's disease are present?
3. What might have caused her Addison's disease—based on health history and therapeutic resolution?
4. What is the most common cause of Addison's disease? What is the mechanism?

Case 2

1. What is the relationship between

central giant cell granuloma and hyperparathyroidism?
2. Are all giant cell granulomas caused by hyperparathyroidism?
3. On what basis were serum calcium and parathyroid hormone tests justified?
4. Can a benign neoplasm of an endocrine gland cause hypersecretion? Can hyperplasia of an endocrine gland cause hypertension?

Case 3

1. Is there an association between NIDDM and atherosclerosis?
2. Is the diabetes well controlled?
3. Do you think there is a relationship between the diabetes and the periodontal disease?
4. Why might an NIDDM patient need to take insulin?

SUMMARY

- Endocrine hormones are secreted by glands or tissues in small quantities and affect target organs or tissues causing regulation of tissue function. Hormonal mechanisms frequently involve feedback inhibition by the stimulated product of the target tissue.
- The pituitary gland produces numerous trophic hormones that in turn stimulate hormonal secretions of target endocrine glands. Pituitary deficiency therefore results in target hormone deficiency, whereas pituitary hypersecretion can cause target gland hypersecretion.
- Growth hormone deficiency and hypersecretion frequently have oral manifestations. Some of these manifestations can contribute toward diagnosis.
- Hypersecretory and hyposecretory diseases exist for each endocrine gland. Clinical signs and symptoms reflect the functional hypersecretion or absence of the hormone.
- Hashimoto's disease is caused by autoimmune destruction of the thyroid gland and is manifest by signs and symptoms of hypothyroidism. Graves' disease is caused by

autoimmune-stimulated hyperplasia of the thyroid gland and is manifest by signs and symptoms of hyperthyroidism.
- The thyroglossal duct cyst and lingual thyroid gland are formed from remnants of the developing thyroid gland. They appear as a swelling of the neck or tongue.
- The papillary adenocarcinoma of the thyroid gland most commonly occurs in patients who have had therapeutic irradiation of the neck.
- The medullary thyroid carcinoma usually is associated with oral benign nerve tumors and MEN syndrome.
- Addison's disease may cause oral pigmentation and hypotension.
- Cushing's syndrome may result from pituitary or adrenal hypersecretion, exogenous corticosteroid therapy, or anaplastic lung cancers.
- Hyperparathyroidism can result from parathyroid tumors or occur secondary to chronic renal disease. Detectable dental bone changes include central giant cell granulomas and loss of lamina dura.
- There are two primary types of diabetes mellitus. The etiology of each type is different.
- Type I diabetes affects younger individuals and is caused by an autoimmune destruction of islet cells. Virus plays a role in the pathogenesis, and a genetically susceptible population exists.
- Type II diabetes occurs in adults and is polygenic in origin. Environmental factors such as stress, pregnancy, and obesity stimulate the onset of type II diabetes.
- Persons with diabetes lack sufficient insulin function because of decreased insulin secretion, increased insulin demand, or reduced insulin target cell receptor formation.
- The course and sequelae of diabetes are related to altered tissue sugar metabolism and cellular starvation. Substitute sugar metabolism mechanisms yield lipids, alcohols, ketones, and high blood sugar levels. These substitute products and high blood sugar levels cause tissue injuries and such pathologic and fatal sequelae as atherosclerosis, neuropathy, infections, and kidney diseases.

- Diabetes may lead to oral diseases and can reduce or slow healing and the inflammatory process. Therefore, diabetic patients are predisposed to oral diseases and complications.

Suggested readings

1. Bartuska DG: Endocrinology. In Rose LF and Kaye D, editors: Internal medicine for dentistry, ed 2, St Louis, 1990, Mosby, section 14.
2. Castano L and Eisenbarth GS: Type I diabetes: a chronic autoimmune disease of human, mouse and rat, Annu Rev Immunol 8:647, 1990.
3. Dunlop D: Eighty-six cases of Addison's disease, Brit Med J 2:887, 1963.
4. Gold EM: The Cushing syndromes: changing view of diagnosis and treatment, Ann Intern Med 90:829, 1979.
5. Jadresic A: Recent developments in acromegaly: a review, J R Soc Med 76:947, 1983.
6. Lamey PJ, Carmichael F, and Scully C: Oral pigmentation, Addison's disease and the results of screening for adrenocortical insufficiency, Br Dent J 158:297, 1985.
7. Moller DE and Flier JS: Insulin resistance: mechanisms, syndromes, and implications, N Engl J Med 325:938, 1991.
8. Petti GH Jr: Hyperparathyroidism, Otolaryngol Clin North Am 23:339, 1990.
9. Roth RN and McAuliffe MJ: Hyperthyroidism and thyroid storm, Emerg Med Clin North Am 7:873, 1989.
10. Silverman S, Ware WH, and Gillooly C: Dental aspects of hyperparathyroidism, Oral Surg Oral Med Oral Pathol 26:184, 1968.
11. Ziegler R and others: Specific association of HLA-DR4 with increased prevalence and level of insulin autoantibodies in first-degree relatives of patients with type I diabetes, Diabetes 40:709, 1990.

20 Forensic Dentistry

IN THIS CHAPTER

1. Dental identification
   - Dental records and charting
   - Example
2. Bite marks
3. Dental malpractice
4. Child abuse
   - Identification of child abuse
   - Reporting
5. Case studies

After studying this chapter, you should be able to meet the following objectives and define the key terms:

- Define forensic dentistry.
- List the reasons for dental identification of unidentified cadavers.
- Use the elements of written documentation necessary for medical-legal purposes.
- Explain the rationale of accurate dental identification.
- Explain bite mark analysis.
- Prepare an adequate dental record.
- Recognize dental signs of child abuse.
- Discuss the legal aspects of reporting child abuse.

The use of dentistry to supply information or evidence to the judicial system is called forensic dentistry. The reliability of forensic dentistry stems from the fact that everyone's teeth and mouth are sufficiently characteristic to allow differentiation and identification of individuals. The dentition is often used to determine the identity of dead individuals when the face and fingerprints are unusable. In similar fashion, well-characterized bite marks inflicted in the skin of victims of violent crime can be analyzed and matched to the teeth of a perpetrator. Forensic dentistry also includes the study of traumatic oral injuries for the determination of child, spouse, or elder abuse. Finally, forensic dentistry is concerned with self-policing and protecting professional standards within the legal system.

Although it may not be immediately apparent, all dental personnel are key figures in forensic dentistry.

DENTAL IDENTIFICATION

Ninety percent of forensic dentistry cases involve the identification of individuals who have died under mysterious circumstances and cannot be identified through other means because of burning, decomposition, skeletonization, or mutilation. In the United States, there are certain legal and moral entitlements for the deceased and their survivors that create a profound demand for proper identification. These rights include the following: (1) notification of kin, (2) determination of cause and manner of death, (3) religious rites, (4) probate of estate, (5) investigation of homicide, (6) other legal and financial consequences, (7) proper disposal and burial, and (8) the humanitarian issue of closure. In most cases of undetermined identity, the coroner or police have the name of a missing person believed to be the victim, but they cannot prove it. Because teeth survive most forms of destruction and are characteristic for each individual, they become a simple, reliable means of identification.

The identification process involves the recovery of the missing person's dental records so that a forensic dentist can compare the recorded dental findings to the teeth of the dead individual. The dental records may include health history and charting of caries and restorations, missing teeth, and pathologic and periodontal findings, as well as radiographs, study models, and photographs. The number and arrangement of missing teeth and restorations, and other recorded findings are all quite characteristic and, in combination, often unique. Therefore, identification is possible when these characteristics are recorded from a cadaver and compared to and matched with those recorded on an accurate dental chart (Fig. 20-1).

Dental Records and Charting

Because the chart reflects only a moment in time when a patient visited the dentist, and because dental changes continually occur, the forensic dentist making the identification might have to do some analytic thinking to arrive at a conclusion.

Some attempts at dental identification result in failure. The greatest number of these failures are due to inadequate or inaccurate dental records. Even in cases where identification is successful, a number of errors, omissions, and illegible entries may be seen in patient dental records. The reason for this, in part, is that ideal record keeping is time-consuming and does not generate income. Often records serve as a historical log and may not be referred to or relied on for subsequent treatment. Therefore, there may be little opportunity to review, and discover and correct recorded errors. Yet, for the forensic dentist, each written entry must be analyzed. If the entry is erroneous, it shows up as a discrepancy and can lead to a misidentification. The recording of accurate, complete, and legible

dental records is a habit that should be developed early in the career of any dental professional. Records should supply patient demographic information, a listing of patient findings, and a narrative explanation of a treatment plan and treatment rendered. Records should reflect that the patient has given informed consent for treatment. This means that the patient has been told of the diagnosis, proposed treatment, risks of treatment, advantages and disadvantages of alternative treatments, and consequences of not having treatment. The record should further indicate that the patient has understood and accepted the treatment plan.

The box on page 324 lists the elements of good record keeping.

Good dental records document thoughtful, complete, and proper patient evaluation and treatment. They protect both the patient and the dental team from misunderstandings that arise between patients and health care providers. Since any dental record may be needed in court, every dental record should be thought of as potential evidence and prepared so as to be explainable and logical. Dental records should never be altered. If a record needs to be corrected, all corrections should be dated and initialed. Deletions should be crossed out so the deleted material is readable. Erasures and correction fluid are not acceptable. In court, poor dental records may be an embarrassment, but improperly altered dental records may constitute an indefensible criminal offense.

The most significant and frequently found deficiencies in dental records include the following:

1. Failure to record the preexisting status of the dentition
2. Incorrect identification of teeth
3. Inaccurate recording of restored surfaces
4. Failure to justify treatment
5. Poor-quality radiographs

New dental patients should have all their existing restorations recorded as baseline

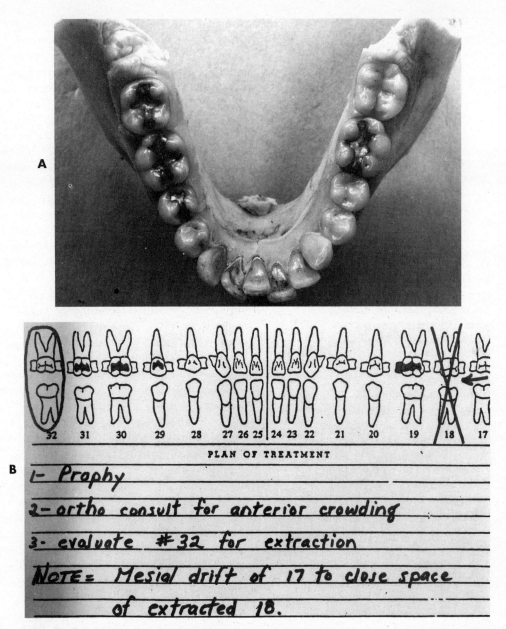

Fig. 20-1 Identification. The teeth and restorations of the cadaver (**A**) can be compared with the dental chart of a missing person (**B**) for possible matchup.

information. It is always disheartening to the forensic dentist when a dental record contains only the restorations that were placed by the current dentist and shows none of the previ-

ously placed fillings. Recording of the preexisting status of the patient's teeth has other, even more practical applications besides forensic identification. The most significant of

Elements of written documentation on dental patients

1. Demographic data
   A. Correctly spelled name including maiden name and nicknames
   B. Address and phone number (updated if changed)
   C. Date of birth, gender, and race
   D. Occupation and place of employment
   E. Name of physician
   F. Name of previous dentist
   G. Person to contact in an emergency
2. Medical history including medications and allergies
3. Recording of patient's complaint(s)
4. Recording of temperature, blood pressure, and pulse
5. Charting of preexisting status of patient's teeth
6. Charting or description of oral disease (caries, periodontal disease, orthodontic abnormalities, soft tissue lesions) and other problems
7. Written diagnosis and treatment plan
8. Informed consent (dated and signed)
9. Narrative description of all work performed including anesthesia given, prescriptions written, and patient instructions
10. Follow-up on previous treatment (patient response to treatment, compliance to instructions)
11. Other communications

these is that if a patient complains about dental work, it is important to know whether the current dentist or a previous dentist performed the procedure.

The misidentification of teeth on dental records may constitute a problem for the forensic dentist but can also create an even greater problem for the treating dentist if the error causes the wrong tooth to be treated. One of the most common errors in dental charting is mistaking right for left. This can occur because of a misoriented radiograph or simple "dyslexia." Another common error is misidentification of a molar when it has drifted following the extraction of an adjacent molar. For instance, tooth No. 17 may be misidentified as tooth No. 18 if tooth No. 18 was extracted and tooth No. 17 drifted mesially. Careful attention to dental anatomy and comparison of right and left sides can usually avert such a mistake. Imagine the repercussions if a dentist refers a patient for extraction of tooth No. 2 but writes tooth No. 3 or tooth No. 15 by mistake, causing the wrong tooth to be removed. In court, the record would be an embarrassment and indicate that the dentist was careless. The patient would have little difficulty convincing the court that the dentist was negligent.

Another common mistake in record keeping is the incorrect recording of carious or restored surfaces. An MO filling may be charted as a DO. The most serious pattern of incorrectly recorded surfaces that we have seen involved a dental record that consistently indicated more filled surfaces than were present in any of the corresponding teeth. In this case, the dentist was charging an insurance company for work he did not perform. This constitutes dental insurance fraud and is a criminal offense.

Because of the errors that can occur in written records, forensic dentists have learned to rely more on radiographs, which are objective and more trustworthy. It is surprising, then, to see a number of radiographs that are rendered useless for identification purposes because of poor exposure, poor development or fixation, cone cut, overlapping, elongation, or foreshortening. Since radiographs are made for diagnostic interpretation, it is also difficult to justify treatment on the basis of such poor radiographs.

Dental auxiliaries frequently record dental findings. Complete, accurate, and thoughtful record keeping is a habit to which every dental professional should aspire and is one of the most important qualities of a competent health care provider. What appears to be a routine, menial chore on a day-to-day basis is one of the most important measures of quality assurance in a dental practice. A seemingly insignificant error or omission can have devastating consequences to the patient and dentist.

Example

Decomposing human remains washed up on the shore of the Ohio River. Although the victim might have been any of several people who had previously drowned or disappeared upstream of the recovery site, the focus of the investigation was on T.R., known to have fallen into the river several weeks earlier. The family of the suspected victim was informed of the body recovery and was asked to help locate dental records on the suspect. The family dentist was contacted, and the dental records of T.R. were requested. The dentist had a diagrammatic chart of work he had performed 1 year earlier and had two bitewing radiographs made at the initial visit. The dentist's chart is shown in Fig. 20-2. The antemortem radiographic findings and the postmortem dental findings recorded by the forensic dentist from the corpse are shown in the box on page 325.

The antemortem diagrammatic chart (Fig. 20-2) gives information only about the teeth that the dentist restored. Older restorations are not recorded so that unless the antemortem radiographs happen to show them, there is no indication of those restorations. Because of this omission, teeth not shown on radiographs cannot be evaluated in the identification process. Fortunately, an identification is still possible. Comparing the antemortem and postmorten records, there are 14 compatible features. Some of those features are somewhat distinctive, such as the porcelain crown on tooth No. 8, B—composite on No. 14 and MO—composite on No. 21. Inconsistencies exist but are explainable. The large number of compatibilities combine to confer uniqueness. The making of postmortem bitewing radiographs would serve to confirm this clinical assessment because they would show the precise morphology of restorations as seen in the antemortem bitewings.

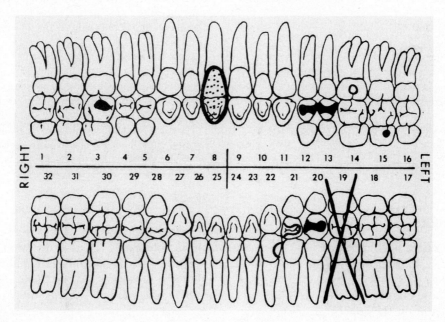

Fig. 20-2 Antemortem diagrammatic dental chart. This record can be compared to the postmortem findings.

Comparison of antemortem records and postmortem findings

Antemortem radiographic findings of patient T.R.

#2: O amalgam
#4: O amalgam
#5: MODL amalgam
#12: distal caries
#13: MO amalgam
#13: distal caries

#14: MOD amalgam
#15: MO amalgam
#17: unrestored drifted mesially
#18: fractured MODBL pin amalgam
#19: missing space closed by #18
#20: mesial caries
#21: MO amalgam

A postmortem charting of the teeth of the corpse reveals the following:

#1: impacted
#2: O amalgam
#3: O amalgam
#4: O amalgam
#5: broken crown
#6: unrestored
#7: L amalgam
#8: full porcelain crown
#9-11: unrestored
#12: DO amalgam
#13: MOD amalgam

#14: MOD amalgam; B composite
#15: MO amalgam; L amalgam
#16: unrestored
#17: unrestored
#18: missing
#19: missing
#20: MO amalgam
#21: MO amalgam
#22: D composite
#23-32: unrestored

Note the following inconsistencies between antemortem records and postmortem findings:

Tooth	Inconsistency	Explanation
5	Antemortem radiograph shows MODL—amalgam; postmortem data shows broken crown	Amalgam restoration might have broken out after the radiograph was taken.
7	No antemortem recording of L—amalgam	Restoration placed by another dentist; bitewing radiographs do not show anterior teeth, and current dentist recorded only restorations performed by him.
18, 19	Antemortem record claims dentist extracted #19, however, radiographs show #19 missing on first appointment. Postmortem data shows both #18 and #19 are missing	Dentist made an error; he extracted #18 and misidentified it as #19. Since #19 was missing on initial radiographs, he couldn't have extracted #19 and is thus inconsistent with his own radiographs.
21	Anterior radiograph shows MO—amalgam; postmortem data shows MO—composite	Dentist replaced the amalgam with a composite restoration (probably as a cosmetic request). This is substantiated in his diagrammatic chart.

BITE MARKS

The presence of bite marks left in skin occasionally accompanies violent crimes such as homicide, sexual assault, child abuse, and battery. Sometimes a defensive bite is inflicted by the victim on the attacker. In either case, the pattern of anterior teeth left in the skin can be compared to the dentition of the suspected biter for purposes of identification. The mere presence of a bite mark indicates a violent encounter, making this evidence significant.

Although a person's bite is unique, skin is a poor impression material and may not display the characteristic features needed for identification. The effects of bruising, healing, and elasticity may cause distortion of the bite mark. For these reasons, a match is much more difficult and occurs with less frequency than with cadaver identification.

The process of bite mark analysis requires the recognition of the oval patterned injury as a bite mark (Fig. 20-3), photographing it with special techniques to allow for precise measurement and analysis, and comparing the mark to study models of a suspect's teeth.

DENTAL MALPRACTICE

Thirty years ago physicians and dentists were not often sued. Health care providers were thought of as exalted healers and were often considered family friends. As health care costs increased and medical and dental care became more depersonalized, the doctor came to be regarded by some as just another repairman. Huge malpractice awards and aggressive legal counsel escalated malpractice litigation. Society has paid for this with higher malpractice insurance premiums and defensive medicine that drives up health care costs. Today, malpractice suits are more commonplace and are literally a statistical phenomenon. If you have enough patients, one day you will probably be sued.

Patients are entitled to appropriate quality care. When a patient sustains damages because the practitioner did something wrong or failed to do something that should have been done, it constitutes *malpractice*. The patient is entitled to a remedy. Sometimes damages occur despite the fact that everything was done correctly. This is called a *bad result*. This terminology indicates that the

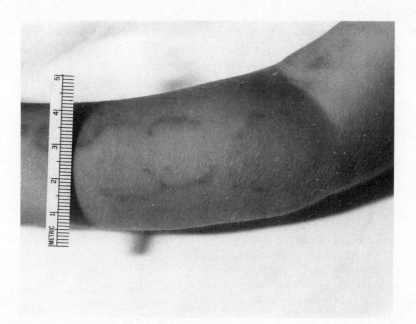

Fig. 20-3 Bite marks. The child was bitten by a sibling. Study model comparisons were necessary to rule out parental abuse.

outcome was not within the practitioner's control. In that circumstance, the practitioner is not responsible for damages and the patient is not entitled to compensation. When a patient suffers a dental problem, the patient may blame the dental professional whether or not the professional was at fault. This is understandable because many patients do not have the professional knowledge to evaluate the reason for the problem and know only that they are displeased with the result. Consequently, some lawsuits are without merit, although some are legitimate. Patient education and assurance, communication, and informed consent should minimize such misunderstanding.

The dental hygienist does not know if the patient he or she is working on today may become tomorrow's lawsuit. Patients must be treated with courtesy, care, and competence, and these attributes should be reflected in dental records. Each record should be written as if it were intended to be used in court. Consider the two examples in the box below.

In the first example, the notation merely serves as a log for bookkeeping. It is not an adequate patient record. If the patient sues because of a problem with the tooth, this

---

Two entries describing the same procedure

Example 1. #18: MOD comp $75.00
Example 2. #18: Pain to cold for last 2 months. Pain lasts only as long as stimulus is present. Old MO alloy is cracked with new decay on distal. Patient desires esthetic filling and does not want amalgam. Patient advised that posterior composite is not as durable and may cause sensitivity. Patient is willing to accept these complications. Local anesthetic (lidocaine with epinephrine) administered (one carpule) MOD   dycal—acid etch/light-cured composite. $75.00

---

record fails to provide answers for many questions. Why did the tooth need a restoration? What were the symptoms? Was a base used? Why was composite used instead of amalgam? Was anesthesia used? Was the patient informed as to the advantages and disadvantages of a posterior composite restoration? In the second example, the record answers all those questions, justifying the procedure with a recording of symptoms, a diagnosis, and patient acceptance of treatment.

CHILD ABUSE

Most people are raised in a protected and nurturing childhood environment and do not imagine the plight of innocent children imprisoned by families that neglect, abuse, and even kill them. The crime is not often observed or reported, yet for the victim, it is unrelenting and inescapable. If the crime goes unrecognized, victims may die or grow up as troubled individuals who may be poorly integrated into society. Any health care professional has a moral and often a legal responsibility to intervene when child abuse is suspected.

Since trauma to the mouth, face, and head is seen in one half of physical child abuse cases, many suspicious injuries pass through the portals of a dental office. Such injuries are often dismissed as accidents. An observant and knowledgeable health professional acting on the conviction of his or her suspicions can save a life. Appropriate action by the dental team depends on an understanding of child abuse, identification of suspicious injuries, medicolegal documentation, and reporting obligations.

Identification

Child abuse is more common than most people realize. Nationally it is estimated that 14% of children suffer maltreatment. The etiology is multifactorial. Child abuse can occur in any community and neighborhood and is not limited to conditions of poverty and lack of education. Certain individuals are predisposed to abusing children and, while it is true that poverty adds to the stresses that make such susceptible people react, no socioeconomic, racial, or religious group is immune to child abuse.

Not every injury is suspicious. In fact, most childhood traumatic injuries are accidental. Bruises overlying bony prominences such as the forehead, knees, and elbows are expected consequences of falls. Active children suffer broken anterior teeth, facial abrasions, and lacerations of the lips and tongue. These are not necessarily indicative of child abuse.

Other injuries, however, are more suggestive of nonaccidental trauma. Multiple bruises over soft tissue areas, or bruises in different stages of healing cannot be dismissed as the result of a single-event accident. Circular bruises on both sides of the chin may indicate "grab" marks where an adult has grabbed the mouth area in an attempt to force-feed or quiet the child. Isolated lacerations on the labial frena may occur as a result of face slapping or lip pulling. Isolated lacerations of the soft palate may follow jabbing of a fork or spoon into the mouth during force-feeding. Of course, a similar laceration can be the result of a fall with a lollipop or pencil in the mouth. Patterned injuries are always suspicious. Slap marks appear as three to four linear parallel red streaks on the side of the face. Belts and cords also leave linear abrasions and contusions (Fig. 20-4). Multiple broken and discolored teeth may indicate repeated beatings if the injuries are all of different ages. Recent dental fractures show sharp edges, whereas old fractures are more worn down. Peculiar malocclusions, especially where groups of teeth are not in occlusion, may indicate old untreated jaw fractures that healed incorrectly.

When such injuries are seen, they should be thoroughly documented in the record and photographed. Keen observation of the child and caretaker can be helpful. Many abused children show unusual behavior. Some are

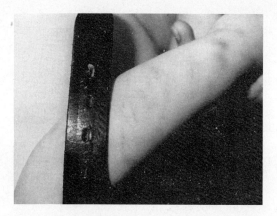

Fig. 20-4 Child abuse. The linear patterned contusions are suggestive of belt marks. (Courtesy of Dr. G. Nichols)

loud, boisterous, uncontrolled, and destructive; but many are quiet and show little affect. They avoid direct eye contact with adults, do not indicate any emotion, and do as they are told. Many are seemingly insensitive to pain. The child will usually not admit to being beaten by a parent and so direct questioning may provide inaccurate answers. The caretaker of the child should be asked about the injury in a nonaccusatory fashion. Questions like "How did the child get hurt?" followed by "Is it possible someone might have hurt the child?" are appropriate. Responses of the caretaker should be recorded in the chart. If the explanation of the injury does not make sense, that fact should be recorded, because such discrepancies between the nature of the injury and the explanation constitute one of the most important means of child abuse detection.

Child neglect is a reportable crime. The outward signs of a child who is not well cared for include lice infestation, uncleanliness, and inappropriate attire. Rampant caries constitutes an important dental sign of neglect but may also represent poor parental skills. Therefore, chronically untreated dental disease should be considered as possible neglect only when the caregiver has been educated and fails to provide treatment for the child.

Reporting

Dental auxiliaries should report their suspicions to the dentist who is responsible for reviewing the case. If the injury is suspicious, the dentist has an obligation to report suspected child abuse to the police or the department of human resources, who will further investigate the case.

The individual who reports will often be plagued with doubt. "What if I am mistaken?" "What if I get sued?" "Shouldn't someone else with more experience do this?" Such thoughts are common, and therefore the law provides for protection from retribution. Most people who have the opportunity to see abuse are unsuspecting and inexperienced and are not expected to make accurate assessments. The legal system understands this and asks only that you direct suspicious cases to professionals who can make the final decision. If your suspicion proves to be erroneous, you do not get in trouble as long as the report was made in good faith. The identity of the reporter is protected and is not given to the parents. Those who report are usually protected from civil and criminal suits, and the confidentiality ordinarily required between doctor and patient (doctrine of privileged communication) is waived. Photographs of the injuries can also be made without consent in many states. In fact, the only way a practitioner can get in trouble is if he or she fails to report. If a child is hospitalized or dies and it is discovered that a dental professional saw the child and missed an opportunity to report a suspicious injury, the professional can be found guilty of a misdemeanor punishable by fines and imprisonment. Additional litigation could then jeopardize the professional's license.

Case Studies

Case 1
The decomposed body of a male Caucasian subject was found in a vacant lot located in a major urban center. The features were unrecognizable, and no fingerprints were available. Dental examination revealed that teeth No. 14, 19, and 30 had occlusal amalgams and teeth No. 1, 16, 17, and 32 were unerupted and developing. Tooth No. 3 was absent. It was determined by a dentist that the patient was between the ages of 16 and 19. The dental records of five missing male Caucasian subjects of that approximate age were compared with the postmortem dental records and radiographs. An identification of C.T. was made based on similarity of restorations and teeth recorded postmortem with those found in one of the dental records. The 3-year-old record of C.T. was considered concordant—even though it recorded the presence and restoration of tooth No. 3.

Case 2
R.B. is a 12-year-old girl who went for routine dental cleaning. On oral examination, a large yellow-brown bruise of the right lower lip and a blue-red bruise of the left upper lip were noted. There was also a recent laceration of the left upper anterior vestibule. Her parent volunteered that the lesions were the result of a bicycle accident 5 hours before. The dental progress notes indicated similar types of injuries 2 years earlier from another bicycle accident. R.B. was referred to a physician, and the child welfare office was notified of possible child abuse. The parent was incensed. However, upon further questioning, one parent reluctantly admitted that the lesions were the result of several assaults by her drunken spouse.

Case 1
1. How can age be determined from dental findings?
2. What would happen if the previous (3-year) record was inaccurate (for example, MOD recorded on teeth No. 14 and 19)?
3. How do you explain concordance when tooth No. 3 is no longer present?

Case 2
1. What is the significance of the differently colored bruises?

2. What is the significance of the previous record of accidental damage?
3. What is the liability of the dental team for reporting suspected abuse?
4. What is the liability of the dental team for not reporting suspected abuse?

SUMMARY

- Dental records and dental information are important in many facets of legal determinations. Dental information is used in identification of the deceased, in determination of criminal bite marks, a identification of child abuse situations, and in settling legal disputes involving dental trauma and dental malpractice.
- Dental records must be systematic and correctly kept because they often serve as legal records.
- Dental identifications depend on comparisons of antemortem dental records and postmortem findings. Comparisons are based on the presence or absence of teeth, fillings, anatomic and pathologic features, and other individual dental characteristics.
- Bite mark situations are difficult to identify and to compare to a perpetrator's dental records. Special techniques and skills are necessary for adequate determinations.
- Careful record keeping is an important factor in dental malpractice considerations.
- Certain types of dental injuries and combinations of injuries should cause suspicion of child abuse. The dental practitioner is required to report suspected child abuse and legally protected from retaliation for reporting such situations.

Suggested readings

1. American Dental Association: Forensic dentistry, JADA 119:355, 1989.
2. Beckstead JW, Rawson RD, and Giles WS: Review of bite mark evidence, JADA 99:69, 1979.
3. Bernstein ML: The identification of "John Doe," JADA 110:918, 1985.
4. Kenney J: Child abuse and neglect. In Averill DC, editor: Manual of forensic odontology, ed 2, Colorado Springs, Colo, 1991, American Society of Forensic Odontology, pp 176-191.
5. Mertz CA: It's the law: professional habits that will protect you in court, Dentistry '85 5:9, 1985.
6. Levine LJ: The role of the forensic odontologist in human rights investigations, Am J Forensic Med Pathol 5:317, 1984.

Index

Note: Page numbers in *italics* refer to illustrations; page numbers followed by t refer to tables.